Social Work Practice

SOCIAL WORK PRACTICE
Treating Common Client Problems

Edited by

HAROLD E. BRIGGS and KEVIN CORCORAN
Portland State University

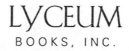

LYCEUM
BOOKS, INC.

5758 S. Blackstone Ave.
Chicago, Illinois 60637

One more time, to Sug Olivetti, the foundation
of all the good changes to come my way and
in memory of Beaudroux Boy-Bob Wilson,
from the partner at the firm of Seigerson,
Olivetti, Moriarty, Wilson and Olivea.
Welcome "O."

Thanks M&M; with all your love and support
I have endured, and together with God, we all
shall prosper. Adam, Giovanni, and Kelijah,
keep the faith and stay with Christ.

© Lyceum Books, Inc., 2001

Published by

LYCEUM BOOKS, INC.
5758 S. Blackstone Ave.
Chicago, Illinois 60637
773+643-1903 (Fax)
773+643-1902 (Phone)
lyceum@lyceumbooks.com
http://www.lyceumbooks.com

ISBN 0-925065-35-8

Library of Congress Cataloging-in-Publication Data

Social work practice : treating common client problems / edited by Harold E. Briggs and
Kevin Cocoran.
    p. cm.
  Includes bibliographical references and index.
  ISBN 0-925065-35-8 (alk. paper)
   1. Social service. 2. Social case work.   I. Briggs, Harold E.   II. Cocoran, Kevin.

HV40.S6195 2001
361.3'2--dc21   00-056338

Contents

List of Figures and Tables

Preface

Graduate students in social work in the twenty-first century are acquiring knowledge and skills from changes that have grown out of a rich past. Many of the common social issues and problems students are exposed to in their field settings are addressed in this book. They are addressed through effective practice technology used by social workers and other helping professionals for more than fifty years. Also, some of the relevant challenges to promoting effective social work practice are addressed in historical context by many of the new authors highlighted in this book, authors such as William J. Reid, Frederic G. Reamer, Christine T. Lowery and Mark A. Mattaini, and Ronald H. Rooney.

Further, what we as social workers use to produce change or the way in which we know how to make an impact are more an outgrowth of the contributions of our previous experiences rather than the results of any systematic effort or planned inquiry. Our foundations in science and the increasing emphasis on evaluation and research are covered in the chapters by Reid and Thyer. These chapters provide students with the background and empirical support of many of the empirical practice methods used in part two.

The legacies of earlier pioneers such as Mary Richmond and her contributions to establishing change technology continue to play an important role in influencing our ideas about change and contemporary social work practice. From our modest beginnings in the latter part of the nineteenth century and early part of the twentieth century up to more recent times, social work practice tools and knowledge have been shaped by a changing society and emerging trends, issues, and concerns. In this second edition of *Structuring Change* (now entitled *Social Work Practice*) we have broadened the foci to accommodate these developments.

All in all, we provided additional chapters to prepare students with a general foundation of the profession of social work as well as the best practice methods for addressing common client problems. In this book, emphasis on change and factors that influence or interfere with it are examined. These include factors such as professional liability and ethics, clinical and community-based social work practice, diversity, and nontraditional approaches to social work practice, such as changes in uses in power between practitioner and clients and paternal involvement in service delivery. Furthermore, additional chapters that emphasize the scientific basis of the profession have been provided, along with their change processes and research methodologies.

This book is about change and effective social work practice. We juxtapose change and effectiveness because we believe that social work is all about change, regardless of whether the focus of change is an individual, a family, or a community. To be an effective social worker, you must be able to facilitate change. Our goal is to help you do this in clinical and community-based social work practice. We will do this by considering the foundations of change and then demonstrating the applications to a number of common problems seen in social work practice.

In part one, the first two chapters introduce social work practice with a broad enough scope to give us two views of clients: a view of those in need of clinical and community services, namely, those who need what is known as goal-directed contracting, and an ecological view, which emphasizes the transaction of the person in the environment. The next two chapters examine the foundations of change for clients in clinical practice and community-based social work practice. Both chapters consider the evidence-based elements and aspects of effective social work practice. Chapter 5 is designed to show how to implement or operationalize the fundamental elements of effective practice by showing how to set goals and contract with clients for change and how to evaluate change over the course of the intervention. As is true throughout the book, evaluation is approached from the perspective of what you should do to set goals and monitor change in clinical and community-based social work. Consequently, the emphasis is more on good social work practice than good research. The goal is to show you how to do evaluation in a practical and informative manner that actually guides your practice. The foundations of clinical and community-based social work are then considered in the context of social work values and ethics in chapter 6.

The chapters in part one, like all those throughout this volume, will use the term "client" to refer to the focus of clinical and community social work interventions. Despite the fact that managed care has replaced all of our "clients" and "patients" with "enrolled members" and "covered lives," we use the term client because it is conventional and fairly well understood as the recipient of services.

Part two of the book presents the foundations of change as applied to a number of common client problems. When we say "common" we simply mean problems frequently seen by a social worker, and these might include the problems of an individual, couple, family, or community. The chapters are organized around common client problems. Each chapter presents at least one problem, shows how you can assess and measure the problem, and delineates how you can use an effective intervention to help facilitate client change. We have tried to assure that each chapter presents at least one intervention in terms that are replicable by readers. After all, we want to show you how to facilitate change in your own social work practice.

The problems covered in this book, of course, do not encompass all those you will encounter in your professional practice of social work. This is also true for the interventions presented here. In fact, most of the problems and practices discussed warrant entire volumes themselves, and the coverage here is limited. In preparing *Social Work Practice* it was necessary to be selective, and we have tried to include a wide range of problems and clinical and community interventions. The specific methods of intervention and problems were chosen to show you how to use a variety of techniques in your practice. Each of the chapters in part two is preceded by a brief editors' note that highlights how the principles presented in the foundations of change are applied in that chapter.

All of the authors hope that you will find this book useful in your efforts to do effective social work. Clearly, we have not covered all of the fundamental and ethical issues, possible clinical and community interventions, or client problems that you will face as a social worker. Those covered, we hope, will provide a good start in helping to facilitate your own change as you learn to use clinical and community interventions.

Acknowledgments

We would like to acknowledge the many people who aided in the completion of this book. First of all, we would like to express indebtedness to the authors of the chapters and recognize their personal efforts. Thanks! We are also grateful to David Follmer of Lyceum Books for his assistance. We would like to recognize Verlea G. Briggs and Lisa Shannon-Joseph for typing and assisting in the preparation of the final manuscript. And finally, it must be pointed out that a flip of a coin determined if the authors' names would appear in alphabetical order or otherwise (a regrettable idea in Corcoran's view).

PART ONE

Foundations of Change in Social Work Practice

CHAPTER 1

Introduction: Implementing the Foundations of Change

Kevin Corcoran

Richard M. Grinnell, Jr.

Harold E. Briggs

How many times has this question been asked by social work students; "What am I supposed to actually do to help clients change?" The process of helping clients requires that someone or some organization change something. In the first edition of this book, we considered some of the foundations of change. In this beginning chapter of the second edition, we direct the reader to consider how to implement these foundational aspects of social work practice. We are using the term "change" to mean planned change—that is, change that is not accidental, change that results from your social work intervention. This book provides students with a framework for how to help their clients change by explaining the main ideas and skills social workers need to effectively assist clients in planned change.

THE STRUCTURE OF CHANGE

We believe that social workers should structure their practices systematically in order to maximize change. The structure of practice, as presented in this book, has seven basic interrelated components: 1) setting client goals, 2) setting client objectives, 3) selecting an appropriate intervention(s), 4) structuring the intervention(s), 5) establishing a contract, 6) monitoring and evaluating the effects of the intervention, and 7) establishing a process for maintaining outcomes of planned change (see chapters 18 and 19; Goldstein & Kanfer, 1979; Pinkston, Levitt, Green, Linsk, & Rzepnicki, 1982; Rzepnicki, 1991; also see Duehn, 1985). By "client," we mean individuals, families, and communities at all levels. We use the term "client" to refer to the recipient of the social work intervention and the target of change.

Setting Goals

The first component of social work practice involves goal setting, which is discussed by Kevin Corcoran, Wallace J. Gingerich, and Harold E. Briggs in chapter 5. Goal setting is the process that maps where you and your client are and where you want to go. Essentially, goal setting involves asking, "What do

I want to accomplish throughout and by the end of treatment?" The importance of setting clearly defined, attainable goals for clinical social work practice cannot be overemphasized. Setting vague or unreasonably high goals subjects your clients to a cruel and destructive experience in disappointment, frustration, and erosion of their confidence (Wood, 1978).

Three important factors should be considered before setting goals with clients (Cordon & Preston-Shoot, 1987; Locke, Sarri, Shaw, & Latham, 1981):

1. Specific and challenging goals are more effective in bringing about the desired client outcomes than are vague or easy-to-achieve goals.
2. Goal setting leads to more effective results when the client is involved in goal selection rather than merely having goals assigned to him or her.
3. Goals should be realistic and attainable.

Why establish goals?   There are three main reasons to establish clear goals when working with clients (Simons & Aigner, 1985):

1. The mutuality of goal selection ensures that both you and your client are engaged in the problem-solving process with the same expectations and are pursuing the same goals.
2. The process of goal selection facilitates the development and implementation of the intervention plan. In short, when goals are specifically stated, the means to attain them become more identifiable.
3. The goal-setting process provides a basis for the eventual evaluation of your intervention plan.

In summary, client goals point all parties involved in the change process in a mutually agreed-upon direction and outcome during the treatment relationship (Anderson, 1989). Some clinical examples of goal statements are

> To be able to cope with a dying child
> To be able to have a happy marriage
> To be able to feel good about oneself

Establishing priorities among goals.   Once the purpose of treatment has been translated into a client's goal statements, the next task is to establish an order of priority for the goals. Austin, Kopp, and Smith (1986) present three criteria that are helpful in guiding the goal selection process:

> The importance of the goal to the client
> The severity or intensity of the problem addressed by the goal
> The potential for successful goal achievement

Each of these criteria should be discussed with your client before deciding which goal to work on first, second, and so on. Once realistic goals have been established and you and the client have set priorities for them, it is important to define each goal operationally in terms of specific client objectives.

Setting Client Objectives

The second component of structuring social work practice is setting client objectives. Although goal statements provide a general set of intervention outcomes, they lack specificity. In contrast, objective statements are specific, concrete, and measurable (Coulton & Solomon, 1977; Sheafor, Horejsi, & Horejsi, 1988). For example, with what specifically would the client be expected to cope if he or she had a dying child? What change is needed and by whom for the client to be happier in a marriage? What must change relative to the client or the social environment in order for him to feel good about himself or herself?

Client objectives address five questions: who, what, to what extent, where, and when?

Who?   Objectives must make it clear who or what specifically is to change. Is it an individual, a family, a group, an institution, an organization, or a community? For example, as Craig Winston LeCroy discusses in chapter 11, is there a need for change in a troubled teenager, or is it the way in which the parents interact with their child that must change?

What?   The question of "what" to change typically refers to the problem areas expressed by the client upon which you both agree to work. However, "to receive family therapy," or "to receive individual counseling" does not adequately address the question. The goal should never focus on the method of intervention, but rather on what you and your client expect to see as a result of the intervention (Howe, 1974). As Nan Van Den Berg illustrates in chapter 8 on working with depressed women from a feminist perspective, objectives might be diverted toward the attainment of more interpersonal control, assertiveness, or political activism in oppressive situations.

Over the years, these "what" questions sometimes have been referred to as client target problems. Social work practice is always geared to changing client target problems. There are three basic types of client target problems that we try to change: behaviors, feelings, and cognitions (which include knowledge levels).

For example, clinical interventions can focus on changing client behaviors, such as school truancy, eating habits, temper tantrums, substance abuse, enuresis, compulsive fire setting, excessive smoking, and physical aggression. As illustrated by Norman H. Cobb and Catheleen Jordan in chapter 10, this change could be in how effectively couples can communicate and negotiate responsibility.

We can also intervene to change clients' affect, that is, the way they feel toward someone, something, or themselves, including emotions such as anger, frustration, anxiety, feelings of personal inadequacies, phobias, social rejection, depression, or self-esteem. Galan illustrates the importance of work with clients' emotions in chapter 15 by showing how to work with identity problems that developed from some Mexican-American family relations.

We also can intervene to change client cognitions, such as inappropriate self-perceptions and inadequacies in processing information about oneself. For example, Corcoran and Keeper in chapter 14 illustrate how to resolve some of the perceptions of emptiness experienced by a person with borderline personality disorder. Also on a cognitive level, we even can help clients change their knowledge levels by, for example, helping them to understand the benefits of safer sex, providing information about various public assistance programs, or educating them about sexual dysfunctions. Gochros in chapter 13 illustrates this in his discussion of the importance of the role of knowledge level when working with persons who are HIV positive.

There are, of course, times when the client change covers more than one target area. For example, in chapter 9, Thyer shows how to work with a client's anxiety (affect) in order to improve specific social behaviors (action).

The important point to remember in changing clients' action, affect, or cognition (including knowledge levels), is that any change must be in a planned and desired direction (Saxton, 1979). In addition to helping clients change their target problems, we also can help them to cope with their target problems, such as by helping them to adjust to their local communities after hospitalizations. In short, we are always working to maintain, increase, or decrease (in the desired direction) some aspect(s) of the client's functioning relative to one or more target problems that involve some specific action, affect, or cognition.

To what extent?   The objectives that are designed to realize the broader goals should also consider the degree of change that is needed. The intent here is to provide you and the client with an idea of the magnitude of expected outcome of the intervention. Both you and the client are trying to determine, in advance of your intervention, what will constitute an acceptable level of change relative to the target problem. Will the decrease of physical abuse of one's spouse by 90 percent constitute success? Will a reduction of a child's truancy from every day to once or twice a week be considered a success? Will the reduction of the number of family arguments from every time they have dinner to only once a month constitute success? How much change, and in what, is needed for a client to be considered successful in coping with a dying child? How much change and by whom will reflect happiness in a marriage? And how much change in what about the client is necessary for him or her to feel good about himself or herself?

Where?   Many of your clients' target problems occur in specific settings or at specific times during the day. For example, Breanne may get aggressive only at school (a setting). Or, Ray may get depressed only during the evening (a time). The answer to this question helps to orient you and the client as to where specifically to look for the expected outcome (Kenmore, 1987).

When?   This question establishes the time frame within which the expected outcome is supposed to occur. A realistic time frame must be established by a negotiation between you and the client. When setting specific dates for resolution of the client's target problem, the motivational levels of everyone engaged in the change process are likely to increase. Although this implies that the goals and objectives should be time limited, it does not necessarily mean that the intervention itself is short term or lacking in continuity. For example, Fischer (in chapter 12) illustrates the need for an ongoing maintenance program with recovering substance abusers. In contrast, certain interventions, such as Nugent's illustration of single-session mediation (chapter 16), are by design time limited. Regardless of the length of the intervention, you and your client should determine when it is reasonable to reach a goal.

Examples of objective statements.   Below are three examples of client objectives that incorporate the characteristics of the above main points:

1. Connie (who), within one month (when), will have decreased her depression (what) at home while caring for her dying child (where) by 25 points (to what extent) as measured on a standardized depression scale.
2. Mr. and Ms. Olivetti (who), within six months (when), will have increased their level of sexual satisfaction and other pleasurable leisure activities (what) at home (where) by 40 percent (to what extent) as measured on the standardized Passionate Love Scale and Index of Sexual Satisfaction.
3. Mr Yachats's (who) emotional swings of fondness and contempt toward women (what) at work and in interpersonal settings (where) will decrease in frequency from daily mood swings to less than once per week (to what extent) within six months (when).

These types of goals and objectives are illustrated in the client target problems discussed in *Social Work Practice*. The problems—and resulting goals and objectives—are typical of those encountered by social workers in a variety of clinical practice settings. The chapters in this book reflect a broad range of client problems, such as suicide, anxiety, phobia, schizophrenia, marital conflict, drug and alcohol abuse, depression, adjustment to living with HIV, disputes, social and interpersonal problems, identity problems, and troubled youth. In addition, each chapter considers a range of related client problems, allowing generalization from a specific application of an intervention to its application to other problems.

The client target problems covered in *Social Work Practice* are presented in various practice settings, including hospitals, residential programs, outpatient clinics, group practices, and just about anywhere that clients are found. Frequently, each client problem is illustrated in terms of various actions, affects, or cognitions specific to the problem. By varying the problems and the settings within which they are addressed, we hope to highlight the important but subtle differences that get played out with respect to the client's specific problem.

Selecting an Intervention

The third component of structuring social work practice is selecting an appropriate intervention that has been demonstrated to work on the client's target problem (Compton & Galaway, 1989). *Social Work Practice* provides directives for working with a variety of different strategies that are appropriate for use with several specific client target problems. The main intent is to show how to actually help clients change by using specific treatment interventions that have been demonstrated to be effective with specific problems. This does not imply that any one intervention is guaranteed to be effective. Even the most proven and apparently straightforward intervention has subtleties that can facilitate or inhibit its impact on changing a client's problem.

Because of the complexity of human behavior, the selection of an appropriate intervention strategy is extremely difficult. Moreover, because no single intervention is appropriate for every client problem, the variety of different presenting problems demands a variety of different treatment interventions. In part, this is why *Social Work Practice* provides so many diverse intervention strategies.

In short, the task of the clinician is to match each client's particular target problem with the most effective and efficient intervention available. The intent is to maximize the fit between the intervention and the client's problem and avoid the temptation to redefine the problem to fit some preferred intervention (Fischer, 1978). Further, a tried-and-true intervention that is applied inappropriately to a client's problem is of little use. The interventions presented in this book are not the only effective means to bring about change in the problems that are discussed. The interventions do represent, however, a variety of structured approaches whose efficacy has been documented in the references that accompany them.

The treatment interventions presented in *Social Work Practice* are derived from a variety of different theoretical orientations. Several are based on a combination of theories. Admittedly, the theoretical orientation implicit in many of the accompanying chapters, or at least some of the specific techniques used in the suggested interventions, are based on social learning theory. This is because there is a lot of research literature available to support the effectiveness of interventions that are based on this theory. Additional intervention perspectives include a feminist view of treating persons with depression, conflict and conflict resolution theory, psycho-dynamics, gestalt, and family theories.

Whenever possible and appropriate, the treatment intervention has tried to avoid relying on a single theoretical perspective. This is important because few interventions are based on one theoretical framework. Planned short-term treatment may be primarily a social learning approach, but it also draws on communication and interpersonal theories, a fact that speaks to its theoretical pluralism. Similarly, the discussion by Cobb and Jordan (chapter 10) concerning the role of social competency in dysfunctional relations reflects a social learning theory perspective tempered by social exchange theory. Van Den Bergh's chapter on feminist intervention with depression draws from several diverse theories and emphasizes the roles of power and politics.

It could be argued, and in fact should be argued, that all of the proposed interventions are "behaviorally grounded," in that each is designed to help clients change behaviors, whether in the form of an action, an affect, or a cognition. It is hard to imagine a clinical social work intervention that is designed to do anything other than to change at least some specific aspect of behavior, either in the client system or in some facet of the broader social environment.

Although the proposed intervention strategies apply to a particular set of social and psychological problems, each chapter also considers the application of the approach to related problems.

Structuring the Intervention

The fourth component of structuring social work practice refers to those identifiable elements of the intervention process that are associated with treatment effectiveness. Reid lays out the scientific and empirical foundations for social workers seeking to employ effective practice, while Thyer highlights examples of evidenced-based approaches to social work practice. Clearly, we have not identified all of the elements related to effective practice. However, there is reason to believe that by incorporating into one's own practice routine those elements that are known, there is a greater likelihood that one will help clients to change (Bloom, Fischer & Orme, 1999).

In general, the structure of effective practice refers to guidelines for using a specific intervention, well-defined and well-organized components of the intervention itself, and the appropriate fit between the intervention and the client's particular problem. Structure is not based on any one specific theory. The theoretical nature of structure, then, makes it possible to enhance the chances of helping the client regardless of the theory or theories behind the intervention.

This is not to imply that theory is inconsequential to social work practice. The theories we employ in practice guide our understanding of clients and their problems; the specific techniques that flow from them, however, can be structured in a variety of ways. For example, even the most dogmatic behaviorist needs to be empathic, and the ego-oriented practitioner uses a subtle form of the behavioral principle of exposure when working with the anxiety associated with narcissism.

We are not suggesting that all theories are equally valid or useful. We simply are asserting that the most effective treatments are based more on what is actually done, within a specific structure, relative to a client system, than on the theory one uses to understand the client. The structure of the intervention should be designed to enhance the probability of effectively helping clients to change, regardless of—and sometimes in spite of—the theory.

All the interventions in the chapters that follow are practical and are considered to be effective with the particular problem with which they are linked. They are presented in a way that will help you to apply them with a variety of clients. Some are presented in a step-by-step fashion to facilitate effective learning and accurate implementation. Interventions that are clearly specified and delineated are not only easier to learn, but also tend to be more effective because they can be implemented with more specificity.

However, not all the interventions covered in the book are highly structured. In part, this is because some techniques are simply less structured and more experiential in nature. Be that as it may, the authors have presented these interventions with specificity and guidelines for their use. When using less-structured interventions, you have to do slightly more of the work of providing the structure. This is not difficult to do and will become routine as you learn to tailor the intervention to the client's problem. Even seemingly less-structured interventions can be defined clearly by delineating what specific techniques are to be used, defining the client's problems and goals, and contracting with specificity. When a less-structured intervention is used, it should be designed to maximize its effectiveness by including the components that have been identified as associated with effective outcomes. By focusing on the available structure and by designing the treatment plan to maximize the structure, you should find that the intervention is not only more effective, but also easier to learn and more readily applicable to a range of social work practice situations.

The client, too, will need to participate actively in the intervention process. This includes not only goal setting, as we discussed above, but also in-session activities and outside homework assignments. The client may need to experience emotional catharsis, practice a new behavior or skill, or restructure a faulty thought process, as well as continue the efforts at change outside the session. Homework assignments are designed to help generalize what is acquired in the session to the client's natural environment. Again, the change that the client is trying to make in the psychologically safe environment of the sessions may include any action, affect, or cognition.

In summary, the treatment intervention must be appropriate for the client's target problem and the client must participate in its implementation. Even the most highly regarded and scientifically sound treatment intervention will not be effective if applied inappropriately to a client problem. For example, individual therapy is rarely effective when applied to marital problems.

Establishing a Contract

The fifth component of structuring social work practice is to formulate a treatment contract. A contract is essentially an agreement between the clinician and the client (Maluccio & Marlow, 1974; Saxton, 1979; Cordon & Preston-Shoot, 1987; Rothery, 1980). It should cover at least the following dimensions:

1. The client's target problem, a solution to which both the clinician and client will work toward.
2. The specific responsibilities of the clinician and client in terms of rights and obligations.
3. The specific treatment intervention to be used in resolving the target problem and achieving the target goals.
4. The administrative procedures and constraints involved, such as when to meet, where to meet, time, costs.

In a nutshell, a treatment contract should spell out *who, will do what, to what extent, under what conditions,* and *when.* The contract should be sufficiently explicit and detailed so that each participant understands clearly what is expected of him or her in the treatment process. The contract enhances a client's motivation to change. Notice how closely the contract relates to the establishment of treatment objectives mentioned above.

Monitoring and Evaluating

The sixth component of structuring social work practice are the monitoring and evaluating of progress toward the resolution of the client's target problem, as Corcoran, Gingerich, and Briggs discuss in chapter 5. When practice is structured to enhance effectiveness, it should include some systematic method of monitoring and evaluating whether progress is being made toward the resolution of the client's target problem (Nelsen, 1988; Howe 1974). Monitoring and evaluating practice are integral parts of effective treatment when they facilitate the change process and assure relevant feedback within a confidential atmosphere (Grinnell, 1993; Grinnell & Williams, 1990; Bloom, Fischer & Orme, 1999).

Maintaining Change

The practice technology for maintaining treatment gains following the removal of treatment is described by Nay in Goldstein and Kanfer (1979). Nay provides criteria for maximizing treatment gains made in clinical programs. Essentially, psychologists believe that the change process used to establish outcomes needs to occur in the environments in which the outcomes are to be sustained and maintained. Adapting these procedures for social work practice, Pinkston et al. (1982) and Rzepnicki (1991) described these methods as generalization and maintenance procedures for extending treatment gains acquired during intervention. They suggest that these procedures need to be defined and included as part of the assessment, intervention, and follow-up methods of social work practice. During assessment, they define generalization procedures for social workers to use as including the 1) selection of behaviors to be increased that exist and occur at a low rate in the client's environment, 2) selection of behaviors to be increased that are incompatible with problem or negative behaviors, 3) selection of behaviors that are not difficult or complex to change, 4) selection of outcome behaviors that occur in at least one environment first to ensure opportunity for reinforcement, and 5) selection of outcome behaviors that are consistent with the client's cultural values, self-determination, and informal system.

Pinkston et al. (1982) and Rzepnicki (1991) recommend four strategies for ensuring maintenance of treatment gains: 1) selection of common stimuli that exist in both the treatment and the client's natural environment settings, 2) availability of desired reinforcement and use of intermittent reinforcement, 3) technical assistance and support for clients to learn skills for changing current and future problem behaviors, and 4) training clients in self-management procedures to address future problem and outcome behaviors. Application of this maintenance of change technology is further described and illustrated through case examples in chapter 18 by Elsie M. Pinkston, Glenn R. Green, Nathan L. Linsk, and Rosemary Nelson Young and in chapter 19 by Briggs.

STRUCTURING CHANGE AND CLIENT MOTIVATION

People seeking social work treatment bring with them widely varying degrees of motivation or commitment to change. Lack of motivation can be problematic with clients who are not voluntary, such as a child on probation or a husband forced into marital treatment. Even voluntary clients may need their motivation enhanced.

Often clients will ask clinicians to "change my husband; make him drink less" or to "get my parents to stop nagging me." Even the voluntary client often asks to change some antecedent condition or a consequence of a behavior, but says "don't change my behavior." It is not until the client comes to terms with the need to change some specific action, affect, or cognition that he or she is motivated.

We believe that one way to help motivate clients is to use structured interventions. This includes setting specific and realistic goals, and you might need to discuss with clients the need to focus on some behavior of theirs rather than of someone else. Moreover, structuring treatment and actively involving clients in the entire treatment process, as this chapter illustrates, will help clients to move forward to realistic change. Monitoring and evaluating, as demonstrated in chapter 5, helps clients see how they are changing. Actively participating in and knowing what is involved in the treatment process, along with seeing that things are getting better, probably influences client motivation. We think that structuring treatment results in more motivated clients.

SUMMARY

This chapter discusses some components of practice that are considered essential to maximizing client change. It is based on the assumption that the effectiveness of practice is in large part a consequence of the extent to which these components are incorporated systematically into the structure of the intervention plan.

One overriding guideline in the structure of change is specificity. An intervention is more likely to be effective if its intended purpose, the client's target problems, and the treatment protocol all are specific. The following questions provide a framework that will help to structure your intervention:

1. What are the client's specific target problems to be changed?
2. What are the specific goals to be pursued?
3. What specific treatment interventions are to be selected in relation to the client's target problems?
4. How, specifically, will treatment interventions be structured? What specific homework will the client do after each session?
5. What, specifically, will the treatment contract include about who will do what, to what extent, under what conditions, and by when?
6. How will it be determined when the client's target problems have been resolved or the goals of treatment have been reached?
7. What will be done to assist the client in maintaining treatment gains following termination of the treatment process?

The client must be actively involved in answering these questions. This client involvement includes not only defining the problem and setting the goals of treatment, but also the actual process of making change within and outside the treatment setting (i.e., client homework). This active participation means that the clinician must be more than a blank screen against which the client reflects his or her feelings. To enhance effectiveness, the clinician also must help the client by problem solving, role modeling, confronting, reinforcing, giving advice; in essence, by actively working toward change with the client.

A Concluding Remark

There are, of course, other salient components to effectively helping clients than those discussed in *Social Work Practice*. We have identified some of the most important ones. It is advisable to incorporate these components into those interventions that are less structured. Although additional components will be identified in the individual chapters that follow and by future research, we believe that interventions that are designed to include these components greatly enhance your ability to help your clients change.

CHAPTER 2

The Foundation of Social Work Practice

Mark A. Mattaini

In this chapter, Mattaini examines the foundation knowledge and perspectives that are central to the conception and practice of social work. He covers the person-in-situation framework as a conceptual lens for developing a critical perspective, as well as organizing and facilitating social work practice. This chapter defines for the reader the distinguishing characteristics of social workers compared with other helping professionals. As a basis for preparing the student in the fundamentals of promoting change, Mattaini lays out the complexities associated with social work practice and defines in detail the person in situation within the larger environmental framework that serves as the setting of the transaction between the social worker and client system. This chapter acquaints the student with the core competency areas for graduate social work practice, including social justice, diversity, ethics, values, and sources of knowledge needed for professional practice. The chapter concludes with a detailed discussion of the ecological systems perspective as an organizing theoretical map used by social workers to facilitate appropriate entry, assessment, intervention, and support to clients. In this chapter, Mattaini helps the student attend to the various relationships, contextual factors, person, situational, and environmental conditions that need consideration in establishing goals and objectives for behavior change through social work practice.

A child suffers from malnutrition with resulting cognitive limitations. A battered woman sinks more and more deeply into depression. A community struggles with what to do about an increasing number of homeless mentally ill people on the streets. An older man despairs of ever breaking free of an addiction to alcohol, despite the loss of his family and livelihood. A school serving minority children lacks basic educational resources and is staffed by unqualified teachers who have long ago accepted that most of their students will fail. Poor, single mothers in a neighborhood live in isolation. All of these situations (and many others), despite their differences, are the province of social work. All involve transactions (or lack of them) between people and their social and physical worlds, and if one looks deeply enough, all involve social justice and basic human rights.

Some view "social work" in narrow terms, as a discipline responsible for child protection (or income maintenance) or as the licensed "mental health profession" requiring the fewest years of education and the least cost. But social work is much more than this. Social work at root involves action to enhance and heal the social fabric, the web of life, in any of innumerable ways. When a practitioner works with an individual client, the purpose of the work is certainly to improve that client's life, but that life always occurs in a social context. When, in contrast, a social worker is involved in community-level practice, not only is the quality of life for the overall community affected, but also that of individuals. While for simplicity's sake we often talk about "practice with individuals," "practice with families," "practice with organizations," and so forth, social work practice is always embedded in, and affects, the transactional web of human relations; that is what makes it "social." There are many ways for social workers to contribute, but the ultimate goal is the same, a community of justice and shared power in which all individuals have access to the resources needed for a satisfactory life and to which all have the opportunity to contribute.

Carol Meyer, a seminal thinker in the profession, describes the socially embedded purpose of social work as follows:

> Social work claims as its central purpose the enhancement of adaptations between individuals, families, groups, communities—and their particular environments (Ewalt, 1979). . . . Every profession has a unique purpose, whether it be carried out in medical, psychiatric, legal, educational, architectural design, or other contexts. Any overlapping among professional disciplines usually occurs in the area of skills or selected knowledge, but not ordinarily in the area of professional purpose. For example, the overlap between psychiatry/psychology and social work is often overestimated. Here we find an example of "sharing" of skills and selected knowledge, but neither psychiatry nor psychology (and certainly not psychoanalysis) focus on the person-in-environment construct, nor stretch the boundaries of the case focus to include psychosocial phenomena." (1993, p. 18)

The purpose of the practice of medicine (including psychiatry) is curing illness and enhancing individual health. The purpose of psychology (the science of behavior or of the mind) is also primarily individual in nature. Social work, in contrast, focuses on the transactional field of which clients are indivisible parts.

In their person-environment practice, which seeks to operationalize social work purpose in an emergent way, Kemp, Whittaker, and Tracy (1997) make a similar point in different terms. As they describe it, this form of practice focuses on

1. Improving a client's sense of mastery in dealing with stressful life situations, meeting environmental challenges, and making full use of environmental resources.
2. Achieving this end through active assessment, engagement, and intervention in the environment, considered multidimensionally, with particular emphasis on mobilization of the personal social network.

3. Linking individual concerns in ways that promote social empowerment through collective action.

As suggested by these functions, social work clients cannot be artificially amputated from their social and physical worlds. The profession is not concerned with either person or environment, but rather with acting on patterns of transaction within which the client (whether that is an individual, a family, or a larger collective) is organically embedded. Consistent with Kemp et al.'s (1997) focus on empowerment, effective social work can only occur within a matrix of *shared power* (see chapter 7), in which the collaborative contributions and responsibilities of worker, client, and others in the ecological field are recognized as essential to process and outcome. As will be seen below, issues of social justice and human rights naturally and constantly emerge in such practice, because they shape the realities within which clients live out their lives.

THE COMPLEXITY OF SOCIAL WORK

Social work is, given what was said above, profoundly complex. Every practice event, whether it be a single word, a touch, a meeting, or the preparation of a report, involves many dimensions—individual, contextual, and transactional. Social workers deal with individuals, families, groups, communities, organizations, and even larger collectives. They collaboratively engage with people of many different social classes, gender identifications, sexual orientations, races and ethnicities, ages and abilities, belief systems and worldviews and grapple with challenges that include personal despair, child rearing and maltreatment, HIV/AIDS, the changes associated with aging, substance abuse, violence, family breakdown, racism, community building, and many others. The responsibilities associated with social work, therefore, are serious, and the burden on professional education and social work students and practitioners to be adequately prepared for practice is substantial. Most of this practice, of necessity, occurs within or in relation to organizations and institutions, for example, in child protective agencies, hospitals, workplaces, nursing homes, clinics, courts, jails, and governmental offices. Those settings and systems must also be considered in case planning, because they shape clients' lives and practices in important ways. Therefore, most social work cases, when seen in their full realities, are complicated, and the social worker in a sense needs to see all of this at once. Every transactional practice event involves multiple dimensions (case specifics, practice models, ethical considerations, and issues of power, for example), and those events are further shaped by additional contextual factors (including agency practices, natural networks, and social institutions, among others). To provide competent service, a social worker needs to know a good deal about each of these dimensions and factors and about how they interlock with and overlay each other. Social work practice requires attention to more transactional variables than any other profession. It is often necessary to learn about the segments shown in Figure 2-1 separately; at any moment, some will be foreground and others will only be background, but all are implicitly present in every practice event. Particularly at the graduate level, the social work professional must not only be prepared to act, but must be prepared to collaboratively and analytically design and supervise service plans and programs that take all of these variables into account. The material that follows introduces each of the segments shown; the subsequent chapters of this volume will gradually fill in the basic map provided here, including the institutional and sociocultural contexts within which practice events occur.

Social Justice and the Sharing of Power

Social work practice nearly always involves issues of social justice and often issues of basic human rights. For example, child abuse and woman battering have traditionally been viewed as "family matters," but, in fact, they involve serious violations of the Universal Declaration of Human Rights adopted by the United Nations in 1948 (United Nations, 1948; Lowery, 1998), which includes the following basic principles, among others: "Everyone has the right to life, liberty and security of person," and "No one shall be subjected to torture or to cruel, inhuman or degrading treatment or punishment." These issues also play out on larger canvases; entire ethnicities continue to be eradicated (Davidson, 1994), and immigrants and refugees face obstacles that few in our society recognize. But justice also is at issue when persons struggling with addictions are viewed as immoral rather than as struggling with biological, behavioral, and social forces beyond their immediate control, or when persons with mental illness are treated as other than fully human. Neither society nor social work (despite its professed values) has a strong history of treating all, especially those who are different than ourselves (or who we feel compelled to see as different for our own comfort), with respect.

Such an authentic commitment requires recognizing the connections among all in the web of humanity, a willingness to value perspectives and worldviews that are truly different from our own, and a commitment to the sharing of power in all areas of practice. "Empowerment" is a term that will be used often in this volume; it is important to recognize that empowerment is an outcome of the process of sharing power. In a shared-power relationship, whether between social worker and client, supervisor and social worker, or among community members, there is a recognition that everyone has something of value (abilities, gifts)—his or her own power—to contribute to collective outcomes and a responsibility to do so. The voice of each person needs to be heard and respected, and access to opportunities to contribute need to be supported.

Friere (1994) indicated that, "we cannot say that in the process of revolution someone liberates someone else, nor yet that someone liberates himself,

FIGURE 2-1   The Dimensions of Social Work Practice in Context

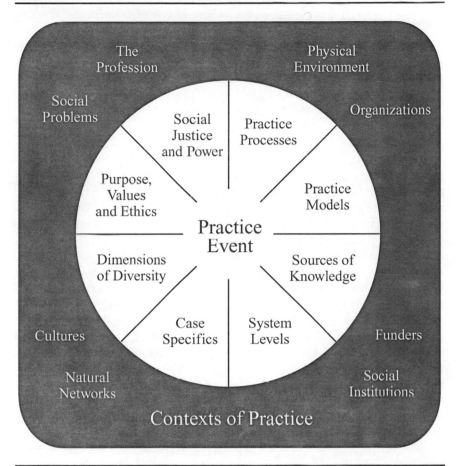

SOURCE: Reprinted with permission from Mattaini, Lowery, and Meyer (eds.) (1998, p. xv).

but rather that human beings in communion liberate each other" (p. 114). This is the process of shared power, which is profoundly different from zero-sum, coercive understandings of power (see chapter 7). It is easy to subscribe to these principles in the abstract, but given the cultural shaping that most people in US society have experienced, it is enormously difficult to operationalize the sharing of power in practice. Can the social worker treat someone who has hurt a child with respect and search with him for his potential contributions, while authentically discussing his obligations and acknowledging with him the need for collective healing? Is the social worker willing to support the voice of clients in the face of systematic oppression, even from one's own employer? Can the social worker let go of self-importance and view herself as one of many contributors to case outcome, one who carries serious responsibilities—not to fix a damaged person, but to contribute as participant to healing damage to the human web of which the social worker is simply a part? These are tests faced every day in practice, tests of the extent to which the social worker recognizes the social justice implications of her or his work and is committed to the sharing of power.

Professional Purpose, Values, and Ethics

Remembering why one is doing social work (professional purpose), even while under pressure, tests the practitioner's commitment. Social work, like every profession, is grounded in a set of core values. Six of these, and the ethical principles they subsume, are specifically elaborated in the introduction to the National Association of Social Workers' *Code of Ethics* (NASW, 1996), as shown in Table 2-1. Even these broad values are probably too narrow, since they do not adequately take into account the collective rights of peoples from cultures in which individual autonomy is not the highest value (see, for example, the UN Draft Declaration on the Rights of Indigenous Peoples, http://www.hookele.com/netwarriors/dec-En.html). Practicing, and living, in concert with such values is the challenge of a lifetime. But this is social work.

The broad values listed in Table 2-1 are elaborated in much more detail in the NASW *Code of Ethics*, which spells out the social worker's responsibilities in many areas, ranging from confidentiality to relationships with colleagues (see chapter 6). Some areas of ethical concern have received particular attention in recent years, including the responsibility to act if the social worker herself or a colleague is impaired (for example, by substance abuse or mental illness) and the risks of dual or multiple relationships. For example, although involvement in sexual relationships with clients or students has been recognized as unethical for many years, it is now clear that social and business relationships also need to be carefully examined for possible risks to the client and to the integrity of the social work relationship. The Code needs to be read often, because different sections become relevant depending on events occurring in one's practice. In addition, in many cases there is a need, and in fact an ethical obligation, to consult with peers and supervisors about how to apply the Code when values conflict and taking action consistent with social justice becomes a challenge.

Dimensions of Diversity

Most social work clients are different from the worker in one way or another. While human beings have much in common, the differences are in fact crucial for practice, because they shape clients', and workers', worlds and worldviews. Individuals, families, and communities are deeply diverse in terms of culture, ethnicity, age, sexual orientation, gender identification, reli-

TABLE 2-1 Core Social Work Values

The following broad ethical principles are based on social work's core values of service, social justice, dignity and worth of the person, importance of human relationships, integrity, and competence. These principles set forth ideals to which all social workers should aspire.

Value: *Service*

Ethical Principle: *The primary goal of social workers is to help people in need and to address social problems.*
Social workers elevate service to others above self-interest. Social workers draw on their knowledge, values, and skills to help people in need and to address social problems. Social workers are encouraged to volunteer some portion of their professional skills with no expectation of significant financial return (pro bono service).

Value: *Social Justice*

Ethical Principle: *Social workers challenge social injustice.*
Social workers pursue social change, particularly with and on behalf of vulnerable and oppressed individuals and groups of people. Social workers' social change efforts are focused primarily on issues of poverty, unemployment, discrimination, and other forms of social injustice. These activities seek to promote sensitivity to and knowledge about oppression and cultural and ethnic diversity. Social workers strive to ensure access to needed information, services, and resources; equality of opportunity; and meaningful participation in decision making for all people.

Value: *Dignity and Worth of the Person*

Ethical Principle: *Social workers respect the inherent dignity and worth of the person.*
Social workers treat each person in a caring and respectful fashion, mindful of individual differences and cultural and ethnic diversity. Social workers promote clients' socially responsible self-determination. Social workers seek to enhance clients' capacity and opportunity to change and to address their own needs. Social workers are cognizant of their dual responsibility to clients and to the broader society. They seek to resolve conflicts between clients' interests and the broader society's interests in a socially responsible manner consistent with the values, ethical principles, and ethical standards of the profession.

Value: *Importance of Human Relationships*

Ethical Principle: *Social workers recognize the central importance of human relationships.*
Social workers understand that relationships between and among people are an important vehicle for change. Social workers engage people as partners in the helping process. Social workers seek to strengthen relationships among people in a purposeful effort to promote, restore, maintain, and enhance the well being of individuals, families, social groups, organizations, and communities.

Value: *Integrity*

Ethical Principle: *Social workers behave in a trustworthy manner.*
Social workers are continually aware of the profession's mission, values, ethical principles, and ethical standards and practice in a manner consistent with them. Social workers act honestly and responsibly and promote ethical practices on the part of the organizations with which they are affiliated.

Value: *Competence*

Ethical Principle: *Social workers practice within their areas of competence and develop and enhance their professional expertise.*
Social workers continually strive to increase their professional knowledge and skills and to apply them in practice. Social workers should aspire to contribute to the knowledge base of the profession.

gion, race, physical and cognitive abilities, health, and many other factors and dimensions. Those differences shape who people are, how they respond to each other, how they experience reality, and how social work services affect them. A worker who does not recognize, respect, and respond to these differences will be at best ineffective and at worst damaging. Deep rifts of credibility and trust, rooted in generations or centuries of oppression, often exist among groups, and it is the social worker's role to bridge those gaps well enough to offer meaningful service.

For example, many traditional models of social work practice with individuals emphasize individual autonomy and individuation. This perspective is inconsistent with more collective cultures, including most indigenous tribal societies and many Asian cultures. Encouraging clients from such cultures to separate in a European American way from family and group may simply discourage them from continuing to work with the social worker because of a perceived lack of empathy or may further alienate clients from essential support networks if they respond to the suggestion. Such advice represents a profound ethnocentric arrogance, which a social worker who is not immersed in multicultural issues would not even recognize. At the same time, every individual lives at the confluence of many transactional dimensions of diversity and is therefore more than an aggregation of traits. Effective social work is deeply sensitized to both collective and individual differences. The practitioner needs to be open to continuous learning in this area and also must be willing to look deeply inside himself to acknowledge and work out the residual biases that we all have been programmed to harbor. By failing to do this, the social worker will only support historic and contemporary oppressive systems.

Case Specifics

Individualizing every case is the traditional role of the social work practitioner (Richmond, 1917; Meyer, 1993). The person or people involved, and the contextual factors that make up their realities, need to inform the practice process from engagement, through assessment and intervention, to termination. Professional, graduate-level social workers often need to coconstruct with the client unique case plans that respond to such specifics. Clients need to have the opportunity to participate deeply in these processes and to have the primary voice in determining focal issues to be addressed in the case. While practice guidelines for, for example, cases of child abuse, potential suicide, or neighborhoods struggling with violence can be enormously helpful, the realities of the lives and systems involved often require additional attention to individualization—in fact, this is usually the situation in the messy world of day-to-day practice. Social workers, therefore, need to be both deeply immersed in the professional knowledge base and highly attentive to factors that make each case different from every other.

System Levels

The Curriculum Policy Statement of the Council on Social Work Education indicates that graduate social workers need to be skilled in working with "systems of all sizes," meaning at a minimum that they must be able to work with individuals, families, formed and natural groups, neighborhoods and communities, and organizations. Some would add cities, states, and nations to this list. Addressing this need clearly requires a tremendous base of knowledge and skills, which this volume, and in fact an entire graduate social work education, can only begin to provide. The responsibility to be competent even at the beginning level in this wide range of work is correspondingly imposing.

Findings emerging from biology and ecology have had a substantial and substantive effect on social work theory in recent decades. These sciences teach us that all living systems, from individuals to communities, have certain characteristics and dynamics in common. For example, general systems theory and recent work on self-organizing systems, discussed in a later section of this chapter, are particularly useful, since they show how to look at living systems in analytic terms, and to some extent also what is required to influence such systems. Some core processes transcend the differences among system levels and may be generally helpful in the analytic work of practice. For example, all organized systems are deeply transactional and interconnected, have boundaries (which may be healthy, overly rigid, or too diffuse), have some form of internal structure or patterning, and operate in nonlinear ways.

Understanding systems requires looking at systemic functioning at the level on which it is organized. All of the processes involved in driving a car or beating one's wife can be studied at the level of cells and neurotransmitters, for example, but neither is organized at that level. Some problems (many struggles between adolescents and their parents, for instance) are rooted in transactional patterns of family culture and cannot be reduced to the individual problems of the people involved. Other issues—poverty, for example—are embedded in larger sociocultural structures, not simply in individual failure. In fact, almost none of the phenomena that social workers deal with can be adequately understood or dealt with if amputated from their contexts. As a result, the social work professional needs to be prepared to work at the system levels that are most likely to make a difference. Doing so requires not only generic skills that are applicable to all practice, but also specific skills that respond to the differential dynamics present in systems of different levels of complexity, for example, the skills of engaging individuals, the skills involved in teaching family problem solving, and the skills required to observe and analyze group processes.

Source of Knowledge

Professions, as opposed to crafts, are based on more than a set of skills and more than a set of values (although both are required). An organized base of knowledge is also characteristic. Since the 1960s, in fact, knowledge has come to be viewed as central to social work practice (Bartlett, 1970). Professional action is grounded in critical analysis, which in turn depends on extensive knowledge. Social work relies on knowledge from a wide range of sources, none of which can safely be ignored. Among these sources are the practitioner's own personal and professional experiences, "practice wisdom" gleaned from other experienced practitioners (often only partially elaborated verbally), quantitative and qualitative research, information obtained from clients, theory, and practice models (Mattaini, 1998a). Each needs to be tempered by the others. One's own experience is more deeply known than that of others, but certainly narrower, for example, and research findings may only partially fit the realities of a case situation. All of these sources may contribute to even micro decisions in practice. For example, at a particular moment in an interview a social worker may say, "Can you tell me more about how you felt then?" (going deeper), or "What happened next?" (moving on); determining the better choice under particular case circumstances is a knowledge-based decision.

Expanding one's professional knowledge and staying current are ethical imperatives in social work. Practice cannot be based on personal preference, convenience, or outdated theory. The social work professional, therefore, has a serious responsibility to be continuously learning, to read books and journals, to reflect with others on one's practice decisions, and to listen to clients to learn how their realities are changing over time. Complex practice requires complex knowledge.

Practice Models

Contemporary social work has sometimes been called "preparadigmatic"—meaning there is no single approach to practice that has been universally accepted. There are multiple theoretical approaches for understanding phenomena at all system levels and multiple practice models that emerge from each. While it may seem easiest to consider oneself "eclectic," random selection of intervention options based on unarticulated preferences of the moment is not professional practice. A social worker needs to have a framework for understanding why people act as they do, how families interact, how communities cope with stresses. Despite occasional claims to the contrary, some practice models and specific interventions have been demonstrated to be effective with some issues, while others have not; therefore, choices among them (which should usually be made in collaboration with the client) have serious ethical implications. One can learn from multiple approaches and models but must finally decide what to do for a reason. The interconnected "reasons" on which practice is based form one's practice model. The chapters in this volume reflect the realities of contemporary practice; multiple practice models are represented. Elaborating one's own practice model and deciding what can be drawn from other models and integrated coherently with one's own are the primary professional challenges. These decisions need to be made based on critical thinking, looking at the options in terms of rigor, applicability to practice realities, effectiveness, and efficiency.

Some contemporary practice models are based on organized theoretical knowledge bases, while others have evolved in a more inductive way. For example, the life model (Germain & Gitterman, 1996) applies ecological principles directly, the psychosocial approach (Goldstein, 1995) is deeply rooted in psychodynamic thought, and the eco-behavioral approach (Mattaini, 1999a, 1999b) relies heavily on the sciences of behavior and cultural analysis. Such approaches come close to the common scientific meaning of the word "model," since they have predictive value. Other practice models, like the now well-validated task-centered model (W. J. Reid, 1992), are structured as a set of practice processes that are not intimately connected with an underlying theoretical framework.

In recent years, it has become more common to find practitioners operating from such different models treating each other with respect and demonstrating a willingness to learn from each other. At the same time, differences among models are real, and they are often deeply rooted in differing worldviews and epistemologies. One of the critical functions of the ecosystems perspective (discussed below) is that it can help practitioners who are taking very different approaches to come to some agreement on what elements, systems, and transactions need to be examined in elaborating a case.

Practice Processes

While every case is different, all social work practice involves a common set of functions that tend to occur as a series of processes. The core processes are 1) engaging the client system, 2) envisioning an improved reality toward which the worker and client work, 3) assessing the case analytically to determine realistic options, and 4) intervening actively to move from the current situation toward the configuration that has been envisioned (Mattaini, 1998b). While these processes tend to occur roughly in that order, they are recursive and interlocking; for example, in the early stages of clinical work, the social worker is often concurrently gathering assessment data and deepening the working relationship. Other important processes overlap with these. For example, professionals bear an ethical responsibility to monitor the progress and outcome of their cases. Monitoring plans should emerge from the assessment, and monitoring itself should occur throughout intervention. When the joint work of client and social worker is completed, they also need to disengage without endangering the maintenance of the progress that has been made. While there is typically more discussion of this termination process near the end of the case, plans and preparation should be established and discussed throughout the process.

Some models of practice tend to emphasize the "problem-solving" process, which can be viewed as consisting of several steps (differing numbers depending on exactly how this process is conceptualized). For example, W. J. Reid's task-centered model (1985, 1992) tends to follow the general framework of clarifying and contracting around problems for work, analyzing those problems in context (examining causes of problems, obstacles that need to be addressed, and resources required), then completing tasks in session or in the client's home, the environment that may be necessary to address causes, obstacles, and resources. Monitoring is continuous through this process, and termination is planned from the beginning, since the task-centered model is a time-limited approach in which the number of sessions is usually determined in the beginning.

Whether operating from the engagement-envisioning-assessment-intervention frame or the problem-solving model, at any point in a case the social worker and client should be able to identify what practice processes they are engaged in. It should be clear, for example, when the focus is on assessment and when it is primarily on intervention. When monitoring indicates that inadequate change is occurring, it may be necessary to shift, for example, to return to assessment, but it should be clear to everyone involved when this is occurring.

Social work practice, then, involves many dimensions, all of which are active at the same time. Practice involves the integration of knowledge from many sources, in the context of values, ethics, and a relationship of shared power. And practice is shaped by a matrix of contextual factors only hinted at in the material above. How does a social worker bring all of this together conceptually? How can social workers who rely on different practice approaches communicate and work together? What ties all of these sources of knowledge together in ways that are consistent with the profession's historic focus on social justice? Over recent decades, a near consensus has emerged that the ecosystems perspective provides a common ground for practice. While originally adopted largely for philosophic reasons, recent scientific advances provide further support for this epistemic choice.

ECOSYSTEMS AND THE WEB OF LIFE

Social work has struggled for a century with how to operationalize the person-in-environment perspective crucial to its purpose (Kemp et al., 1997; Meyer & Mattaini, 1998). Because of the complexity of this view, it is tempting to focus primarily on either the person or the environment, rather than on the entire transactional field. In particular, social workers have often emphasized the individual—which is easier to grasp, and about which much is known—to the extent that many have narrowed their vision of the profession to the practice of psychotherapy (Specht & Courtney, 1994). Practitioners, however, regularly rediscover that working only with individual dynamics (particularly with an emphasis on pathology) is not adequate for addressing the socially embedded issues that define social work (Reynolds [1934] 1982; Germain, 1968; Meyer, 1983; Kemp et al., 1997). The ecosystems perspective, now over thirty years old, has become an almost universally accepted response to this problem. Two bodies of knowledge, in particular, were originally integrated in the ecosystems perspective, general systems theory (GST) and ecological science (Meyer, 1983; Meyer & Mattaini, 1998). More recent findings from the scientific study of biological ecosystems (Capra, 1996), described below, have the potential to further expand the utility of ecosystemic thought in social work.

General Systems Theory

GST was originally developed by Ludwig Von Bertalanffy, a biologist and member of the "Vienna Circle," as a general science for understanding self-regulating systems in transaction with their environments, for example, cells, organisms, and ecosystems. Social work theorists, in particular Germain (1968) and Meyer (1983), recognized how the principles of GST seemed to apply to the systems with which social workers practice. Several characteristics of GST that have been particularly important to social work include the following:

1. A shift from linear (cause → effect) to systemic thinking, in which events multiply and are reciprocally caused. Family dynamics, in which mutual, transactional effects are common, are an example. As a result of such nonlinear influences, there are often multiple equivalent routes to an outcome, a principle called *equifinality*. This can be particularly useful in practice, since some approaches for addressing an issue may not be accessible, but others may be. A corresponding principle, multifinality, indicates that many possible outcomes may result from a particular initial case configuration, frequently depending on the amplification of often very subtle factors within the system. This is a hopeful principle, since it contradicts strong determinism; a person who has experienced severe abuse, for example, may or may not achieve an adequate emotional state, depending on events later in life. It also suggests the need for social workers to abandon a sense of certainty, to remain open to possibilities and humble about what they know.

2. Systems are enclosed by boundaries that define what is inside and what is outside the system, and they exchange energy with the environment across that boundary. Systems that are overly closed, in which the boundaries are too rigid, are unable to obtain enough energy, and gradually run down (a process known as entropy). Those systems whose boundaries are too diffuse tend to lose their identities and dissipate into the environment (for example, a household in which people move in and out relatively randomly, leaving it unclear to anyone who really is the "family"). Recent research indicates that systemic boundaries are not artificial, but rather are naturally constructed by the processes that make up the system

(Capra, 1996). The social worker, then, cannot define boundaries as he or she wishes, but rather needs to recognize and work with such natural boundaries.

3. Living systems have structure, but that structure is dynamic rather than static. Patterns that organize the system remain in dynamic balance, even as the elements change. The structure of a living system is more like that of a whirlpool, in which the water molecules continually change but the pattern remains, than they are like the static equilibrium of a mobile (Capra, 1996). Only by continual renewal (which requires energy) does such a structure survive; if that renewal were to cease, the structure would dissipate. (Such "dissipative structures" were first described by Ilya Prigogine, a Russian Nobel laureate; see Capra [1996] for further details). The structure of a culture, be it the microculture of the family or the more complex culture of a community, is found in patterns of consistent practices.

The structure of systems in GST is viewed as hierarchical, with larger systems, organisms, or families, for example, being constituted of smaller systems like cells or family members. The focal system may shift at different times; for example, at one point transactions between an individual and her environment may be the focus of assessment and intervention, but at other points in the case the focus may shift to transactions between her family system and its environment.

4. Interactions among elements of a system are reciprocal; a change in one—whether positive or negative—reverberates through other parts of the system, and its effects may in fact be amplified in this process. A social work intervention directed toward one individual, for example, a single student in a classroom, will in some way affect the teacher and the child's classmates. If the intervention results in greater job satisfaction for the teacher, this may also have an effect within her own family system, and so forth. The importance of such transactions has become even clearer in recent years, as discussed below.

The other major force that shaped the ecosystems perspective in its early years was the then emerging science of ecology. GST theory alone often seemed quite abstract and somewhat difficult to apply; Carel Germain in particular identified metaphoric similarities between ecological theory and social work practice that could help to further operationalize this perspective (Germain, 1979).

Ecology

The core of ecological thought is the recognition of the organic interdependence of living things on each other, within a dynamic of mutual adaptation. People and their environments in the social world similarly adapt to each other, and the life model of social work practice developed by Germain and Gitterman (1980, 1996) directed the practitioner's attention to those transactions, focusing on the following dimensions:

1. Coping with environmental stressors.
2. Coping with life transactions.
3. Changing dysfunctional interpersonal processes.

Many ecological concepts, including adaptation, habitat, niche, predation, pollution, and diversity, can be useful in social work practice (Germain & Gitterman, 1986). Perhaps most important of all is the clear awareness that ecological science has of the transactional relatedness of all things within an ecosystem. Contemporary ecosystems science, which has emerged from years of ecological research, now has much more to offer to social work practice theory, particularly in refining our view of the core phenomena that need to be examined and with which practice is engaged.

Emerging Ecosystems Science

Fritjof Capra, in his volume, *The Web of Life* (1996), provides a readable introduction to emerging scientific findings that have the potential to further expand the utility of ecosystemic thinking for practice. Space permits only a brief sketch of this material here. Capra, a physicist and philosopher now working in the field of ecological science, summarizes several interlocking programs of research that indicate the organic interconnections among physical, biological, ecological, and social phenomena. Some of the material discussed remains controversial, but much of it has strong empirical support and is also heuristically useful.

There are three core principles from Capra's work that have a direct application to social work theory and practice: the shift from objects to relationships as the basic elements of reality, the central importance of self-organization in those networks, and the crucial place of diversity in such interlocking systems. A fourth related principle, consistent with this work, but emerging from behavioral science, is the central place of interlocking cultural practices in shaping human systems. Researchers have not yet determined the extent to which findings that are clearly applicable to biological systems at all levels from the cell to the ecosystem also apply to social and cultural systems, but the research from which this fourth principle derives suggests that they do. Some of this work may advance ecosystemic thinking in social work from a philosophic stance and metaphor toward practical prediction and application.

The primacy of relationships.   As summarized by Capra, emerging perspectives from both physics and biology recognize that reality does not consist of a collection of objects, but rather an "inseparable web of relationships" (1996, p. 37). The primary components of this web are patterns of relationships; objects are secondary and have reality only in the relationships. See Figure 2-2 for a depiction of this epistemic shift. The key organizational pattern is now seen to be the network or, more precisely, the network of transactions. Cells, organisms, ecosystems, all are organized in this network pattern. The parallels with "web thinking" in Native American thought (see chapter 7) are striking, and the two might be seen as different ways of describing the same processes. Human action, including social work practice, consists of transactions that either contribute to and strengthen networks of relationships or damage them. "Hierarchies" in these forms of systems thinking consist of levels of networks rather than of dominance hierarchies; for example, a community may be seen as a network of families, which in turn are themselves networks of people, which in turn are organic networks of biological organs and so forth. In fact, however, it is the network of richly interconnected and nonlinear transactions that is central in each, rather than the "entities."

The level of interdependence in such network thinking is core and organic. Capra indicates that "members of an ecological community are interconnected in a vast and intricate network of relationships, the web of life. They derive their essential properties and, in fact, their very existence from their relationships to other things" (1996, p. 298). This premise is also descriptive of human collectives, not just metaphorically, but actually. Einstein described individual autonomy from a scientific perspective as a delusion and indicated that, "The individual is what he is and has the significance that he has not so much in virtue of his individuality, but rather as a member of a great human society, which directs his material and spiritual existence from the cradle to the grave" (1979, p. 8).

Social work practice, in fact, can be seen as action that influences the pattern of transactions that form this web. All of social work practice, even when working primarily with an individual client, is about changes in transactional networks. The social worker is part of the web, the client is part of the web, and any changes (or positive conditions that the client wishes to maintain) will be supported, opposed, or both, by transactions elsewhere in the web. Practice with families involves work with transactions within the family and between the family and other systems; group work involves shifts in transactions among group members; and community practice involves work with higher-level networks.

Self-organizing networks.   Contemporary science extends our understanding of the structure and boundaries of such transactional networks as well. These networks, described by the term *autopoietic*, are self-organizing and "self-making." The dynamic patterns of transactions that structure the network

FIGURE 2-2   Figure/Ground Shift from Objects to Relationships

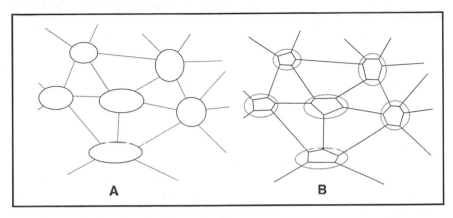

A   B

SOURCE: Reprinted with permission from Capra (1998, p. 3).

are organized by the network itself, and these richly interconnected networks of transaction establish their own natural boundaries. For example, cells are self-organizing networks of cellular components, organs are networks of cells, organisms are networks of such organs—each is in fact an ecosystem, connected with other ecosystems in higher-order networks. The boundary of each occurs as an inherent and natural result of its organization.

This material may seem very esoteric, but in fact it has significant practical applications to social work. First, social workers and their clients need to determine by observation where the natural boundaries of the case may be. A household, for example, is a network; the boundaries of that network are not determined by defining who should be considered a member of the family, but rather by paying attention to transactional patterns. If someone participates as a consistent actor in household transactions, they need to be included; if they do not, they are not part of the autopoietic system.

Second, networks "couple" with their contextual environments, but those environments do not ordinarily become parts of the network. How a network responds to an influence from outside is determined by the state and structure of the network. For example, two families may both be influenced by aversive pressure from a dangerous neighborhood. One may respond by collapsing, with its boundaries diffusing and members being lost to the street or to death. Another may respond with great resilience and may take collective steps to minimize contact with aversive events and to couple to the extent possible with healthier networks (churches and youth organizations, for example). Simply knowing the family's environment does not mean that the response of each family is predictable; the structure (enduring patterns of transactions) of each family makes a profound difference.

The social work practitioner may, therefore, need to work specifically with those patterns, and may in some sense need to "join" the family network (see Minuchin, 1974) in order to do so. Simply suggesting that the children living in such neighborhoods participate in an after-school program, for example, may not be enough. The social worker may also need to spend time with the parent, grandparent, and/or fictive kin to ensure that the family network supports that plan and is prepared to take the additional steps that may be necessary to address obstacles like finding or creating a "safe corridor" for the children to take to the program.

The role of diversity.   The crucial importance of diversity is a basic tenet of ecological science, of course. As Capra notes, "A diverse ecosystem will also be resilient. . . . The more complex the network is, the more complex its pattern of interconnections, the more resilient it will be" (1996, p. 303). Unfortunately, many in contemporary society regard respect and appreciation for diversity as primarily a matter of "political correctness" or as a way of placating minority groups, rather than as key for cultural and spiritual survival. For example, European American cultural practices have resulted in a continuously increasing number of persons incarcerated, who then become a drain on rather than contribute to society, and whose value as human beings and members of the collective is often lost. Solutions to this new and critical sociocultural challenge have not been easy to find. Indigenous groups, however, have developed entirely different responses from their very different worldviews, responses that are much cheaper, more effective, and more humane (Ross, 1996). Sadly, cultural diversity is disappearing as rapidly as biodiversity (Davidson, 1994), and the results are likely to be equally serious not only for members of endangered cultures, but for the human collective as a whole.

Interlocking cultural practices.   One question not answered by ecological scientists is whether the principles they have identified are applicable to "social systems" as well as biological systems. An emerging science of cultural practices indicates that they are. In the past two decades, behavioral scientists have recognized that much of human behavior is shaped by cultural level selection (Skinner, 1981) and that organized human groups are, in fact, dissipative structures that are organized by networks of interlocking transactions; each is a culture organized by its own cultural practices (Biglan, 1995; Glenn, 1991; Lamal, 1991, 1997; Mattaini, 1996). A family is not a coherent system because people are legally related, but rather because of regular patterns of exchange among the individuals, for example, and will dissolve if those exchanges stop. Professionals working with issues like violence, child maltreatment and child rearing, substance abuse, and community mental health systems increasingly recognize that the crucial variables are not so much individual behavior, but rather transactional networks of practices that organize family, neighborhood, community, ethnic, and other cultures (Biglan, 1995; Mattaini & Thyer, 1996).

Social problems cannot be understood or influenced if amputated from their ecological context, and that context consists primarily of interlocking supporting and opposing practices. If, for example, one wishes to reduce violent crime and death among high-risk youth, community organizations like Jesse Jackson's Rainbow Coalition have recognized that the interlocking practices of groups including parents, teachers, police, business, and churches need to be addressed, not merely the behavior of the youth involved. Understanding the underlying science of autopoietic networks can be helpful for operationalizing the actions that need to be taken (Mattaini, 1996; Mattaini, Lowery, Herrera, & DiNoia, in press). Not surprisingly, the results prove to be consistent with a commitment to shared power, in which the unique voices and varying contributions of all involved in the social web surrounding the behavior of interest are important, and all carry responsibility for the outcomes.

MAPPING THE TRANSACTIONAL WORLD

Whether working at a community or an individual level, the complexity of this view of practice realities, however, can be overwhelming. As is true in many other disciplines dealing with complex phenomena (meteorology, medical imaging, and theoretical physics, for example), visual images can be enormously helpful for organizing the data. The most common method of graphically conceptualizing social work cases is the ecomap (Hartman [1978] 1995; Mattaini, 1993b; Meyer, 1976; Meyer & Mattaini, 1998). Consistent with the discussions above, to be maximally useful, ecomaps should emphasize not so much the systems depicted as the transactions among them. Transactional ecomaps like that shown in Figure 2-3 are designed to do just that and are useful in ensuring that transactional interventions are privileged in case assessment and planning.

This image portrays a case from rural Alaska. The household consisted of a single Alaska Native mother (Julia), her 9-year-old son (Sam), and her 4-year-old daughter (Jessie) and came to the attention of the service system when one of Sam's friends reported that the two of them and two other boys had "had sex" with Jessie and another small girl. The social worker's first response, thinking in a linear way, might be to engage Sam in therapy, perhaps play therapy given that his verbal skills were very weak. Before jumping to that conclusion, however, it was critical to examine the transactional networks in which Sam was embedded. The social worker considered the household: Julia had a very severe drinking problem (drinking every day and very heavily on weekends with her boyfriend, one of a few white professionals in the community, with whom she often stayed overnight at those times). She had very few economic resources, and her friendship network consisted primarily of other heavy drinkers. As a result of these patterns, the children were often left to fend

FIGURE 2-3   A Transactional Ecomap Depicting a Social Work Case

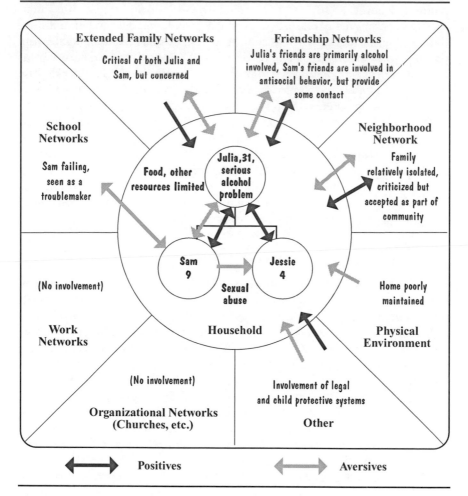

for themselves, spending a good deal of time at the homes of their grandmother or aunt and uncle; these relatives were highly critical of Julia. While Julia clearly loved her children, when she was intoxicated her treatment of them could shift from very punitive to largely nonengaged. Sam was one of a small number of students in the local school who had consistently failed in his schoolwork and was regarded as a troublemaker by the entire school staff. His father had died some years earlier. He had no close friends but was associated with a small network of children who occasionally got into trouble, primarily for using alcohol and vandalizing property.

   The transactional ecomap, in capturing these exchanges, provides many far more powerful points of intervention than individual child therapy, although this may be crucial for educational work with the child and for preparing him for family healing. Changes in the transactional network within the household certainly require attention (including parental monitoring and support and protection and healing for the daughter); other important possibilities involve the school and the extended family. Identifying specifics of the multiple possibilities for work in this case is a useful exercise for the reader, but a few words about the outcome of the case are instructive. The most powerful intervention proved to be the mother's serious engagement in substance abuse treatment, prompted in large part by Sam's involvement with the justice system resulting from the sexual abuse incident. Julia's treatment relied on engaging with networks of recovering persons, and reengaging with family and alternative friendship networks in a healing process. Her boyfriend also acted on his drinking problem. Julia found the strength, when sober, to work with the school to address her son's learning disabilities. Over the course of a few months, Sam's behavior in turn dramatically shifted; substantial family healing around the drinking, sexual abuse, and other areas occurred. The social worker's role was not simply therapeutic, but rather involved connecting clients with new networks, performing healing work within the family network, working with extended family and other natural networks, and conducting individual consultations with both Julia and Sam. A new ecomap prepared six months into the case would show extremely different transactional patterns than the original, and this is the key in practice. (The preparation of sequential ecomaps is one useful approach to monitoring practice, particularly if the observations recorded are gathered relatively rigorously.)

A FINAL WORD

Social work is a profoundly complex profession, with a profoundly crucial mission and purpose. Those who enter social work, therefore, take on serious responsibilities, involving the balance and care of the human web. As a result, social work professionals need to take seriously the core professional values of service, social justice, and competence, as well as the others discussed earlier, and respond by staying current with emerging knowledge and living a commitment to social justice and shared power. Social work, if it is done in a good way (chapter 7), is not a career—it is something much closer to the core of being human. Social work is not about taking care of those less fortunate, rather it is about caring for the web of which we are all part.

CHAPTER 3

The Scientific and Empirical Foundations of Clinical Practice

William J. Reid

In this chapter, Reid examines the contributions of the developmental research paradigm to clinical social work practice in community settings. The chapter highlights the relevance and principles of model-development research and how practitioners should use these guidelines to facilitate knowledge development and therapeutic gains through social work practice. Reid describes the early beginnings and contributions of science to clinical social work practice. He covers the early paradigms used to establish effective social work practice and describes the evolution from the influence that the scientific revolution had on social work practice from the early days to the modern contributions of behavioral psychologists and social workers. The reader is presented with an exhaustive analysis of the research knowledge base for social work practice and the conceptual support for social workers as practitioner-researchers. The reader of this chapter is shown once again the role of the behaviorist and of single-subject research and how they serve as a basis upon which social work practice can accrue more sophistication and methodological rigor. Reid lays out a convincing argument that at the beginning social work practice should be thought of as an empirical set of routine events that correspond to the scientific process. The chapter reminds students of their responsibility to advance the body of knowledge for the profession of social work. It includes a discussion about the role of agency-based practitioners and their use of empirical methods in practice and in controlled environmental settings. This chapter gives the student seeking knowledge about whether or not science has any place in social work practice arguments for and against empirically supported social work methods as the optimal choice for practice.

In the course of its evolution over the past century, clinical social work has made increasing use of empirical research to inform its practice. Reference to "the scientific base" of clinical social work is no longer simply rhetoric. Its empirical foundations have a substantial reality, one that has the increasing power to increase the effectiveness of what social workers do.

These foundations are most fully articulated in practice that is scientifically based or empirical. Historically, this form of practice has been characterized by three major components: 1) employment of a scientific orientation and scientific procedures in work with clients; 2) use of knowledge derived from research; and 3) contributions to knowledge through research carried out in conjunction with one's own practice. In this chapter, I shall examine the beginnings and development of scientifically based practice, its current characteristics and variations, and issues relating to it.

ORIGINS AND EVOLUTION

Since its earliest beginnings in "friendly visiting" among the poor, social work has aspired to be "scientific." The notion of "scientific charity" was developed in an effort to weld the methods of nineteenth-century science to the art of almsgiving. As C. S. Loch (1899), an early pioneer, succinctly put it, charity work is "not antagonistic to science: it is science" (p. 11). However, it was science more in imagination than reality, since there was little research on charity and no research-based interventions for practitioners to use.

Early Paradigms of Scientific Practice

The idea of a scientific base for social work became less rhetorical in the work of Mary Richmond (1917). Richmond spelled out an essential component of scientific practice: how scientific principles could guide social workers' efforts in their work with clients. In her formulation, a social diagnosis was the product of a scientific process of gathering facts, developing hypotheses based on the facts, and obtaining evidence to test the hypotheses. The psychoanalytic movement that began to dominate clinical social work in the 1940s and 1950s brought with it a commitment to the scientific study of psychological phenomena and treatment processes. Although it introduced theories and concepts that made such inquiry extraordinarily difficult, in many ways it represented a further advance in social work's aspirations to be scientific. At the very least, a whole new terrain—the hidden processes of the psyche—had become the object of scientific scrutiny, and new methods of case study had been introduced. The continuing commitment to scientifically based practice was well expressed by Hollis (1963), a leading advocate of psychoanalytically oriented casework: "Casework is a scientific art. Certainly since the days of Mary Richmond we have been committed to objective examination of the facts of each case. We draw inferences from those facts, we diagnose, we view the individual against a frame of reference which is itself the product of informal research. We constantly alert ourselves to sources of error" (p. 13).

The Behavioral Revolution

Beginning in the 1960s, these earlier paradigms were challenged by the behavioral movement, which introduced a new view of the integration of science and practice. With its focus on behavior and its environmental determinants, behaviorism came equipped with an empirically grounded terminology, objective measures, and a distinctive methodology for conducting experiments on behavior change. The occurrence of change could be documented, and interventions responsible for it could be isolated through the rigorous study of single cases. Moreover, behavioral approaches seemed to be demonstrably effective with a growing range of problems. For many social work practitioners, it offered a framework for scientific practice that was superior to the then reigning psychoanalytic model with its opaque theories, its difficult-to-measure concepts, and its lack of feasible experimental methods for linking interventions with change.

Although a distinctly behavioral social work began to emerge in the late 1960s (Thomas, 1967), practitioners were reluctant to embrace the behavioral paradigm as the framework for scientifically based practice. This paradigm was not selling all that well in the practice community, where there were concerns about its narrow focus on behavior, lack of attention to underlying issues, reliance on external rewards, and relative neglect of the clients' inner lives and larger social contexts.

What emerged was essentially a broader conception of empirical practice that made use of the research methodology used in single-system studies of behavioral approaches, such as careful delineation of the targets of intervention, collection of baseline data on their frequency of occurrence, monitoring change during the course of intervention, and constructing graphs of change over time to demonstrate intervention effects (see chapter 19). Incorporated into these methods was the use of standardized paper-and-pencil tests to assess and track changes in client problems (Corcoran & Fischer, 2000a, 2000b; Hudson, 1982). This methodology, it was reasoned, could be applied to any form of direct social work practice, whether or not it made use of behavioral methods of intervention. Its use would make practice more effective and accountable. A literature explicating this methodology soon developed (see, for example, Bloom, Fischer, & Orme, 1999; Howe, 1974; Jayaratne & Levy, 1979; Nelsen, 1978; Tripodi & Epstein, 1980; Wodarski & Thyer, 1981).

The Research Knowledge Base

From the earliest days of social work, a key part of scientific practice was to make use of existing research to inform work with clients. For many years there were few studies of any quality that could serve this function. Although assertions were made that social work had a base of scientific knowledge, this base was still almost as illusory as the "scientific" underpinnings of nineteenth-century almsgiving.

Beginning in the 1950s, this picture began to change as a growing number of relevant studies began to emerge from such fields as psychiatry, psychology, and the social sciences, and as experimental tests of social work programs were begun in earnest. It would take a while, however, before this fledging research base would be of much help to social work practitioners. For example, experimental studies of social work programs conducted in the 1970s tended to produce discouraging results, namely, that professional social work intervention could do no better than lesser services or no service at all (Fischer, 1973, 1976). Such studies could provide little guidance to practitioners. However, by the 1970s, experimental research, fortified with better methodology and perhaps better programs, started to document the effectiveness of a range of social work models (Reid & Hanrahan, 1982). These experiments were a small part of a growing body of research in the helping professions generally, much of it involving tests of behavioral and cognitive behavioral models. Over the past two decades such research has demonstrated effective interventions for a wide variety of clinical problems, perhaps most types that social workers are likely to encounter (Gorey, 1996; Reid, 1997).

At the same time, research on human behavior and psychosocial problems has continued to accumulate in the helping professions and the social sciences. Any number of examples could be given. In their work with parents and children, social workers make use of research-based knowledge of the norms and variations in human development and behavior, such as when, on average, infants and children reach developmental milestones (Bloom, 1975), as well as knowledge of the effects on children of different kinds of trauma, such as divorce (Zaslow, 1989). Although research has produced few fully developed explanations of problems of psychosocial functioning, it has identified risk and protective factors for many problems, such as schizophrenia relapse (Anderson, Reiss, & Hogarty, 1986), suicide in special populations (Clark & Fawcett, 1992; Ivanoff & Reidel, 1995), and adolescent drug use (Smith, Lizziotte, Thornberry, & Krohn, 1995). For numerous problems there is credible and useful scientific knowledge concerning onset, prevalence, natural course, and variation according to class, gender, and other factors.

A part of the scientific knowledge base available to practitioners has always consisted of "in-house" studies or databases produced by what might be referred to as "operations research." Such knowledge is developed to serve particular agencies or programs. Although it is usually not disseminated, and hence not a part of general knowledge available to the profession, it has always had a role in agency programs. In the earlier years of the profession it consisted largely of agency statistics on numbers and types of clients served and so on and was of little use to practitioners. Larger and better-funded agencies, such as the Community Service Society of New York, established their own research units, which conducted evaluative studies designed to inform agency practice, as well as studies for more general dissemination. However, the results of in-house studies were often ignored by the staff, who was likely to see them, rightly or wrongly, as dated and not relevant to practice decisions. In most agencies, operations research seldom rose above the "routine statistics" level.

Nevertheless, agency operations research continued to grow. Requirements by funding agencies for needs assessments and program evaluations were major factors. Computerized agency information systems, which began to evolve in the 1960s, were another. With their capabilities to store and retrieve routinely collected data on clients and on service operations, costs, and outcomes, such systems became capable of generating information of use to clinical staff. However, the development and utilization of information systems for clinical purposes was delayed by problems of data quality and their emphasis on administrative rather than service needs.

The Practitioner as Researcher

Finally, there has been a long-standing tradition that practitioners should be involved in the production of scientific knowledge. The role model that many social workers sought to emulate was Freud himself, who was seen as both an eminent practitioner and a contributor to scientific knowledge. Freud's celebrated cases were regarded not only as therapeutic *tours de force*, but also as building blocks of the scientific base of psychoanalytic knowledge. Case studies by social workers were aimed at building a fund of practice-relevant knowledge (see, for example, Frailberg, 1977; Hollis, 1939; Nicholls, 1956). However, it was recognized that such studies, including Freud's own masterpieces, could not be regarded as rigorous scientific work. While insightful and stimulating, they lacked the kind of methodological rigor needed to determine causal relationships, especially the role of intervention in effecting change.

The single-system designs (SSDs) introduced by the behavioral movement provided much stronger vehicles for research by practitioner-scientists. SSDs not only made use of rigorous methods of measurement, such as objective observations of behavior, but they provided controls to enable determination of intervention effects as discussed in chapter 5. Preintervention baselines could provide information about change prior to intervention. In more complex versions of SSD, even more powerful controls could be begun, stopped, then begun again, to determine if positive change was more likely to occur when intervention was "on." In the multiple-baseline across-clients design the beginning of intervention could be staggered across clients. For the first client, the baseline period might be two weeks; for the second client, it might be a week longer, and for a third client, an additional week could be added. One could then determine if positive change was more likely to take place after intervention was begun. Such controls could permit practitioner-researchers to rule out various extraneous variables that might be contributing to change such as "spontaneous remission" and nontreatment factors in the client's environment. Advocates of SSDs, such as Briar (1977), envisioned a "clinical scientist" who would use complex designs to test the effectiveness of social work interventions. These designs, it was hoped, would usher in a new era of practitioner involvement in research and contribution to the scientific knowledge base of the profession.

CHARACTERISTICS OF CONTEMPORARY EMPIRICAL PRACTICE

Three of the main components of scientifically based practice involve employing the use of scientific viewpoints, tools, and knowledge in work with clients. These components can be used routinely in virtually every case. The third component, the practitioner as producer of knowledge, has a much more selective application. I shall first describe routine empirical practice that involves the first two components. I will then consider the third.

Empirical Practice as a Routine Activity

In the everyday application of empirical practice, practitioners try to think like scientists, which does not mean that they are cold or detached. They combine scientific thinking with the capacity to understand, nurture, and care. Indeed, scientific thinking can enhance practitioners' empathy since it enables them to gain a truer picture of the client's plight.

To think like a scientist means a number of things. It means having a healthy skepticism toward all knowledge and a conviction that suppositions should be backed up with evidence. It also involves making use of scientific methods of inquiry and decision making; systematic data gathering; forming and testing hypotheses in light of the available knowledge and data provided by the case; using language defined by empirical realities; developing and evaluating alternative explanations of phenomena; and selecting interventions based on the best knowledge available.

Ron Harris, age 22, was recently discharged from a psychiatric facility with a diagnosis of schizophrenia and is currently living with his parents. The social worker, Nancy Stowe (an empirical practitioner), is attempting to help Ron and his parents, who are African-American, cope with the illness. One problem concerns conflict between Ron and his parents, who complain that he does nothing but sit around and watch TV. They nag him about getting a job, but to no avail. Another is that he has been acting strangely, and they fear he may be headed for a relapse. Ron himself is not very communicative with either his parents or the practitioner, but he mutters that he does not like his parents "being on my case."

As Ms. Stowe gathers facts about these problems, she begins to form hypotheses. One hypothesis is that Ron may indeed be on his way to a relapse. The behaviors he has been exhibiting appear to be prodromal signs of a relapse. Ms. Stowe has acquired this knowledge from research on schizophrenic relapses (Anderson et al., 1986). Another hypothesis is that his parents are unintentionally creating an atmosphere in which "expressed emotion" is high. Expressed emotion refers to a pattern of criticism and overinvolvement on the part of caretakers toward their schizophrenic charges. There is a well-developed theory, supported by numerous studies, that high levels of expressed emotion in the home are predictive of relapse (Leff, 1989; Leff & Vaughn, 1985). As can be seen, facts are not simply amassed, but rather are pursued to test hypotheses derived from research-based theories. Any practitioner might make use of theory to seek out assessment data, but one who is empirically oriented does so systematically through the use of hypotheses to be tested and the use of theory supported by research.

In formulating and testing these hypotheses, Ms. Stowe attempts to use terms that are clearly defined and are connected to empirical referents. Thus, the indicators for expressed emotion need to refer to specific actions, and these need to be applied to the case at hand. For example, Mr. Harris's criticism of Ron for being lazy might meet her definition of the term. But Ms. Stowe is not wedded to these particular hypotheses. She is not only willing to consider alternative explanations for Ron's prodomal signs but actively seeks evidence that might disconfirm her suppositions. A practitioner not using a scientific practice model might be more likely to ignore or misinterpret evidence running counter to his or her hypotheses. In this case, an alternative explanation for Ron's distressing symptoms might be failure to take his medication as prescribed, a well-established predictor of relapse. Accordingly, data on this possibility are gathered.

Let us assume that the evidence points to expressed emotion as the main factor in Ron's symptoms. As an empirical practitioner, Ms. Stowe would attempt to make use of a research-based intervention for dealing with the expressed emotion. Here she might employ the family treatment model developed by Anderson et al. (1986). Among other goals, the model was developed in an attempt to reduce expressed emotion. Controlled experiments have found this approach, and others similar to it, to be effective in relapse prevention (Hogarty et al., 1991; Hogarty, 1993; Penn & Meuser, 1996). However, in selecting and using the model, Ms. Stowe would be alert to the possibility that populations in which the model has been tested might differ in important ways from the case at hand. For example, the Harrises are African-American, whereas the research base Ms. Stowe has been using was built largely from samples of white subjects. How does this affect the validity of applying the research to this particular family? Is there additional research that bears on this question?

Empirical practice is not restricted to work with the individual client or family. It can be used with intervention involving any type of system. Michael Stevens, a school-based social worker, uses an empirical approach in group treatment of children who have problems of aggression as part of a schoolwide antiviolence program. In his work with the children, Mr. Stevens makes use of an empirically based group treatment model developed by Feindler and Gutterman (1994). The model that Mr. Stevens and his colleagues use in the school was further evaluated in an in-house study. The study found that children who participated in the program showed a decrease in suspensions and disciplinary reports, both indicators of aggressive behavior. In addition, Mr. Stevens is attempting to develop other antiviolence programs in his school and school district. His efforts are being facilitated by Astor, Behre, Wallace, and Fravil's (1998) study of such programs.

As might be surmised from the description above, empirical practice is a matter of degree. At some level, all responsible social work practice makes use of principles and procedures consonant with a scientific paradigm. Any good practitioner gathers data, forms hypotheses about possible causal factors, and makes use of existing knowledge. As practitioners accentuate the scientific component of their practice, they will carry out these operations in ways that will be in even greater conformity with a scientific paradigm, for example, by forming hypotheses whose terms can be empirically defined and by giving precedence to research-based knowledge.

Also, the kind of empirical practice I have described and illustrated thus far is an articulation of the orientation and methods that preceded the behavioral movement. Scientifically inclined practitioners of the Mary Richmond era, perhaps Mar Richmond herself, might have practiced this way, if they had had at their disposal the research-based knowledge and theory that is now available. It is still a very viable model of scientific practice, one used by many practitioners and one that a good number of researchers would endorse.

SSD methodology has added to this framework by providing ways of assessing client problems, monitoring their change over time, and evaluating outcomes in relation to the interventions used. However, as I have tried to make clear in the foregoing analysis, it should not be seen as the only form of empirical practice.

When using SSD methods, the practitioner begins by helping the client formulate a specific, measurable problem. A preintervention measure of the problem is taken in the form of variations in the frequency and severity of the problem over time. Ideally, intervention should be delayed until such baseline data are collected prospectively. To illustrate the distinction, a man whose problem consists of panic attacks at work might be asked to keep a log for a week to record the occurrence of each attack. From the log, a prospective baseline could be generated, one showing how often the attacks occurred, with perhaps a rating for each attack according to severity. Intervention could then begin. Alternatively, the client could estimate retrospectively, say, in the initial interview, how often such attacks occurred in the previous week and describe their nature; intervention could then begin immediately. A prospective baseline is likely to be more precise but at the cost of a delay in intervention. A variety of measures can be used to obtain baseline data. One of the more common types, client self-monitoring, has been illustrated. Other types include client self-report in the form of brief standardized instruments or responses to questions in a clinical interview, direct observation of the client by the practitioner or caregivers, and archival data, such as a record of absences from school. Repeated measures of the problem are obtained, permitting both the practitioner and client to chart changes as the case continues. These data, which can be put in graphic form, can be used to evaluate whether expected changes are occurring and to make decisions about a change in the intervention if they are not. The extension of such data collection through the end of the case provides the basis for an evaluation of outcome at termination. The evaluation helps clients see graphically—possibly in both the figurative and literal senses of the word—what they have accomplished. In general, the application of the SSD methods I have described provides practitioners with feedback about the possible effectiveness of their interventions. Finally, they also serve to document the practitioner's accountability to the agency and the community. (More detailed discussions of this methodology can be found in Bloom et al., 1999.)

Practitioners and the Production of Knowledge

Agency-based practitioner-researchers.   The hope that practitioner-researchers in agencies will contribute to intervention knowledge through the use of SSDs has achieved only limited realization. Only a small number of studies, perhaps three or so a year, have appeared since SSDs began to be used for this purpose. (See, for example, Briggs, 1996a; Broxmeyer, 1978; Besa, 1994; Jensen, 1994; Pinkston, Levitt, Green, Linsk, & Rzepnicki, 1982; Tolson, 1977). The rate of production does not appear to be increasing. For example, in his comprehensive meta-analytic review of social work effectiveness studies, Gorey (1996) found only nine published SSDs during the 1990 to 1994 period. There has been little evidence of the use of replication series (Barlow, Hayes, & Nelson, 1984) as a means of establishing generality of results. Lack of agency support for practitioner research, practitioner reluctance to use intrusive, complex SSDs in service contexts, and lack of practitioner skill in the use of such designs appear to be among the main reasons why agency-based practitioner-researchers have not become a major factor in the experimental testing of social work interventions.

However, there is evidence (discussed subsequently) that social workers are making greater use of less complex SSDs or at least elements of them. There is little reason to suppose that much of the data collected is used by anyone but the practitioner. But as Benbenishty (1996, 1997) has suggested, data from such simpler SSDs could be collected systemically following agency guidelines. The data could then be fed into the agency's computerized information system. The result would be a continually updated fund of agency-based knowledge concerning how different kinds of interventions used in the agency's programs have fared with different types of clients and problems.

Another role for practitioner-researchers in the agency would be to use small-scale experiments in design and development (D&D) projects. The main purpose of D&D is to use research to test and improve innovative intervention methods (Rothman & Thomas, 1994; Fortune & Reid, 1999). The D&D paradigm sets forth a systematic way of accomplishing this goal. In brief, the practitioner-researcher analyzes the problem, reviews the literature relating to the problem and the intervention for it, designs an intervention, tests it out with a single case or small group of clients, and collects quantitative and qualitative data on how intervention processes were implemented and on outcomes. The data have two functions: 1) to provide a basis for assessing whether the intervention shows sufficient promise to warrant implementation or further testing; 2) to provide a basis for improving the intervention. For example, the trial may identify shortcomings in the intervention that may need to be corrected or may reveal creative and apparently effective variations of it that should be built into the service design. Practitioner logs and critical incidents, tape recordings of sessions, feedback from practitioners and clients, and brief standardized instruments are among the data collection methods commonly used. If the intervention appears promising, it can be put to more general use in the agency with the knowledge that it has been systematically designed, tested, and modified in the light of that test. Further and more rigorous testing prior to general use is always ideal but may not be feasible.

Initial field trials may consist of single case studies or "exploratory experiments" (Fortune & Reid, 1999) involving six to ten clients. Because their research components are small scale and nonintrusive and do not require sophisticated statistical analyses, the field trials can be readily managed by agency practitioner-researchers who may not have special funding or high levels of expertise in research methodology. Yet they can yield products of immediate benefit to the agency, not in the form of findings that need to be utilized before they matter, but rather in the form of research-improved interventions that can be put to work at once. Examples of such small-scale D&D projects may be found in Bailey-Dempsey and Reid (1996), Naleppa and Reid (1998), and Kilgore (1995).

Practitioner-researcher in academia.   Much of the experimental testing of social work treatment methods during the past three decades has taken the form of group designs carried out by academic practice-researchers (see, for example, reviews by Gorey, 1996; deSchmidt & Gorey, 1997; Mac-Donald, Sheldon, & Gillespie, 1992; Reid & Hanrahan, 1982; Rubin, 1985; and Videka-Sherman, 1988). Typically, these researchers test models that they themselves have helped develop. Often they are involved in practice in other ways, such as teaching practice courses, contributing to the nonresearch practice literature, or seeing clients. While not the kind of practitioner-researchers originally envisioned, they have combined a well-grounded knowledge of practice with research expertise to create a mode of experimental work that is perhaps more productive than the traditional mode in which researchers were cast primarily in the role of evaluators with little involvement in the design and operation of the service programs. The intervention approaches tested in this newer mode of experimental research have been better developed with more realistic goals than in the older mode and are more likely to yield positive outcomes. Although the effects have been often limited—modest changes in circumscribed problems—and investigator allegiance (experimenter bias) is a particular concern in the practitioner-researcher model, the studies have added considerably to social work's storehouse of demonstrably effective interventions.

EXTENT OF USE

The question that is frequently asked in one form or another is, to what extent is scientifically based practice used? The answer, of course, will depend entirely on how one defines this form of practice. If, as I have suggested, it is seen as a continuum and as appearing in different forms, the question can be rephrased as, what kinds of scientific orientations, procedures, and knowledge do practitioners make use of, and to what extent?

Most of the research on this question has concerned practitioner implementation of one form of scientifically oriented practice, the use of the SSD methodology (Cheatham, 1987; Gingerich, 1984; Kirk & Penka, 1992; Marino, Green, & Young, 1998; Milstein, Regan, & Reinherz, 1990; Penka & Kirk, 1991; Richey, Blythe, & Berlin, 1987). In these studies, samples of graduates of particular programs or of practitioners in general were asked to respond to questionnaires that explore the extent to which they have used SSD methods. By and large, the studies have reported substantial use of such components as specifying target problems and goals, describing goals in measurable terms, and monitoring client change over time, but only quite limited use of more intrusive or time-consuming procedures, such as more complex SSDs or graphing.

The studies also point up some of the ambiguities in efforts to determine how "scientific" practice might be. For example, Penka and Kirk (1991) found in their national study of NASW members, two-thirds of whom had little or no exposure to SSDs in their graduate education, that subjects reported using such components as "operationalizing target problems" or "monitoring client change" with over three-quarters of their clients on average. The subjects may have given these procedures different definitions than the researchers had in mind (Richey et al., 1987). Thus, affirmative responses to "monitoring client change" might have included not only the use of systematic repeated measurements but also informal inquiries about the client's progress in the course of a clinical interview. Studies of actual samples of practice are needed if we are to get a clearer picture of the empirical dimensions of the SSD.

Currently, there is even less knowledge about the extent to which practitioners might use a more generic scientific approach, one that might not be grounded in SSD methods. For example, some of the practitioners indicating use of empirical methods in the Penka and Kirk survey might have fallen into this category.

Another question concerns practitioners' use of research-based knowledge in their practice. There is a good deal of research that suggests that practitioners make little instrumental use of research: they seldom read practice studies and apply the results (Kirk, 1990). However, utilization of research other than practice studies may be more common. A good deal of such utilization can be thought of as "conceptual" (Rich, 1977; Weiss & Bucuvalas, 1980). In conceptual utilization, research information is joined with such other factors as the practitioner's own impressions of effectiveness, informal case reports, general knowledge, available alternatives, and cost factors. For example, suppose our Ms. Stowe attends a workshop in which there is mention of studies that suggest that the use of time limits may motivate clients. This information makes sense to her since it jibes with her own clinical observations. As a result, she decides to make more use of limits.

There is also indirect utilization, which involves not the use of research studies or tools per se, but rather the use of products of research (Reid & Fortune, 1992). In social work, indirect utilization involves the use of theories, knowledge, or interventions that have been produced, shaped, or validated by research. Thus, the practitioner who employs a form of parent training that was developed through a series of experimental studies is utilizing research, albeit indirectly. Indirect utilization requires that the practitioner's application be reasonably close to whatever was developed or tested by the research. For example, the case for indirect utilization would be strong if the practitioner followed substantially the procedures used in an empirically supported intervention. It would become questionable if he or she used only some of the procedures, or used them differently.

Unlike other forms of utilization, indirect utilization requires no direct exposure to research. The practitioner's interface is not with the research itself but with the practice approach or knowledge based on it.

Although we have little hard data on the extent to which conceptual and indirect utilizations occur, there is evidence to suggest that social workers are making use of research-based practice methods, such as cognitive-behavioral interventions. (While interventions from other approaches may also be empirically based, cognitive and cognitive-behavioral approaches are more likely to be). For example, in one survey (Jensen, Bergin, & Greaves, 1990), the vast majority of social workers identified themselves as eclectic. Of those who did so, about half reported use of "cognitive" and "behavioral" methods. Of course, we do not know to what extent their use conformed to methods actually supported by research.

Although instrumental utilization of the traditional kind—social workers reading research reports and using the findings—has had limited influence, a new kind of instrumental utilization is growing in importance: the utilization of data from agency information systems. For example, federal and state initiatives for the development of information systems in child welfare (Depart ment of Health & Human Services, 1998) provide social workers with the answers to such questions as "Are the African-American children in my district who are in foster care more likely to be placed in institutional settings than children from other ethnic groups?" Answers to such questions, which may involve the use of complex cross-tabulations generated by the system, are clearly examples of research utilization. Even though such systems may be used for nonresearch purposes, such as case review, they can bring research information literally to the social worker's fingertips.

IS EMPIRICAL PRACTICE THE BEST PRACTICE?

The relationship between science and clinical social work raises a host of issues, some of which have already been alluded to. Most of these issues relate to one central question: Is scientifically based practice superior to alternatives? That is, is it the kind of practice the profession should foster or is it best considered as just another model, one that should take its place alongside the myriad of approaches that clinical social workers use? In the earlier days of the profession, the question would have been regarded as rather naïve. "Of course we want practice to be scientific!" would have been the answer. But that was before empirical practice was a reality. Now that it has become one, not everybody is so sure that it is the way to go. In examining the various facets of this issue, I shall consider some of the criticism of empirical practice that has emerged in recent years. Most of this criticism has been directed at forms of empirical practice that makes use of SSD methods, but much of it also applies to more generic forms.

Epistemological Controversies

Over the past two decades, there has been a good deal of criticism of the epistemological foundations of empirical practice. These criticisms have challenged the assumption that empirical practice and the scientific viewpoints and procedures on which it rests are the best way to determine the truth about the world, including human beings and their social relations. Some of the critics have taken the stance that the epistemological base on which empirical practice rests, supposedly logical positivism, is outmoded and untenable (Heineman, 1981; Tyson, 1992). Others have taken the stance that science, like other human inventions, is a social construction, a form of discourse, if you will. It has no special lock on getting to the truth about anything.

There are many ways of knowing, as Hartman (1990) put it. The empirical approach represents one, but there are others as valid or perhaps more valid for certain purposes. From these "postmodern" philosophical perspectives, more specific criticisms have emerged. The scientific paradigm on which empirical practice rests encourages inappropriate quantification, reductionism, and context stripping, and denies the value of intuition, tacit knowledge, and other "nonrational" ways of learning about the world. The critics have proposed alternative paradigms that, they claim, offer research strategies better suited to the study of much of the social phenomena with which social workers are concerned. The heuristic approach, critical theory, and some forms of constructivism are among them (Atherton, 1993; Franklin, 1995; Heineman, 1994; Tyson, 1992; Morris, 1994).

In my view, this criticism and the resulting alternatives have many more shortcomings than the paradigm they oppose. To begin with, much of the attack is directed not at the paradigm that empirical practitioners and mainstream social work researchers actually use, but rather at caricatures and distortions of them. A prime example is the assertion that these paradigms are cemented in the canons of logical positivism, a long-abandoned philosophical movement that was simply one rather problematic attempt to articulate the foundations of science. It never became any kind of meaningful foundation for scientific practice (Phillips, 1990; Schuerman, 1982).

The epistemologies underlying contemporary scientific practice, whether used by empirical practitioners or mainstream researchers, do share certain features. They tend to be realist in orientation, that is, they hold that "the external world exists independently of our sense experience, ideation, and volition, and that it can be known" (Bunge, 1993). Although the nature of this world, which includes human behavior, may be difficult to discern exactly, it is possible to obtain knowledge about it that is at least approximately true. Truth is viewed as a "regulative ideal" (Phillips, 1990, p. 43). Inquiry is aimed at determining what the truth is, even though one may fall short of revealing it completely. The position that phenomena exist independently of human perceptions makes it possible to obtain knowledge about them that is reasonably objective, that is relatively free from human bias. Even though our perception of reality may be filtered through our theories (Hanson, 1958) and may not always be based on observational data, it is possible to achieve close approximations to what is real through rules of logic and inference.

Although it is recognized that phenomena can be construed in many different ways by different observers, these constructions are regarded as differing viewpoints, not "multiple truths." Although what is true can be extraordinarily complex, it should be contrasted with what is false rather than with "alternative truths." Truth or valid knowledge must ultimately be backed by evidence that can be appraised through such standards as corroboration and freedom from error (Reid, 1994). Although scientific knowledge can be built in many ways, incrementally or through paradigm shifts (Kuhn, 1970), its building over the long term is progressive (Kitcher, 1993). That is, we know more about the world and its human inhabitants now than we did a century ago, and we will know much more than we do now a century from now.

However, progress in the study of human behavior and its social environments must necessarily be slow. The phenomena in question are difficult to study and in constant flux; much of the knowledge gained may be outdated by the march of events. Moreover, the main vehicles for advancing this kind of knowledge—behavioral and social theories-are difficult to put to definitive tests. It is recognized that theories are "underdetermined" by the evidence (Hesse, 1980), that is, they can be endlessly adjusted to avoid disconfirmation in the face of negative findings. Still, with continual testing over the long term, some theories will prove to be superior to their rivals with respect to their predictive and explanatory powers; as various examples in the history of science have demonstrated, these superior theories will survive, and their rivals will be discarded (Brekke, 1986; Lakatos, 1972; Reid, 1994).

The basic ideas that researchers use have evolved not from logical positivism or any other "ism," but rather from the rational, problem-solving capabilities of the human mind. As Dewey (1938) once put it, "Scientific subject-matter and procedures grow out of the direct problems and methods of common sense—but enormously refine, expand, and liberate the contents and the agencies at the disposal of common sense" (p. 66). That philosophers are needed to provide foundations or rationales for the practice of research is, as Rorty (1979) said, an invention of the philosophers themselves.

There are of course many ways of knowing and most of the knowledge that we have is not derived from scientific inquiry. Nevertheless, I would argue that science has always been directed at developing superior ways of obtaining knowledge and it has done so with considerable success. When appropriately applied, scientific methods can surpass their rivals as a means for acquiring knowledge that may not be possible to acquire through simple observation or other ready means. For example, a well-designed controlled experiment in social work is indeed the best means of determining if one intervention is superior to another with respect to agreed-upon outcomes. If there were a demonstrably better way, then *that* way would be the preferred scientific procedure. In other words, science is all about the most effective ways of extracting truths from often recalcitrant realities. If certain scientific methods are preferred for certain problems, it is because those methods appear to be the most effective in the light of what is currently known, but better ones might come along tomorrow.

The principle is to make the best fit between the question and the method of inquiry. Qualitative, holistic methods may be the most appropriate for certain questions. These methods certainly have a place in mainstream research. It is not necessary to invent new epistemologies to justify them, although that impression is often given (Morris, 1994). But it is also assumed that all methods of inquiry, whether qualitative or quantitative, need to be examined against common standards for determining truth and error. The epistemologies of mainstream research may clash with the alternatives if these standards are denied. It is hard to say how often this may happen. Only a limited amount of research has been conducted under the banner of constructivism or other postmodern epistemologies, and in most such studies it is not clear where the epistemological conflict might be found.

The Utility of Research-Based Knowledge

A core assumption of empirical practice is that the use of research-supported interventions will yield better results than those lacking research support. Issues arise around the following questions: 1) How does one determine which interventions might be considered to be empirically supported or better supported than others? 2) How can one be sure about the ability of a supported intervention to be generalized, that is, it may have worked in the studies, but will it work in a situation that may differ in various respects, such as the type of client or practitioner training? Witkin (1991) and Chandler (1994), among others, have argued that lack of objective criteria for determining empirical support and limits on generalizing findings nullify the presumed superiority of research-based content.

There is no simple way of resolving these issues. It would be difficult to develop agreed-upon criteria to decide what is, in fact, "empirically supported." It is always a matter of judgment, with considerable possibility for error, whether or not an intervention that was effective in one or more research studies will also be effective in a given application. However, progress has been made on these issues. For example, based on the work of the Task Forces of the American Psychological Association, Chambless and Holon (1998) have developed criteria for different levels of efficacy for psychological interventions. In the light of this ongoing work, it is possible to make informed judgments about which methods may have more empirical support than others and the likelihood of applying them to specific cases.

In some cases, the efficacy of an intervention is so well established across so many studies, that it is reasonable to assume that it would also be efficacious in the case at hand. Even if it turns out not to be, it would at least make sense to try it. The use of exposure to the outside world for treatment of agoraphobia is a well-documented case in point (DeRubeis & Crits-Christoph, 1998). In the much larger number of situations in which there would be considerably less certainty, one could make use of the principle of using the "best available knowledge" (Klein & Bloom, 1995; Reid, 1994). Suppose for a given situation that a social worker knows of three kinds of interventions that might be applicable. One of these has some research support, for example, it was found to be effective in a controlled experiment. The others are untested. Even though the clients who participate in the experiment might differ from the client in the case and even though the social worker might wish to see more studies, the tested intervention may be considered as offering the "best knowledge" of the set because at least it has been tested and found to be effective. In this and in other situations, we do not have to be certain that an intervention has been proved to be efficacious, simply that it has better evidence on its side than possible alternatives.

Research Methods in Practice

A third issue concerns the use in practice of research methods associated with the SSD, such as baselining, standardized instruments, repeated data collection over the course of a case, graphing progress, client self-recording, and questionnaires. Advocates of empirical practice have argued that such procedures can provide practitioners with data for guiding interventions and evaluating outcomes, thus helping to make practice more effective and accountable. Not all agree.

Sources of opposition have been diverse. As might be expected, some of the critics are those who reject what they view as the epistemological foundations of empirical practice (Heineman, 1994; Tyson, 1992; Witkin, 1996). But there are others who appear to have no quarrel with the epistemology of mainstream research or with scientifically based practice in the more generic sense described above (Bronson, 1994; Wakefield & Kirk, 1997; Rubin & Knox, 1996). These latter "inside" critics have argued that SSD methods have not proved their value, that is, they have not demonstrated any contribution to effectiveness that might compensate for the time and effort they consume. In fact, by confounding research and service objectives, they may actually have adverse consequences for clients. They do not satisfy accountability requirements since they cannot determine if the practitioner was responsible for change or used appropriate methods. Finally, they place a behavioral stamp on whatever intervention they are used with. As a result, practice may be overly restricted if not distorted. Those critics with epistemological objections to empirical practice agree, of course, with these criticisms and add others of a more philosophical nature (Witkin, 1996).

The sharp edge of some of these criticisms has been blunted by a redefinition among the advocates themselves of how SSD methods might be used by students or by practitioners in everyday agency practice. There has been a deemphasis on the use of more complex, intrusive designs, the kind that might be used for research purposes (Ivanoff, Blythe, & Briar 1997). What has been stressed is their efficacy in gathering data that would serve immediate clinical goals as well as accountability purposes.

It is true that there is little evidence that practitioners using SSD methods are more effective than those who do not. However, such evidence would be difficult to obtain since one would have to disentangle the effects of these methods from those of the interventions used with them. One of the few studies that have addressed the question (Slonim-Nevo & Anson, 1998) did show some positive effects. Israeli juvenile delinquents who received treatment accompanied by SSD methods (for example, targeting of specific problems, collection of baseline data, tracking change through scales, self-monitoring, and graphing) were compared with a group that was treated similarly, but without the addition of the SSD methods. The group treated with SSD methods showed statistically better outcomes on self-reports of arrests and school or work participation than the control group at a 9–12 month follow-up. Although a possible lack of comparability between the groups limits the findings, the study demonstrates the feasibility of testing the efficacy of an empirical approach and provides at least some evidence that it may enhance practice.

The critics make some valid points concerning accountability. It is more than measuring client change, which is about all that an empirical practitioner can accomplish. Accountable practitioners need to show that they have used the best possible methods for the case at hand in the most suitable way. If it meets these criteria, practice can be properly accountable, even if the case is not successful. A more inclusive concept of accountability, such as "appropriate practice" is needed (Ivanoff et al., 1997).

Single-case evaluations can contribute to establishing accountability in this broader sense, but to do so they need to be obtained in a systematic manner, for example, following Benbenishty's (1996, 1997) notion of pooling evaluation data in an agency database. If such accountability data can be collected systematically, they should prove far superior to traditional agency practices of presenting "success stories." They may also satisfy the demands of funding and managed care organizations that insist on performance-based evaluation systems for accountability purposes.

One aspect of the use of SSDs that has been glossed over in the debates about their efficacy, contribution to accountability, and so on is their role in student and practitioner self-development. Accurate feedback from one's own cases can be an important source of learning for both beginning and experienced social workers. It is reasonable to suppose that SSDs can facilitate this process through the case data they provide, although evidence needs to be gathered on this point.

Finally, what can be made of the criticism that empirical practice inevitably carries a behavioral stamp that may distort the practitioner's efforts? Here it is important to be clear about what kind of empirical practice one has in mind and what that variant requires.

The kind of empirical practice most widely advocated and taught today requires, among other things, specifically defined problems at the outset and data on the frequency of their occurrence over time (Bloom et al., 1999). This configuration reflects a blend of practice theory—behavioral or something similar—and certain measurement procedures. One does not have to claim that this brand of empirical practice is "theory free" (Bloom, Fischer, & Orme, 1995; Blythe, Tripodi, & Briar, 1994). Rather it can be seen as a "perspective" with its own assumptions and requirements (Reid & Zettergren, 2000). As such, it can be used in conjunction with a range of intervention models, just as a feminist or generalist perspective might be. Certain accommodations may need to be made, however. For example, combining this form of empirical practice and narrative therapy may affect the way the therapy is conducted as the Besa (1994) study illustrates. But such hybrids can have their own rationales and, if effective, can be justified. They do not have to be seen as distortions of practice.

A theme of this chapter is that empirical practice can come in different forms and gradations. SSD methodology is flexible and can be modified to meet the requirements of a given intervention, even at the cost of less precise data. For instance, a particular form of couples' therapy might preclude a specific definition of the problem at the outset. This requirement of the methodology might be set aside, but one might still track changes in marital adjustment through repeated administration of rapid assessment instruments. A more generic form of such practice, such as the kind illustrated earlier, may have fewer assumptions or requirements that would need to be modified.

CONCLUSION

Over the past century, the scientific foundation of clinical social work has been transformed from an illusion to an influential reality. Granted, it is only one source among many that shape practice and is not yet the dominant one. But it should continue to grow in importance, as research on human behavior and practice continues to accumulate, as computerization and other technologies advance, and as societal forces, such as the managed care movement, place increasing stress on research-based knowledge and methods.

This foundation has achieved its major expression in the form of scientifically based or empirical practice. Historically, this kind of practice has taken different forms and different forms exist today. There are many ways of scientific knowing, to paraphrase Hartman (1990). Variation in empirical practice is a healthy development and should be fostered. The leading form of such practice, based on the SSD methodology, represents a major advance and may with justification (and perhaps modification) continue to lead. But it should be recognized as just one perspective among many others.

CHAPTER 4

Evidence-Based Approaches to Community Practice

Bruce Thyer

In this chapter, Bruce Thyer shows how integrating the scientific process, critical thinking, and practice research techniques creates a basis for teaching practitioners evidence-based practice methods. The chapter offers a framework for practitioners to use in planning and evaluating accountable social work practice in community settings. Inquisitive students who are seeking an answer to the question, "How do I know that what I do makes a difference?" will find Thyer's perspective useful because it gives them a rationale for preferring the use of data-based methods over others. Thyer gives a clear critical perspective and conceptual lens for students who are attracted to practice methods and approaches that include data collection and analysis. Students not drawn to this way of thinking may also find this information useful, although their reasons for reading this chapter may be different. They may read this chapter to reinforce their preconceived notions about evidence-based approaches. However, it may surprise even these readers that they appreciate Thyer's perspective. The basis for their appreciation may stem from Thyer's detailed analysis of the problems and challenges to evidence-based approaches. Despite the fact that these skeptical students may be zealously searching for justification for not using a data-governed treatment approach, this chapter will impress them with case examples of successful community practice evidence-based approaches. The students who are wondering, "What's in this for me?" and "Why learn about evidence-based approaches anyway?" are going to have their questions answered as they acquire the foundation knowledge that Thyer provides about the science, research foundations, and scientific criteria that are used to judge whether a treatment is reliably effective. All in all, what the reader will come to know from reading this chapter is the purpose of science and community practice, the limitations and challenges to evidence-based approaches, the American Psychological Association's standards for treatment effectiveness based on empirical support, the role of evaluation research in community practice, and detailed and empirically supported examples of evidence-based approaches established in social work practice.

There are a number of interesting developments occurring within professional social work practice today. A major one, stimulated by a variety of forces, revolves around making greater use of scientific research findings in the design and provision of human services. Within social work, this initiative has been labeled "empirical clinical practice" (Siegel, 1984); within clinical psychology, it has long been known as the scientist-practitioner model of training (Turnbull & Dietz-Uhler, 1995), and within the health care professions as "evidence-based medicine" (Sackett, Robinson, Rosenberg, & Haynes, 1997). While these and other human services have long paid lip service to the notion that practitioners need to incorporate research findings into their delivery of services, it has only been within the past couple of decades that a sufficiently robust body of scientific findings has emerged that justifies actually attempting to apply them to practice. The central tenet of this movement was summarized by Thyer (1995) as follows:

> Clients should be offered as a first choice treatment, interventions with some significant degree of empirical support, where such knowledge exists, and only provided other treatments after such first choice treatment have been given a legitimate trial and been shown not to work. (p. 95)

For many years, the qualifying phrase "where such knowledge exists" applied to very few areas of practice, but sufficient advances have now occurred within the domain of clinical practice to make the application of this standard justifiable. For example, a task force of the National Academy of Sciences has noted

> The knowledge base in the behavioral sciences has reached the point where effective utilization of its findings by physicians, clinical psychologists, nurses, and social workers can have a very significant impact on health-related problems in our society. (Committee on National Needs for Biomedical and Behavioral Research Personnel, 1994, pp. 38–39)

Even the venerable National Association of Social Workers has begun collaborating with members of other disciplines in the development of practice guidelines for various disorders, guidelines constructed largely on the basis of empirical research on effective treatments (see *Work on Clinical Guides Begins*, 1998). A growing number of textbooks have been recently published that summarize the present status of evidence-based services across the field of direct practice (e.g., Thyer & Wodarski, 1998; Hibbs & Jensen, 1996; Seligman, 1998; Nathan & Gorman, 1998; Giles, 1993; Ammerman, Last, & Hersen, 1993). These books are invaluable resources for social work practitioners who need to learn about psychosocial interventions that really are demonstrably effective in helping clients, small groups, couples, and families. One can anticipate, perhaps optimistically, that over time evidence-based training will supplant graduate course content, which often lacks credible evidence of efficacy.

Research-based therapies initially tested and validated under carefully controlled conditions are being replicated in community-based agencies and clinics and in many instances proving to be similarly efficacious (DeRubeis & Crits-Christoph, 1998; Kazdin & Weisz, 1998; Wade, Treat, & Stuart, 1998; Westbrook & Hill, 1998; Shadish et al., 1997). This is wonderfully encouraging news for social workers practicing in various clinical arenas such as in the mental health professions, in hospitals, and in school settings, but an examination of the literature on evidence-based services would not seem to uncover much to offer the social worker engaged in community practice. In fact, it could be contended that the empirical literature does not offer much to the social worker engaged in community practice social work, but this contention would be a mistake. Actually, some parallel developments have transpired within the domain of community practice, consisting of well-crafted controlled trials of psychosocial interventions applied in community settings and demonstrating positive results. The balance of this chapter will review selected examples of these developments, with some preliminary remarks on the nature of "community practice," and of evidentiary standards.

COMMUNITY: DEPENDENT OR INDEPENDENT VARIABLE?

The use of the term "community" in community practice can have at least two meanings. In one meaning, the focus is on improvements in some aspect of community functioning (a social problem, racial injustice, unfair hiring practices, crime), that is, "community" as a dependent variable or outcome measure. In the second meaning, "community" refers to the modality of service delivery, with services occurring in community contexts such as local neighborhoods, usually involving small groups of stakeholders or constituents. In this use of the term, "community" is an independent variable or intervention. Where does this leave services that are provided within community contexts but that are focused on the concerns of individuals, such as substance abuse, smoking prevention, crime reduction, or unemployment? In my opinion, these services are squarely within the purview of traditional community practice as provided by social workers (see also Poole, 1997). Even the most intimate of personal problems has community sequelae; witness the carnage on the road caused by drunk drivers (leading to the establishment of community groups such as Mothers Against Drunk Driving). Although it may seem odd to view intervention aimed at individuals as a valued component of "community practice," such a view is consistent with the sociological theory which contends that, "Social structure is nothing more than the processes of action and interaction among individuals" (Turner, 1986, p. x).

Thus, for the purpose of this chapter the definition of "community organization" as provided in *The Social Work Dictionary* will be applied to our use of the term "community practice":

> An intervention process used by social workers and other professionals to help individuals, groups, and collectives of people with common interests or from the same geographic areas to deal with *social problems* and to enhance social well-being through planned *collective* action. (Barker, 1995, p. 69; italics in original)

THE PROBLEM OF "EVIDENCE"

In these times, everyone wishes to jump onto the empirical bandwagon. All approaches to social work intervention seem to enjoy defining themselves as empirical, but they twist the meaning of the term to suit their own purposes. For example, some approaches choose the most liberal meaning of the term, as in "relying upon or derived from observation . . . relying solely on practical experience and without regard for system or theory" (Berube, 1991, p. 449). This view basically contends the following: "If my personal experience justifies my belief, then that belief is empirically supported." This ignores other essential, more conservative, aspects of the meaning of the term empirical. Arkava and Lane (1983) provide the following definition: "Empiricism is the process of using evidence rooted in objective reality and gathered systematically as a basis for generating human knowledge" (p. 11). Further, Grinnell (1993) defines "*empirical* knowledge [as] derived from observation, experiences, or experiment" (p. 442; italics in original). These additional elements of "systematic" and "experiment" elevate scientifically credible knowledge to a higher standard of empirical justification than the common observations of everyday life by laypeople or the qualitative impressions of even highly trained professionals.

For the behavioral and social scientist, empirically based knowledge relies upon evidence gathered systematically, in a manner that tends to reduce or control for bias, is potentially replicable, and whose findings have actually been replicated by different researchers in different settings using different clients. The ultimate evidentiary standard is commonly seen as the multisite, randomized, controlled trial, a very rare animal indeed in social work literature. As a practical matter, we must settle for less than ideal standards of evidence, recognizing that the building of a credible foundation of empirical support can be begun by conducting a number of single-system research studies and finding positive results. A randomized no-treatment control group design conducted in one community presents a higher standard of evidence than an uncontrolled pretest-posttest design conducted in the same community. A well-controlled study with long-term follow-up data documenting the maintenance of community improvements is methodologically superior to a similar study demonstrating positive change only in the short term, and so on.

How much evidence is *enough*, sufficient to justify labeling an approach to practice as empirically supported or as evidence based? Ideally, we can never have enough. There will always remain new communities and more diverse groups of clients or practitioners for whom additional evaluation research is needed. But in the short term, we must settle for a lesser standard of proof. Some guidance has been provided by clinical psychologists, who have been wrestling with this problem for some years with respect to individual and group therapies. The Task Force on Psychological Interventions (Chambless et al., 1995) of the American Psychological Association's Division 12 (Clinical Psychology) has provided the following standards as some criteria to be used in classifying a treatment as "well-established" in terms of its empirical support:

1. There are at least two published, well-designed, outcome studies using group research designs that have demonstrated the efficacy of the experimental treatment by showing it to be superior to or equivalent to another psychological treatment.
2. Experiments must be conducted with treatment manuals.
3. The positive effects must have been demonstrated by at least two different investigators or investigatory teams.

Now, there is no positive assurance that an intervention that meets the above standards is genuinely efficacious, but these minimal criteria (*only* two published outcome studies!) certainly act as a coarse sieve that we may use to sift the wheat from the chaff. A few bugs may remain in our meal, but the resulting loaf will surely be more wholesome than making bread from whatever other (less rigorous) scrapings of evidence we can throw into the mixing bowl.

It is a well-kept secret, but a surprisingly large number of community-based interventions have been developed and subjected to rigorous empirical testing. The results have been most encouraging in that a growing number of community practices have been shown to be quite effective in ameliorating some very serious social problems. The balance of this chapter will provide an overview of a selected number of community interventions that have been subjected to experimental research of sufficient rigor to justify labeling these approaches as evidence based.

ASSERTIVE COMMUNITY TREATMENT FOR CHRONIC MENTAL ILLNESS

Assertive community treatment (ACT) is a well-tested model of care and support for individuals with chronic mental illnesses (CMI; e.g., schizophrenia), wherein the locus of services consists of the communities in which these individuals reside, often following discharge from a psychiatric hospital. ACT models make use of a core team of service providers, frequently headed by a social worker, dedicated to providing the client with whatever is necessary in order to sustain them for living outside the hospital, e.g., "medications, supportive and problem-solving therapy; crisis intervention; and assistance with housing, work rehabilitation, and daily living activities" (Test, 1998, p. 422). It is not simply a "case management" model, with a key professional providing linkage to needed services. Rather, the ACT team is available seven days a week, twenty-four hours a day. The use of an interdisciplinary team ensures that clients receive a wide range of needed services expeditiously (from help in fixing a lock or finding employment in the community to quickly adjusting medications in the face of unpleasant side effects). Services are mobile—team members come to where the client is in the community, not the other way around, that is, the client is not required to come to the professional's office (hence the term "assertive")—and highly individualized. Services also include client and family education about the nature of CMI with a strong focus on building adaptive skills (e.g., personal hygiene, cooking, cleaning, shopping, money management).

There are two other characteristics about ACT worth noting. One is that quite literally dozens of well-controlled outcome studies have been published on this model of community practice, with strikingly positive effects in terms of reduced hospitalizations, reductions in symptoms, and improvements in life skills, working, and quality of life. The model has been applied by diverse groups of professionals, in diverse settings with diverse clientele (e.g., the poor, homeless persons, minorities of color, etc.). The second is that social work practitioners and academics have been at the forefront of developing and testing the ACT model in community settings. Social work professors Mary Ann Test of the University of Wisconsin at Madison, Carol Mowbray of the University of Michigan, and Phyllis Solomon and Jeffrey Draine, both of the University of Pennsylvania, are four of the leading figures in this regard (e.g., Mowbray, Plum, & Masterton, 1997; Test, 1998; Solomon & Draine, 1995).

Another prominent researcher in the field of CMI who is a social worker is Gerald Hogarty, Professor of Psychiatry at the University of Pittsburgh School of Medicine and developer of family psychoeducational approaches to helping clients and their families (see Hogarty et al., 1991). Community-based social workers dedicated to helping individuals with CMI should obtain comprehensive training in either ACT or family-based psychoeducational models, inasmuch as these are two approaches with substantial and credible empirical evidence of efficacy to support their use.

THE JOB-FINDING APPROACH TO UNEMPLOYMENT

The problem of unemployment and its consequences is a central issue of concern to social workers. The ramifications (financial, societal, familial) of not having a steady job and deriving sufficient income from it are immense, and many community problems are either directly or indirectly linked to unemployment (crime, drug abuse, alcohol abuse, domestic violence, child abuse, etc.). Certainly, providing social work services intended to help the unemployed find productive jobs can be seen as a crucial element of community practice.

Almost twenty-five years ago, Azrin, Flores, and Kaplan (1975) reported on their development and experimental evaluation of a comprehensive approach to helping the unemployed labeled the Job Finding Club (JFC). The JFC initially consisted of the following elements, all provided in the context of community-based small group meetings: assistance in preparing resumes and job applications; interviewing skills training, including language (body and verbal) coaching; proactive efforts to obtain job leads and to share them with others belonging to the JFC; access to a telephone and mail drop (where potential employers could contact the applicant, especially useful for persons without a telephone at home); transportation assistance to attend interviews; and the development of a buddy system, whereby applicants were paired with each other for purposes of mutual self-help and support.

The initial positive results of the JFC have been replicated many times (see Richman, 1982; Stidham & Remley, 1992; Rife & Belcher, 1994), even with so-called hard-core cases (e.g., long-term welfare beneficiaries) and physically and psychologically disabled individuals receiving SSI benefits (Murphy & King, 1996; Corrigan, Reedy, Thadani, & Ganet, 1995), and the model has been adopted in a large number of states. Individuals participating in a community-based JFC typically obtain work earlier, retain employment longer, and earn more money than persons receiving alternative forms of job counseling. It is a multielement approach that follows a fairly structured intervention protocol available in a manual format. Community-based social workers who assist unemployed persons in obtaining employment can consider the Job Finding Club as one evidence-based service that they should become trained in themselves and make available to their clients.

COMMUNITY REINFORCEMENT APPROACH TO ALCOHOLISM AND SUBSTANCE ABUSE

Like poverty caused by unemployment, alcoholism and the abuse of illegal drugs is a pervasive community-based social pathology that causes untold pain to millions of abusers and their families. A large proportion of crime (e.g., theft) is caused by the quest for money to purchase drugs, and the medical costs for alcohol and substance-abuse related illnesses is immense. Reliably effective clinical or community-based interventions for these problems are not widely provided to alcoholics and drug abusers. This is unfortunate, since a fairly effective community-based intervention has been available for over twenty-five years (another well-kept secret!).

The model to be presented here is called the community reinforcement approach (CRA) and was initially developed and tested by Hunt and Azrin in 1973 using a small-scale randomized controlled trial. Positive findings with alcoholics have been replicated by Azrin (1976) and others (e.g., Azrin, Sisson, Meyers, & Godley, 1982), and the model was refined and extended (e.g., Mallams, Godley, Hall, & Meyers, 1982; Sisson & Azrin, 1986; Smith & Meyers, 1995) using experimental designs of increasing sample size, internal validity, and sophistication. Most recently, the CRA has been tested and found efficacious with cocaine abusers (Higgins, Budney, Bickel, Hughes, Foerg, & Badger, 1993), heroin abusers (Abbott, Weller, Delaney, & Moore, 1998), and homeless individuals (Meyers & Smith, 1995; Smith, Meyers, & Delaney, 1998).

By any reasonable standard, the CRA to alcohol and substance abuse can be considered a viable evidence-based method of community practice. Given that alcohol and drug abuse are complex, multiply determined problems, the CRA is similarly complex and multifaceted. In its early stages, the CRA included providing standard AA-oriented groups, job counseling, social and leisure counseling, assistance in accessing nondrinking reinforcers, an alcohol-free social club, and relapse prevention, involving, in part, home visits by the community workers (again note the theme of proactively providing services to clients in the communities in which they live, as opposed to an office-based consulting mode). Later variants of the CRA included disulfiram therapy to deter drinking, a buddy system for mutual support, the use of small groups to convey services, refusal skills training, and relaxation training. With drug abusers, the use of urine screens was another added element, which incorporated the provision of added reinforcers contingent on submitting a drug-free urine test.

Dramatic reductions in alcohol and drug use, longer periods of complete abstinence, and decreases in alcohol/drug-related hospitalizations, all things related to standard alcohol and drug treatment services, are the typical outcomes of using the CRA model. It is clearly incorrect to view these problems as intractable community plagues not amenable to reliably effective community-based services. The CRA is one of strongest examples of an evidence-based service that can be provided by social workers engaged in community practice.

THE TEACHING-FAMILY MODEL FOR TROUBLED ADOLESCENTS

What is to be done with troubled kids, those who require some form of out-of-home placement because of emotional disturbance and/or delinquent behavior? There are many options, ranging from boot camps, incarceration in conventional prisons, foster care, respite services, and surrendering custody to the state, to traditional orphanages. The empirical literature on the long-term effects of such residential placements, particularly in terms of their success in promoting a healthy transition to adulthood, free of significant emotional or behavioral disorders or additional criminal activity, is sparse.

One evidence-based community service for these adolescents involves the teaching-family model (TFM) of care. In the TFM, an extensively trained married couple lives in a regular home located in the community and cares for six to eight adolescents. The kids are involved in a token economy system wherein they earn points (earned for prosocial, adaptive behavior) redeemable for privileges, receive extensive social skills training, and participate in the quality of care they receive from the couple managing the home. As reviewed by Friman (in press), the TFM has a formal certification training program in place, which trains couples, and over twenty-two programs across the country are so certified. In addition, perhaps another one hundred programs use a modified version of the TFM, as, for example, the Boys Town Family Home Program, associated with Father Flanagan's Boys Home, in Boys Town, Nebraska, which involves over 1,200 youths, of whom about 36 percent are females and about 41 percent are minorities (Friman, in press). However, the majority of TFM homes are located in regular communities, not within larger institutional campuses. The teens attend regular schools within the community and are indistinguishable from their community peers in terms of social life, access to community resources, and so on.

The TFM was originally reported over twenty years ago in a manualized protocol by Phillips, Phillips, Fixsen, and Wolf (1974) and in a journal article by Wolf et al. (1976). Follow-up studies of adolescents residing in TFM homes, both in the United States and in European countries, reveal dramatic improvements in their behavior and school performance, a reduction in psychiatric symptoms, a reduction in criminal activities, and, surprisingly, extremely positive appraisals from the youth themselves on the quantity and value of the care they received (e.g., Friman et al., 1996; Slot, van Bilsen, Henck, & Kendall, 1995). Moreover, the TFM program seems to be extremely cost-effective (Weinrott, Jones, & Howard, 1982) and to yield positive effects, which are well maintained for years after the youth leave the TFM home (Thompson, Smith, Osgood, Dowd, Friman, & Daly, 1996). A comprehensive review of the TFM can be found in Wolf, Kirigin, Fixsen, Blase, and Braukmann (1995).

OTHER EXAMPLES OF EVIDENCE-BASED COMMUNITY PRACTICE

Without going into as much detail as in the previous case examples, a few other citations of evidence-based community-focused interventions are listed in Table 4-1. It is hoped that this listing accurately conveys the fact that a very diverse group of community problems are amenable to effective psychosocial intervention using community-based services. Many additional examples could have been provided, but space limitations preclude a more comprehensive listing. The collection of reprinted articles by Greene, Winett, Houten, Geller, and Iwata (1987) is a highly recommended resource for further illustrations of evidence-based community practice, as are a couple of the author's recent books (see Mattaini & Thyer, 1996; Thyer & Wodarski, 1998) and an early bibliography (Thyer, Himle, & Santa, 1986).

THE ROLE OF THEORY IN COMMUNITY PRACTICE

The role of theory is vastly overrated in social work research and in evaluation studies in general. Most evaluation occurs on programs that have been in operation for some time and are at best only very loosely tied to any partic-

TABLE 4-1   Selected Examples of Additional Evidence-Based Community-Focused Psychosocial Intervention Programs

Problem	Intervention	Citation
Adolescent smoking	Refusal skills training in schools	Biglan, Sverson, Ary, & Faller (1987)
Depression	The Life Satisfaction Course	Breckenridge, Zeiss, Thompson, & Munoz (1987)
	Community-based prevention program	Vega, Valle, Kolody, Hough, & Munoz (1987)
Juvenile delinquency	Multisystemic therapy	Borduin, Mann, Cone, & Henggeler (1995)
Failure to use child safety seats in automobiles	Increased citations (fines)	Lavelle, Hovell, West, & Wahlgren (1992)
Failure of drivers to use safety belts	Prompting signs	Williams, Thyer, Bailey, & Harrison (1989)
Home burglaries	Helicopter patrol	Schnelle et al. (1978)
Malnutrition in the elderly	Assertive outreach	Bunck & Iwata (1978)
Increasing charitable giving to a senior center	Public feedback	Jackson & Mathews (1995)
Socially isolated people with physical disabilites (1995)	Home access modifications	White, Paine-Andrews, Mathews, & Fawcett
Drunk driving	Promoting a designated driver program	Brigham, Meier, & Goodner (1995)

ular theory of human behavior. Many, for all practical purposes, are "theory free." Ask the community practitioners the question, "What theory is your program based on?" and you will likely draw puzzled looks. Evaluation research can be profitably conducted with minimal recourse to theory, in an attempt to answer relatively modest questions such as, "Did the community indicators improve following implementation of this intervention?" Evaluation research is a very poor vehicle to try and demonstrate that a particular theory's propositions are "true" (see Thyer, 1998).

However, despite these sentiments, it will not have escaped the notice of the keen-eyed reader that many, if not most, of the evidence-based community interventions described in this chapter are derived, directly or tangentially, from social learning theory. As in the domain of clinical practice, in community practice the psychosocial interventions with the greatest degree of empirical support are, so far, those based upon social learning theory. Many publications extending the principles of social learning theory to the field of community practice already exist, and the numbers of these are likely to grow (e.g., Mattaini, 1993a; Biglan, Glasgow, & Singer, 1990; Weisner & Silver, 1981; Rothman & Thyer, 1984). To the extent that training in one or more theoretical models of human behavior is deemed necessary for community practitioners, graduate-level course content in social learning theory and applied behavior analysis would seem highly recommended (see Thyer, 1992).

THE ROLE OF EVALUATION RESEARCH IN COMMUNITY PRACTICE

The only way in which the evidence-based practice agenda can be advanced within social work and its sister human service disciplines is for community practitioners themselves to proactively build an evaluation research component into every service plan. This is best done prospectively, not retrospectively, or as an afterthought some years after a community program has been in operation. The type of research being advocated here is fairly simple program evaluations. Using rudimentary group (such as the O-X-O) and simple single-system (such as the B and A-B) research designs, most community practitioners can gather data credible to others in support of the hypothesis that the community improved following the implementation of some human service initiative. Thyer (1998), Thyer and Larkin (1998), and Royse and Thyer (1996) provide some practical suggestions on conducting program evaluations of community-based services. Community practitioners need to break free from the conventional theory-testing model of scientific inquiry, whose aims are to test theory and to produce generalizable knowledge, in favor of simply seeing if one's local community interventions are being following by improvements in community well-being. The aim is not to test whether knowledge is generalizable to many other communities, but to see if something is apparently working in your community. This can be done locally, using available resources, and with very limited funding. You do not usually need externally funded grants to have the capacity to conduct small-scale evaluations of local community programs.

Social workers and other human service professionals must take it upon themselves to generate the empirical evidence in support of the effectiveness of community-based programs if we expect local citizens, the government, or the private sector to fund our efforts. It is becoming increasingly ethically incumbent that we take into account the evidence-based foundations of the interventions we seek to apply within our communities and adopt empirically supported ones in favor of programs lacking credible scientific support. Once implemented, we need to be proactive in empirically evaluating the outcomes of our services and be courageous enough to be guided by the results. These features are the hallmarks of a mature profession. There is a term for those who disregard scientific evidence regarding proposed interventions and who decline to systematically evaluate the effectiveness of the services offered. The term is charlatan!

CHAPTER 5

Practice Evaluation: Setting Goals and Monitoring Change

Kevin Corcoran

Wallace J. Gingerich

Harold E. Briggs

This book describes a range of approaches for working with a variety of client problems and shows how you can use them in your social work practice. Although the approaches differ in important ways, they are all goal-oriented in the sense that they specify a particular change in the client's behavior or situation that becomes the focus of intervention. Progress toward the goal should be monitored continually throughout the intervention to determine whether it is working and to decide when services should change or are no longer needed. Thus, evaluating change is an integral process in all of the social work practice approaches presented in this book.

WHY EVALUATE YOUR PRACTICE?

Although social work interventions incorporate evaluation implicitly, it is important for several reasons to make evaluation an intentional and systematic part of your practice.

Probably the most important reasons are that both you and your client have a stake in the client getting better and you need reliable information on the status of the client's problem to tell you whether this is taking place (Nelsen, 1993). Think of your clients as consumers who need to have some way of telling whether they are getting their money's worth. Good evaluation procedures will provide accurate information on this. Knowing that things are getting better probably is an important factor in motivating clients to continue in treatment, and it is an important component of client satisfaction with social work intervention.

Systematically evaluating your practice gives you important feedback on whether your intervention is having the desired effect, which is becoming increasingly common with managed care (e.g., Corcoran & Vandiver, 1996). If so, you will continue until the goal is reached; if not, you will need to analyze the situation and revise your intervention or perhaps modify your original goal. Reliable ongoing evaluation should help you fine-tune your intervention, leading to a more efficient outcome for your client.

Another reason for evaluating your practice is that over time you will learn a great deal about which interventions work best with which clients in which situations. In other words, you are likely to become an increasingly effective social work practitioner. Practitioners report that their own practice experience is their most frequent source of knowledge about practice (Morrow-Bradley & Elliott, 1986), and systematic practice evaluation is one important source of such information.

Although we believe that evaluation will improve your practice, it is important to note that there is little or no empirical evidence to date to support this assumption (Levy, 1981; Hudson, 1987; Hayes, Nelson, & Jarrett, 1987). There is general consensus, however, that evaluation is a necessary part of practice, for reasons of professional accountability (Bloom & Fischer, 1982; Blythe, 1995; Briar, 1973) as well as for improved practice. In fact, schools of social work are now required by accreditation standards to include content on practice valuation in their curriculums (Council on Social Work Education, 1988). Clearly, research is needed to determine how practice evaluation contributes to improved outcomes.

EVALUATION VERSUS RESEARCH

What we are describing in this chapter is practice evaluation, not clinical research (Barlow, Hayes, & Nelson, 1984; Blythe & Rodgers, 1993). Practice evaluation is a practice process used to determine whether a desired client outcome was achieved. Although practice evaluation uses research methods and procedures, its primary goals are to provide feedback about client change and enhance the client's outcome (Corcoran, 1993). In contrast, clinical research uses rigorous research procedures to develop scientific knowledge. Requirements regarding measurement error and design validity are much more rigorous for research than for evaluation. The distinctions between evaluation and research, then, are primarily purpose, rigor, and emphasis.

It is important to remember that evaluation is a practice activity, done to provide feedback on your work with your client. Evaluation will tell you whether your client improved and may provide some clues as to whether your intervention was responsible for the improvement. However, because the methods used in practice evaluation are not as rigorous as those for research purposes, you will be limited in what you can conclude about the effectiveness of your intervention.

We freely admit that this version of evaluation can be criticized as weak in terms of research methodology; this weakness prevents you from proving scientifically that an independent variable (your social work intervention) caused change on a dependent variable (a client symptom or set of problems). The purpose, however, is not for you to conduct research, but rather to monitor your client's change over the course of intervention and facilitate your understanding of how effective you were with your clients. Other methods for evaluating your work with clients include intake assessments, family histories, diagnostic work-ups, and your ongoing experiences and clinical judgment about your client. To reiterate, practice evaluation methods are simply another source of information to use along with other data about your client and your intervention.

As the practice chapters of this volume frequently illustrate, it often is necessary and helpful to establish intermediate and instrumental goals (also see Nelsen, 1984, 1993; Rosen & Proctor, 1978). In family treatment, for example, an intermediate goal might be to resolve a particular family crisis. An instrumental goal, one that is necessary to bring about the outcome, might be to establish communication skills, which should help improve the family cohesion. In terms of practice-based evaluation, intermediate and instrumental goals provide feedback about whether you are effectively helping your client. Monitoring how you reach these goals not only serves to establish your accountability, but also has practice utility, because these goals are designed to enhance the likelihood of obtaining your final goal.

HOW TO DO PRACTICE EVALUATION

Simply stated, practice evaluation requires that you 1) satisfy the target behavior and set the desired goal, 2) select a suitable measure of the behavior and use it systematically for treatment, and 3) analyze whether change has occurred and the goal has been reached (Corcoran, 1993; Corcoran & Gingerich, 1994). We use the term "behavior" broadly to refer to any change that you and your client have identified as the target of intervention. This could include changes in action, affect, or cognition of your client or others.

Specify the Target Behavior and Set a Goal

As should be clear by now, practice evaluation is basically a determination of whether there has been useful improvement in the problem situation that brought the client into treatment in the first place. Accordingly, the most important part of the evaluation is specifying clearly the problem situation and how the client would like things to be different at the end of treatment. Note that this involves specifying both the target behavior in the amount of change that is desired.

Specifying target behaviors and setting treatment goals are integral parts of social work practice (Hepworth, Rooney, & Larsen, 1997). However, different treatment approaches tend to emphasize somewhat different target behaviors, reflecting their different understandings of human behavior and behavior-change interventions. The authors of the client problem chapters in part two of this book give you a good idea of the types of behaviors to focus on in their respective approaches. Therefore, we will not deal here with what behaviors you should select, but rather with how you should specify the target behavior and state the goal.

Specification of target behaviors and goals always should be based on a thorough assessment of your client's situation and the kind of changes your client desires. In other words, target behaviors and goals should reflect your client's real, practical concerns and should flow naturally and logically from the assessment you have conducted. We emphasize this point because historically the tendency has been to select outcomes for which standardized research measures existed, instead of outcomes that seemed clinically important. With the use of individualized measures, which we will discuss shortly, this problem is less serious than it once was.

Questions to consider.   The six questions discussed below should be considered when specifying goals. They are derived from procedures described by a number of writers (Mager, 1972; Gottman & Leiblum, 1974; Bloom, Fischer, & Orme, 1999; Hepworth et al., 1997). Fortunately, there is good consensus on the characteristics of good goals.

1. Why?   The reasons for goal setting and practice evaluation are similar. These reasons should be known to the person doing the evaluation as well as understood by the people who are the subject and beneficiaries of the evaluation. For social workers, goal setting and practice evaluation are important to all levels of practice, such as individual, family, and agency practice. Goal setting and practice evaluation provide social workers with benchmarks, indicators, and means to obtain relevant information about the usefulness of treatment strategy, program methodology, or an agency's approach to behavior change or problem solving. Also, goal setting and practice evaluation provide the ongoing means by which practitioners can refine, further develop, and enhance their capacities to do a better job (Cherin & Meezan, 1998; Pinkston & Linsk, 1984a, 1984b; O'Looney, 1997; McCready, Pierce, Rahn, & Were, 1996). Further, goal setting and practice evaluation are methodologies to use in ensuring professional accountability. They give client subjects and funders of programs and services a basis for judging the aims and accomplishments of the staff and management of clinical and community-based programs and services (Au, 1996; Auslander, 1996, 1998; Martin & Kettner, 1997).

2. Who?   Be clear about whose behavior is to be the target of intervention. This is not always as obvious as it may seem. Sometimes it is the person you are seeing, as in the case of the depressed client who wants to feel happier. Sometimes your client will ask you to help bring about change in another person's behavior; for example, a mother might like her child to stop misbehaving, or a wife might like her husband to be more attentive and loving. In such cases you might help your client to specify the desired change in the other person's behavior, but you probably also would direct your client to specify changes in his or her own behavior that would facilitate or bring about the desired change in the other person's behavior (Rosen & Proctor, 1978; Nelsen, 1984, 1993; Reid, 1993).

3. Will do what?   State what the client will be doing, in observable terms, when the goal has been reached. What actual behaviors will be different? This sometimes is difficult when the client presents the problem in mental or psychological terms, such as depression, lack of trust, lack of love, and so forth. Many times, however, you can enable the client to be more specific by asking such questions as: How will things be different when the problem is solved? If you were to make a videotape, what would you see that is different? What would another family member or someone who knows you well notice? If you have ever before felt the way you hope to feel, how were things different then?

Occasionally clients are not able to specify observable behaviors or indicators of their goals, in which case you can have them make ratings on a simple scale that you construct for them. Procedures for observing behaviors and constructing self-rating scales will be discussed later in this chapter.

4. How well?   This is where you make a desired level of performance explicit. In other words, once the client has specified the target behavior, he or she decides how well or how often the behavior must occur to signify success. Usually goals can be stated along the continuum of performance. The idea here is to identify what level your client would consider satisfactory. You may need to negotiate this with your client, because some clients underestimate what they can achieve and others may be overly optimistic. In any case, discussing the range of possible performance conveys to your client that the concept of goals is negotiable into the outcome achieved may indeed be somewhat different than planned.

5. Is it realistic?   Treatment goals must be realistic if they are to be useful. There is no point agreeing to goals that you or the client know are not possible. The guideline here is whether the goal you have set is viable, given your client's ability and willingness to work for change, the availability of other people necessary for the change, your ability to bring about the desired change, and the time and resources that are available.

6. Is it important?   Sometimes, in the process of making your goal specific and observable, it changes from the original complaint. Therefore, once your goal statement answers the previous four questions, you should ask yourself if indeed this is the goal that is important to your client. Assuming that your client achieves the goal, will he or she consider treatment a success? This is critical to good evaluation because we assume that attaining the goal means intervention was successful. If it turns out that the goal selected was inappropriate, achieving it would be meaningless.

Specifying the goals. The questions discussed above for consideration when specifying behaviors and setting goals may seem more like clinical concerns than research concerns. That is because this is an area where the purpose of practice and research come together. From a practice standpoint, you want your clients to be working toward goals that are meaningful, realistic, and that will make concrete differences in their lives. And from a research standpoint, you want your indicators of change to be ones that signify real changes there were accomplished; therefore, they must be related directly to the actual goals that you and your clients are working toward with your specific social work intervention.

We have described a rather generic procedure for specifying target behaviors and setting goals. Kiresuk and associates have developed a specific technique known as goal attainment scaling (GAS) that incorporates most of these ideas and is widely used in mental health settings to set treatment goals and evaluate change (Kiresuk, Smith, & Cardillo, 1994; Mintz & Kiesler, 1982). We highly recommend GAS as a way to structure the goal-setting process and incorporate it into your normal clinical practice.

GAS is a simple procedure for observing change in relation to treatment goals (Kiresuk & Sherman, 1968; Kiresuk et al., 1994). It can be used to establish goals by specifying the behaviors where change is to occur and delineating outcomes, such as those reflecting the attainment of the goal or failure to meet the goal. A conventional GAS specifies in observable terms five levels of outcome: 1) the least favorable outcome, 2) a less-than-expected outcome, 3) the expected outcome if the intervention is successful, 4) a more-than-expected outcome from a successful intervention, and 5) the most favorable outcome. Each outcome should be described briefly and in such a fashion that it is observable by others, such as your client, yourself, or another relevant other (e.g., spouse or coworker).

Table 5-1 shows the five levels of outcome established for a mother and son who sought clinical social work services because of the very complex-ridden and occasionally combative relationship. The GAS is designed to reflect the expected outcomes from the mother's perspective, with her rating her son's behavior. The scoring system here ranges from 0 to 45, although any set of numbers can be used, provided that the same ones are used each time the GAS is completed. For example, some writers recommend using -2 -1 0 +1 +2, so that the less-than-expected outcome is expressed by negative numbers. You should select a numbering system that is meaningful to you and your client.

Once you have established your goal and developed the GAS, you can start rating your client's attainment of the goal. An advantage of the GAS is that the behavioral description allows for relevant others, such as a field supervisor, to interview the client and rate the goal state. In fact, the GAS was originally designed so that someone other than the social worker could conduct a follow-up interview and complete the measure. Although this is, indeed,

TABLE 5-1   Goal Attainment Scaling for Mother-Son Conflict

Outcome	Behavioral Description	Score
Most favorable	Talks almost daily. Expresses fondness toward mother.	4
More favorable	Talks several times per week. Does one fun activity each week.	3
Expected	Has at least one good talk per week. No big arguments.	2
Less than expected	Son yells at mother and verbally assaults her.	1
Least favorable	Son yells at mother, verbally and physically assaults her.	0

important for research purposes, for a practice evaluation it is acceptable for you or your client to evaluate the attainment of the goal. You may decide to do this toward the end of the intervention process (see discussion below). If you have one or two intermediate goals (such as improved communication skills, as reflected in the GAS in Table 5-1) you should develop a separate GAS for each intermediate goal as well as one for final goal.

Select a Measure and Use It Systematically

The first crucial decision you must make in monitoring the progress of a client or a particular outcome is how to measure the characteristic or attribute. In technical terms, measurement is the process of assigning a number to some thing according to some rules. In social work practice, the "thing" is probably a major symptom your client is experiencing or a goal of intervention. In essence, you are observing the magnitude, intensity, or frequency of a problem or goal. The fact that the method of making the observation is standardized means that it is made the same way each time. Standardization thus means that you can be fairly certain that you are measuring pretty much the same thing each time you see it. Researchers call this "thing" the dependent variable, because it is expected to change as a consequence of an independent variable, which presumably is the social work intervention. Assigning numbers to the attribute or variable allows the use of mathematic procedures to monitor a client's progress. As we will discuss below, you can plot your observations on a graph and monitor whether the behavior changes; for example, a patient with borderline personality disorder may display a decrease in magic thinking, or a dual-career couple might show an increase in the sharing of household responsibilities as part of a fairer and more equitable relationship.

For practice-based evaluation, the basic measurement issues are deciding what measure to use and deciding where and when to make the observations.

Deciding what measure to use.   We recommend that you use both individualized and standardized measures of the client problem or treatment goals. Individualized measures are tailored to the unique complaint and situation of the client (Mintz & Kiesler, 1982). These often are referred to as idiographic or tailored measures. By their nature, individualized measures usually are suitable for obtaining daily feedback on the target behavior. Standardized measures are scales that have known reliability and validity and often have been normed for clinical populations. Standardized measures usually are given only a few times during treatment (for example, before and after treatment) and are used to verify the findings obtained from the individualized measure (Jordan & Franklin, 1995).

Many times the target behavior is a discrete behavior or event, such as having an argument, failing to complete homework, waking up at night, having headaches, or thinking negative thoughts. In each case, the client is describing something he or she does or does not do. Even if the client's initial description of the problem or goal is not in behavioral terms, you should explore with him or her whether it can be so described. The goal-setting steps and GAS procedure outlined above are useful tools in this regard. Most client outcomes can be stated in behavioral terms, and doing so has the advantage of making them more explicit and concrete and more easily observed by social worker and client.

Individualized measures.   The two individualized measurement procedures we recommend are direct observation and self-anchored rating scales (SARSs). Observations made using these techniques then can be substantiated with standardized measures, such as a rapid assessment instrument (RAI).

When using direct observations, you should write out a description of the target behavior. After both you and the client have agreed on the description, it should be included in the client record. Your description should be clear, objective, and complete. *Clear* means that someone else using your description would agree with you on occurrences of the behavior. *Objective* means that the behavior is directly observable and requires little or no inference. For example, "in-seat behavior" (defined as having one's buttocks in contact with a chair) is objective, whereas "studying" is not objective. *Complete* means that your description encompasses the likely range of behavior and excludes those behaviors that may only be similar. For example, when describing a temper tantrum, you would exclude those times when a child cries because of a hurt finger or a bad dream.

Behaviors and discrete events can be observed and counted in a variety of ways. The most common method is a simple frequency count, in which the client (or other observer) keeps a tally of the number of times each day that the target behavior occurs. Occasionally, you might be interested in the latency of a behavior; for example, the length of time it takes a child to go to bed after he or she has been asked to do so. Sometimes the duration of the behavior is of primary interest, such as how much time a couple spends talking with each other each day. There are other, more specialized observational procedures (e.g., time sampling and discriminated operants) that you may want to explore (Barlow, Hayes, and Nelson, 1984; Ciminero, Calhoun, & Adams, 1986). In any case, it is crucial, that you have a clear, objective, and complete description of the behavior that can be observed and reported by the client on a regular basis, perhaps daily or weekly.

When the target problem is an internal state, such as fear, depression, or self-esteem, we recommend the use of a SARS. Direct observation is not appropriate in these situations because the complaint does not correspond to an observable behavior; only the client is able to observe these situations.

A SARS is so flexible and easy to use, regardless of the client situation, that it has been called the "all-purpose measurement procedure" (Bloom, 1975). To develop a SARS, establish a range of the client problem that defines the extreme ends of the problem from, say, most intense to least intense. Then determine the number of points on the scale, from say, 0 to 15 or 1 to 7, with the extreme ends of the problem reflecting the lowest and highest numbers. The number range should be based on your client's ability to discriminate the levels of the problem. With younger clients, you might use 1 to 5, or even 1 to 3. It is helpful to then define the middle range of the problem to correspond to the numbers between the lowest and highest.

The crucial point with SARS is to develop clear anchors. Do this by having your client imagine a recent time when she or he felt very low on the scale. Then ask him or her to describe what was happening along three dimensions: what he or she was *doing, thinking,* and *feeling.* For a client who complains of low self-esteem, reported behaviors could include procrastinating on her work, spending most of the day in the house, and turning down a request from a friend to go out. Along the second (cognitive) dimension, the client may report recurrent thoughts that she is not competent in her job, that she will not get the promotion she would like, and that her boss thinks she is not performing adequately. The third dimension, feelings, is best captured with word pictures that describe physical sensations that go along with strong emotions. For example, the client might report a "sinking" feeling or a "heavy" feeling, or perhaps simply feeling "down" or "blue" or "like the bottom is dropping out."

Once you have elicited anchors at each end of the scale and at the midpoint, ask the client to select the three or four anchors that best represent the numbers on the scale. The client then rates herself on the scale according to whether she is experiencing those anchors or not, rather than by making a global judgment.

Figure 5-1 displays a SARS for the son in the above-mentioned mother-son conflict. Here the son is able to rate his feelings toward his mother. Because the SARS is so simple, it is possible that the client could complete the SARS daily or even several times a day at meaningful periods, such as when his

FIGURE 5-1   Self-Anchored Rating Scale of Son's Feelings toward Mother

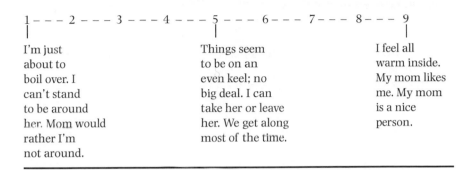

mother is instructing him to do something (e.g., take out the trash, do his homework).

Standardized measures.   Direct observations and SARSs, of course, have limitations when it comes to reliability and validity. This is more troublesome for research purposes than for practice evaluation purposes. However, you can minimize some of the limitations by corroborating individualized measures with a standardized measure. For clinical evaluation, we recommend that you use rapid assessment instruments (RAIs) (Levitt & Reid, 1981; Corcoran & Fischer, 2000a, 2000b). Because standardized scales may be time consuming, even when they are as short as twenty items, they are useful primarily to substantiate the observations made with a direction observation or a SARS.

As is illustrated in many of the chapters in this book, RAIs are available for most client problems. They can be used regardless of theoretical orientation to practice. In addition to personality traits (e.g., the Trait Anger scale [Spielberger, Jacobson, Russell, & Crane, 1983]) and problem states (e.g., a measure of phobia, such as the Fear Questionnaire [Marks & Mathews, 1979]), RAIs are available to observe treatment satisfaction, beliefs, and many affective and cognitive states.

Choose standardized scales that are easily administered and scored; they also should have published data on reliability and validity. Any short, easily comprehensible questionnaire has the potential to be used as a secondary measure. Several books are available that reprint scales that are appropriate for practice evaluation or that contain subscales from lengthier instruments that could be used to observe a particular characteristic of your practice (Corcoran & Fischer, 2000a, 2000b; Robinson & Shaver, 1973; Schutte & Malouff, 1995). There also are numerous books that describe various instruments, such as Sweetland & Keyser (1983), and journals that frequently publish new instruments, such as *The Journal of Personality Assessment* and *Journal of*

Behavioral Assessment and Psychopathology. For a more detailed list of these books and journals, see Jordan, Franklin, and Corcoran, 1997. In addition, computerized measurement systems are available, the best of which is Hudson's Computer-Assisted Social Services (1990).

The problems and benefits of reactivity. All of the observation methods we have recommended are subject to reactivity (reactivity refers to how the process of observing something can change what is being observed). For example, if you ask a client to monitor his or her cigarette consumption, it is possible, even likely, that consumption will change as a result of self-monitoring. Consumption may go up or down, depending on a number of factors (Bloom et al., 1999).

Most writers advise using procedures that reduce reactivity—so-called nonreactive measures (Webb, Campbell, Schwartz, Sechrest, & Grove, 1981). This is sound advice for research purposes, but it often is not practical in social work settings. Most nonreactive measures do not involve the client directly (for example, someone else may observe the client without his or her awareness). Helping the client to observe his or her own behavior and change it if desired usually is an important component of clinical social work. Self-observation (and hence reactivity) is an integral part of the intervention.

Because reactivity is likely to be a factor for many clients, you should use this effect to your client's advantage by designing your measurement procedure so that the anticipated effect of reactivity is to move your client closer to his or her goal. Accordingly, you should design the measurement procedure so that it heightens your client's awareness of undesired behaviors *before* he or she engages in the behavior (for example, the client could count the number of cigarettes in the pack before smoking the next one). Better yet, have him or her record the desirable counterpart of the unwanted behavior; for example, the number of times he or she had the urge to smoke but did not. Reactivity also argues for working toward positive goals, such as increasing the positive talk time between spouses. This often has the effect of drawing the spouses' attention to the positive aspects of their relationship rather than the negative.

Summary. There is a wide variety of ways to measure client problems and treatment goals. We recommend GAS, SARSs, and standardized instruments. However you decide to measure the problems and goals, the measurement process should be an integral part of treatment that helps accomplish the desired change.

Deciding where and when to make the observations. The purpose of your practice determines where and when you should make observations. If, for example, you were helping parents to manage an acting-out adolescent, it would be important to measure the problem in the family home or wherever else it occurs. On the other hand, if the problem is a more enduring characteristic of the client and does not occur in a specific situation, then you probably can make the observations at your office or some other place.

The point to keep in mind is that the observations should be made in the environment in which the problem is apparent, such as at home, school, or work. When the problem is not situation specific, you have more flexibility in terms of where the measurement should occur.

Whatever place is used to make the observation, it is important to be consistent. If, for example, your client's problem occurs only at work, he or she should complete the SARS or standardized scale while at work. The issue here is standardization. Your measurement will be more valid (that is, accurate) if done the same way and in the same circumstances each time. You and your client should decide at the beginning of your intervention where she or he will observe the problem or goal state.

In terms of how often to make the observations, we suggest daily, if feasible, for the individualized measures. The standardized scales should be completed at least three times—before, during, and after treatment—although they can be used more frequently. More frequent measures may be necessary for certain types of client problems, such as suicidal tendencies. When the practice focus is on more enduring traits, such as personality disorders or identity problems, then less frequent observations may be appropriate. It is important not to make observations too frequently or too infrequently. You should make observations at regular and meaningful intervals after the problem occurs and in the same circumstances. In essence, the decision of when to make the observations is the basis on which you will analyze change.

Analyze Whether Change Has Occurred and the Goal Has Been Reached

Specifying the target behavior and measuring it systematically over time provide the basis for practice evaluation, but another important step is needed: deciding whether there was change, or whether the treatment goal was met, or both. These really are two different questions. The first question—was there change?—requires some notion of how the client would be if there were no change and usually is referred to as statistical or experimental significance. The second question—was the goal reached?—compares the client's behavior at the end of treatment with the goal that was initially set. This kind of analysis is called clinical or practical significance. Each analysis requires a different basis for reaching a conclusion. Before we can analyze change, however, we must gather observations according to a systematic plan or strategy.

Strategies for collecting observations.   In social work treatment clients usually hope to achieve some change in their targeted behaviors. They want to be less depressed, more relaxed, more loving, less suspicious, more cooperative, and so forth. Usually clients expect change to occur gradually during the course of intervention. If change is going in the direction of the treatment goal, the client will be satisfied, but if there is no change or if change is in the opposite direction—that is, the client is getting worse—it is time to reevaluate the intervention.

Assessment of change requires, at a minimum, observation at two points in time using the same measurement procedure, namely, direction observation or standardized scale. If the second observation is different from the first, we say there has been change. In practice evaluation we carry this idea further to include repeated observations over time, sometimes daily, but usually at least weekly. As mentioned above, frequency depends on the client problem or treatment goal. Traditional research terminology refers to these systematic ways for observing behavior as research designs.

Designs are nothing more than the procedures by which you decide to make your observations. Although there are a variety of different designs available (see, for example, Bloom et al., 1999; Jayaratne & Levy, 1979), most have two basic components: observations made when intervention is occurring and observations made when there is no intervention. Observations prior to intervention are called baseline, or A phase, and observations during intervention are referred to as the treatment phase, or B phase. In research parlance, this is referred to as the AB design. As we will discuss in the section on graphing, the purpose of collecting these systematic observations is to compare the client's performance during treatment with a time when treatment was not occurring.

One of the easiest ways to collect baseline observations is during the initial intake and assessment periods. If, for example, the client is scheduled for an intake assessment, it is a good idea to develop a SARS and start measuring the problem at that time; if the same client is scheduled to come in the next week to start work on the problem, this time also can be used for baseline observations.

To analyze change, plot the observations on a graph and compare the B phase with the A phase. This is illustrated in Figure 5-2 where the baseline phase is composed of three observations. By plotting the observations on a graph, you are able to monitor your client's progress by comparing the observations made during your intervention with those collected during the baseline. Failure to observe change in the A and B phases would then warrant a reconsideration of the appropriateness of your intervention. For example, if your client's SARS scores did not change, you might decide to use a different social work intervention. Your original B phase then stops, and a new intervention, the C phase, begins, giving you a slightly different design, the ABC design, where the new intervention is compared with the A phase and the B phase (Figure 5-3). An example appears in Corcoran (1997), where systematic communication skills training was not helping a distressed family and was then replaced with structured family therapy techniques.

FIGURE 5-2   AB Design for Analyzing Change

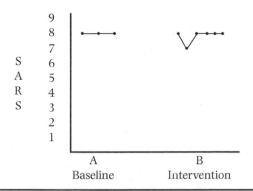

Retrospective baseline observations. Sometimes clinical considerations prohibit collecting baseline observations before you must begin intervention (Reid, 1993), for example, in the case of a suicidal client. There are two solutions to this problem. One is to have your client report retrospective observations, that is, observations that your client makes based on his or her memory. Although these are less valid than observations made as the behavior is occurring, they generally are better than no baseline at all. Retrospective baseline observations usually are collected by asking your client to recall as accurately as possible the frequency of the target behavior on each day of the preceding week or two. If this is not feasible, you can ask your client to estimate the average frequency for the week prior to treatment, or perhaps for the month prior to treatment. For clear, specific, salient behaviors (such as drinking, for example), clients sometimes can provide useful information for a period of three to four weeks prior to the start of treatment. A set of retrospective observations that is particularly useful is to have the client recall the problem "last week," "in general," and "at its worst."

Postintervention retrospective baseline. A second solution to the problem of not having actual baseline observations is to collect them after the intervention has occurred. This is called a postintervention retrospective baseline (Howard, 1980), which involves asking the client, at the conclusion of treatment, to estimate the level of the behavior prior to treatment. Some kinds of client problems, such as extreme pessimism or paranoia, may affect the client's perception or judgment. In such cases, the client may give a more accurate and comparable baseline estimate after treatment than he or she could have before. There is no reported use in the social work literature of postintervention retrospective baseline, but when a prospective baseline is not possible, this may be a useful substitute.

FIGURE 5-3   ABC Design for Analyzing Change

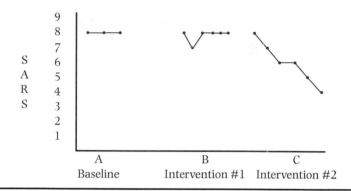

Follow-up observations.   In addition to the baseline and treatment phases, you should have your client observe the target behavior periodically after you have stopped treatment. These follow-up observations are quite valuable because they enable you to determine whether the improvement in your client's target behavior is continuing after treatment or whether it is deteriorating. It is advisable to have at least one or two follow-up contacts, either through an actual session or by telephone or mail. Giving your client a self-addressed, stamped envelope increases the likelihood that he or she will report the follow-up observations.

Intervention-only designs.   In rare instances you may not be able to collect baseline or retrospective baseline observations. When baseline of any type is not possible, it is useful nonetheless to observe and analyze the target behavior during the intervention. Observing during intervention allows you to evaluate whether the client is progressing toward the goal and whether the goal is achieved. You can monitor your client's change in relation to the target behavior's level, magnitude, or frequency from week to week, or at the middle and end phases of practice in relation to the earlier sessions.

Many clients terminate treatment before clinicians believe that they are ready; therefore, you may not have the immediate opportunity for follow-up observations, which might leave you with an intervention-only design. Often, however, such clients will contact you when the problem again becomes distressful. The use of retrospective observations for the time between interventions enables you to develop a more accurate design to evaluate whether your intervention is indeed helping your client change.

A variation on the intervention-only design is the repeated pretest-posttest experiment proposed by Thyer and Curtis (1983). This design strategy can be used when pretreatment baseline in the usual sense is not possible and where some of the treatment effect may be expected immediately following a therapy session, as is true in desensitization and social skill training. In this design, measures of the target behavior are taken immediately before and after each treatment session to see whether there has been change in the target behavior, presumably as a result of the intervention techniques. This strategy is repeated with each treatment session, hence the pretest-posttest designation. In essence, you do a series of pre-post observations for each session of your social work intervention.

Summary. There are a number of strategies for observing the target behavior in order to provide a basis for analyzing change. Deciding when to make your observations sets the bases for your design. In each instance, the idea is to observe the target behavior systematically under various treatment and no-treatment conditions. With a little creative work, you will be able to develop your own variations of the above designs to monitor clients' progress.

Assessing change. Once you have collected systematic observations of the target behavior, you will need to analyze them to decide whether they reflect real change. This is not as obvious a decision as it may seem. When the change is dramatic and consistent, there is little doubt that change has occurred. But frequently the observations do not present such a clear-cut case, and the analysis of change becomes more difficult.

There are two general approaches to analyzing change: visual analysis using graphs and statistical analysis. We will discuss only visual analysis here, because it is the most practical approach and should always be used. Sometimes statistical analysis also can be helpful when visual analysis is inconclusive. Statistical and quasi-statistical techniques for assessing change are discussed in Bloom et al. (1999), Gingerich (1983), and Jayaratne (1978).

To conduct visual analysis, plot the observations on a line graph so that you can see the pattern (Jayaratne & Levy, 1979; Kazdin, 1979).The vertical axis is used to plot the target behavior, such as scores on a SARS or standardized scale; the horizontal axis is used to represent time, usually in days, sessions, or weeks (see Figures 5-2 and 5-3). The observations within each phase are connected by a line, and a vertical line is drawn between phases. As the above discussion suggests, you will be comparing the treatment observations with baseline observations to see whether there is a difference.

The standard for analyzing change in visual analysis is "clearly evident and reliable"; that is, the differences in target behavior between baseline and treatment phases is unequivocal and consistent. Operationally, there are several guidelines to follow in reaching this conclusion. First, there should be little or no overlap in target behaviors between phases. This means that there should be a clear change in the level of the target behavior between baseline and treatment. Second, if the target behavior shows a trend during baseline, it should be in a direction opposite from the goal. This is because if baseline behaviors are moving toward the goal, it will be difficult to show that there is an added improvement during treatment. In fact, you may be well advised not to implement treatment at all in such cases, because the client may achieve the goal on his or her own.

Assessing goal attainment.   As noted earlier, analyzing change involves two questions: first, is the target problem any different now than it was before treatment; and second, did the client reach his or her goal? This second question is addressed here. Although change per se is not the issue, reaching the goal almost always implies that there has been some change. One exception to this is if you are working with a client to prevent further deterioration in functioning, in which case enabling the client to stay the same could be considered a worthwhile goal in comparison to further deterioration.

To assess goal attainment, plot on a line graph the level of the target behavior that you hope to achieve at the point in time that you have set. In other words, graph your goal right on the chart before intervention begins; as intervention proceeds and you graph the target behavior, you can see whether it meets or exceeds the goal.

From a graphing standpoint, assessing goal attainment is a simple matter. The critical issue is deciding upon a realistic goal. In the research literature this usually is discussed in terms of assessing clinical significance or applied significance (Gingerich, 1983). From a more practical standpoint, you might use the criteria discussed above under setting realistic treatment goals. The issue here is, how much change must there be for you and your client to conclude that treatment was a success? Unfortunately, there are no objective standards or empirical tests to tell you this. It is largely a subjective, clinical judgment, but an important one, because this is in a sense the criterion for success that your client will use.

INTEGRATING EVALUATION INTO PRACTICE

For evaluation to become an integral part of your routine practice, it must be conducive to what you do as a social worker; in other words, it must have practice utility (Gingerich, 1990). Moreover, practice evaluation must be easily accomplished. With this in mind, we suggest that observation and graphing become part of your regular progress or case notes. Figure 5-4 provides an example of a practice evaluation form. The left and right axes have been left blank so that you can use any set of scores from a SARS, GAS, or standardized scale. For example, the left axis could be set from 1 to 100 in order to use one of Hudson's (1987) scales; or you might set it from 1 to 9, or whatever set of scores are appropriate for a SARS. The right axis could be set to a different scoring system on perhaps another measurement, such as a GAS. Figure 5-4 is set up for twenty-one assessment periods, which could be days, weeks, or

FIGURE 5-3   Practice Evaluation Form

CLIENT/CONSUMER:

PROBLEMS: 1.	2.	3.
GOALS: 1.	2.	3.
TX: 1.	2.	3.

PLANNED NO.
OF SESSIONS: 1. | 2. | 3.

SCORES

1 2 3 4 5 6 7 8 9 10 11 12 13 14 15 16 17 18 19 20 21

SCORES

DATE   NOTES

whatever is meaningful for your client, and has space for brief notes under each observation.

Using the practice evaluation form thus enables you to chart two types of observations, such as a SARS and a GAS, on the left and right axes as well as record the date of the observations and any salient qualitative information that might facilitate your understanding of the client. If this form, or one that you develop yourself, is used as part of your standard case notes, you will find that doing practice evaluation not only is relatively easy and nonintrusive on your routine practice, but also helps you to be more thorough in observing your client's progress and evaluating your effectiveness.

SUMMARY

Practice evaluation has three primary components: 1) specifying the target behavior and setting the treatment goal; 2) selecting a measure and observing systematically over time; and 3) analyzing behavior change and goal attainment.

Until recently, single-case evaluation has seemed more compatible with behavior therapy than with other therapeutic approaches (Corcoran & Gingerich, 1994; Hersen & Barlow, 1986; Nelsen, 1993; Reid, 1993). This is especially true when it comes to the research purpose of asserting causality. Practice evaluation as we have described it, however, is more flexible than evaluation for the purpose of research. We hope that this discussion and the following chapters will convince you that practice evaluation is quite conducive to most social work interventions, especially because the purpose is to have more empirical bases for observing client change, as opposed to concluding a causal relationship between an independent variable and a dependent variable.

Many of the requirements of practice evaluation already are fulfilled in traditional clinical social work (Blythe, 1995; Corcoran, 1985). We recommend, however, that practice evaluation become a more intentional and systematic part of your practice. We advocate more specificity in your observation of the client and more standardization—structure, if you will—in your intervention. As we discussed in the first chapter of this book, the more specific you are about what you are going to change, and the more standardized you are in how you try to change it, the more effective you will be in helping your client to change. We suggest that you use systematic measures of the target behavior and observe before, during, and after you help your client so that you can monitor client change and evaluate your effectiveness. Doing so not only will give you additional information to use in helping your client, but also will enable you to adjust your intervention according to the observations and be more effective in helping clients change.

CHAPTER 6

Ethics and Values in Clinical and Community Social Work Practice

Frederic G. Reamer

In this chapter, Reamer presents the thinking and conceptual support for the National Association of Social Workers (NASW) revised *Code of Ethics in Social Work Practice* (1996). He examines the historical development of ethics in social work and the practice principles and other assumptions that guide ethical thinking and judgment in the profession; Reamer then presents a problem-solving method to use in resolving ethical dilemmas and challenges for practitioners. This chapter provides the reader with foundation knowledge regarding the ethics of the profession of social work and shows how ethics in social work evolved. Reamer, as one of the authors of the profession's *Code of Ethics*, describes the historical context and revolutionary periods of the ethics and professional standards that govern social work practice and presents an up-to-date version of where the profession is and what the current vulnerabilities are with respect to ethical standards. Reamer goes on to describe the ethical dilemmas facing social workers in practice in the twenty-first century. The chapter provides the reader with a decision-making model for considering the challenges to clinical social work practice. Also, Reamer draws the reader into a discussion about the theoretical basis that underlies ethical development during historical and current times. The chapter gives the reader an up-to-the-minute portrayal of the state of the art with respect to the ethics, values, and practice principles that drive the professionally governed social services. The chapter ends with a discussion and hints for managing professional liability as social workers conduct and maintain their practice.

Contemporary clinical social workers face a wide range of daunting ethical issues. Many of these issues stem from clinical social workers' customary counseling, casework, or psychotherapeutic duties. As in other clinically oriented professions—such as psychology, counseling, and psychiatry—clinical social workers encounter ethical decisions and challenges related to client confidentiality, informed consent, self-determination rights, intervention approaches, and termination of services.

However, clinical social workers, especially those practicing in community-based settings, face additional ethical issues by virtue of their status as social workers. As I will discuss more fully below, the traditional values and mission of social work, along with specific mandates in the profession's principal code of ethics (the NASW's *Code of Ethics*), create a set of ethical duties and obligations that distinguish clinical social workers' ethical responsibilities from those of other clinically oriented professionals.

The purpose of this chapter is twofold. First, I will provide an overview of ethical issues in clinical social work. Second, I will describe the resources and conceptual tools clinical social workers can use to address these issues. Where appropriate, I will compare and contrast social workers' ethical responsibilities with those of other clinically oriented professionals.

TRENDS IN THE DEVELOPMENT OF CLINICAL SOCIAL WORK ETHICS

Most clinical social workers are familiar with ethical issues concerning such phenomena as client confidentiality, privileged communication, and informed consent. Education and literature on these subjects have been staples in the social work profession for decades. In recent years, however, especially since the early 1980s, knowledge related to clinical social work ethics has burgeoned. This exponential growth is the result of a number of complex historical and contemporary factors that have profound implications for today's clinical social workers.

Social workers' assessment and understanding of ethical issues have changed dramatically during the profession's history. Our current understanding of ethical issues is the product of several stages of development. More specifically, social work's approach to ethics spans four major, sometimes overlapping, periods—the morality period, the values period, the ethical theory and decision making period, and the recent ethical standards and risk management period (Reamer, 1998c). When social work began formally in the mid-nineteenth century, practitioners were much more concerned about the client's morality than about the morality or ethics of the profession, its intervention methods, or its members (Leiby, 1978; Lubove, 1965; Reamer, 1987a, 1995a; Reid & Popple, 1992). During this "morality period"—typically associated with the charity organization society era—many social workers focused their efforts on people living in poverty and promoted paternalistic efforts to rehabilitate the "shiftless," "indolent," or "wayward" moral character of the poor (Paine, 1980; Siporin, 1992).

This preoccupation waned during the early twentieth century, when many social workers—especially those involved in the settlement house movement—became especially concerned about the harsh social consequences of industrialization and turned their attention to environmental causes of the problems of individuals and of society (such as poverty, unemployment, poor sanitation, public health risks, substandard housing, alcoholism, and mental illness). During this period, the center of gravity for many social workers was the profession's moral duty to confront social injustice and promote social reform (Brieland, 1995; Lee, 1930). Also during this period, social workers produced the profession's first ethical standards. For example, as early as 1919 there were attempts to draft professional codes of ethics (Elliott, 1931;

Frankel, 1959; Joseph, 1989). In addition, there is evidence that in the 1920s at least some schools of social work were teaching courses on values and ethics (Elliott, 1931; Johnson, 1955).

During the next phase, the values period, social workers were especially concerned about developing intervention theories and strategies, training programs, and education models innate to social work, partly in an effort to distinguish social work from professions such as psychology and psychiatry. Nearly half a century after its formal start, social work took several ambitious steps to develop and publicize ethical standards and guidelines. In 1947, the Delegate Conference of the American Association of Social Workers adopted a code of ethics. In addition, during the 1950s several important books and journal articles on the subject were published (Frankel, 1959; Hall, 1952; Johnson, 1955; Pumphrey, 1959).

The turbulent 1960s and early 1970s marked another significant turning point. Along with major segments of the broader society and many professions, social workers were especially concerned about issues of social justice, social reform, and civil rights. Enrollments in social work education programs burgeoned, in part because students were attracted to the profession's social justice values and ideological commitment to social advocacy related to human rights, welfare rights, equality, and nondiscrimination (Emmet, 1962; Keith-Lucas, 1963; Levy, 1972, 1973; Lewis, 1972; McDermott, 1975; Plant, 1970; Vigilante, 1974). Significantly, NASW adopted its first code of ethics at the beginning of this period, in 1960 (Reamer, 1997a).

This period in the profession's evolution produced what have turned out to be many classic statements on social work's values. These included discussions of the profession's core values (Arnold, 1970; Bartlett, 1970; Bernstein, 1960; Biestek, 1957; Biestek & Gehrig, 1978; Gordon, 1962, 1965; Hamilton, 1940, 1951; Keith-Lucas, 1977; Levy, 1973, 1976; Lubove, 1965; Perlman, 1965, 1976; Plant, 1970; Pumphrey, 1959; Reynolds, 1976; Stalley, 1975; Teicher, 1967; Timms, 1983; Towle, 1965; Vigilante, 1974; Working Definition, 1958; Younghusband, 1967); critiques of social work values (for example, Keith-Lucas, 1963; McDermott, 1975; Whittington, 1975; Wilson, 1978); and reports of empirical research on values held or embraced by social workers (e.g., Costin, 1964; McCleod & Meyer, 1968; Varley, 1968). Especially important were discussions highlighting the need for social workers to examine, critique, and clarify their own personal values (see, for example, Hardman, 1975; McCleod & Meyer, 1968; Varley, 1968), based on the belief that a social worker's personal values with regard to, for example, people living in poverty, race relations, abortion, homosexuality, marriage, civil disobedience, and drug use may have a profound effect on their approach to and relationships with clients.

A particularly influential phase in the development of social work ethics began in the early 1980s, influenced significantly by the creation in the 1970s of a new field known as applied and professional ethics (Airaksinen,

1998; Callahan & Bok, 1980; Winkler, 1998). The applied and professional ethics field began primarily in medicine and health care—what is now known as bioethics. The emergence of the applied and professional ethics field was itself a product of several factors, including ethical challenges created by new health care technology (e.g., the debates about organ transplantation and termination of life support), widely publicized ethical scandals (especially the Watergate scandal), and the widespread cultural emphasis on "rights" during the 1960s (e.g., patients' rights, consumers' rights, prisoners' rights, welfare rights; Callahan & Bok, 1980; Reamer, 1995a, 1995b). Scholars and practitioners active in this new field developed a variety of conceptual and practical tools, along with pedagogical models, to help professionals who encounter ethical issues and dilemmas, especially by applying principles, concepts, and theories of moral philosophy and ethics to the ethical challenges faced by professionals.

Influenced by this trend, a small group of social work scholars began to write about ethical issues and challenges while drawing explicitly on literature, concepts, theories, and principles from the traditional field of moral philosophy and the newer field of applied and professional ethics (Loewenberg & Dolgoff, 1996; Reamer, 1982; Rhodes, 1986). An important component of these discussions was the development of decision-making strategies that social workers can use when they encounter difficult ethical judgments (as will be discussed more fully below).

The most recent phase involves the active, ambitious development of more explicit ethical standards to guide practice and strategies to prevent ethics complaints and lawsuits, focusing on issues such as client confidentiality, informed consent, dual and multiple relationships (or boundary issues), conflicts of interest, culturally competent practice, and termination of services. The most significant event during this period was the 1996 ratification of a new *Code of Ethics* (1996), which significantly expanded ethical guidelines and standards for social work practice (Reamer, 1998a).

Based on the knowledge that has evolved during these phases of the profession's history, clinical social workers (those who serve individuals, families, couples, and small groups) must be prepared to address several sets of ethical issues that arise in practice: the nature of core values in the profession and ethical dilemmas involving conflicts among them, ethical decision-making tools, and risk management strategies designed to prevent ethics complaints and lawsuits.

ETHICAL DILEMMAS IN CLINICAL PRACTICE

Ethical dilemmas in clinical practice occur when social workers encounter values or professional duties and obligations that conflict. This can occur no matter what one's clinical role or setting. Caseworkers in community mental health centers may encounter ethical questions concerning a client's right to refuse psychotropic medication. School social workers may encounter problems related to the disclosure of confidential information about students to parents, teachers, or administrators. Counselors in hospice programs may encounter clients who want to take steps to end their lives. Psychotherapists in private practice may be uncertain about what kind of post-termination social relationship they can have with clients.

Here are several concrete examples of ethical dilemmas involving clinical social workers:

1. A social worker employed by a major hospital provided counseling services to a young couple whose baby was born severely impaired. Medical staff did not expect the baby, who could not function without life support equipment, to live long. Despite the grim medical prognosis, the parents wanted the doctors and hospitals to take aggressive steps to prolong the baby's life, claiming that, "God will perform a miracle for us." The social worker, however, along with the medical staff, believed that the parents had unrealistic expectations. The social worker was unsure about the extent of her obligation to advocate on behalf of the parents in accordance with a social worker's obligation to promote a client's right to self-determination.

2. A social worker in private practice provided counseling services to a young man who was struggling with a number of self-esteem and family-of-origin issues. During the professional-client relationship, the client decided to change careers and enroll in graduate social work school. After the client graduated from social work school, which occurred eighteen months after the social worker's professional relationship with the client ended, the former client contacted the social worker and asked him to provide clinical supervision while the former client worked toward licensure. The social worker was unsure about whether it would be appropriate for him to enter into this new relationship with his new colleague and former client.

3. A social worker at a psychiatric hospital provided individual and group counseling to patients diagnosed with chronic mental illness. She had been employed at the hospital for nearly four years. The social worker learned that the hospital's custodial staff, kitchen workers, and clerical workers were about to declare a labor strike, after protracted labor-management negotiations failed to yield a satisfactory new contract. The social worker was torn between her obligation to the hospital's patients and her ideological belief that she should respect picket lines set up by striking workers.

4. A school social worker provided counseling to a fifteen-year-old student who had been referred by his teacher. The teacher reported to the social worker that the quality of the student's work had deteriorated recently and the student seemed depressed. After several counseling sessions, the

student disclosed to the social worker that he had started using cocaine and was "losing control" of his life. The social worker continued to work with the student and helped to arrange for substance abuse services. One day the teacher who referred the student to the social worker encountered the social worker in the school's hallway. The teacher asked the social worker for an update on the student's situation. The social worker was unsure about whether she could or should disclose this confidential information to the teacher.

Social work ethical dilemmas occur in direct practice (involving work with individual clients, couples, families, and small groups) and indirect practice (for example, in social work organizing, policy work, social advocacy, administration, education, and research). Common ethical dilemmas in clinical practice—the focus of this chapter—concern confidentiality and privacy; a client's right to self-determination; boundary issues; conflicts of interest; conflicts among the competing values of clients, social workers, agencies, and society; social workers' obligations to address colleagues' unethical conduct, incompetence, or impairment; and service delivery (Reamer, 1998b, 2000).

Confidentiality and Privacy

Social workers have always appreciated the central importance of confidentiality and privacy in the clinical relationship. However, social workers also understand that confidentiality has its limits and that circumstances sometimes arise requiring difficult decisions about disclosure to third parties (Dickson, 1998; Reamer, 1994). Examples include social workers' decisions about the following issues:

1. Disclosing confidential information, without the client's permission, to protect third parties who have been threatened by clients.
2. Disclosing confidential information to law enforcement or protective services officials without the client's permission.
3. Informing parents of confidential details about their children, over the objections of the minor clients.
4. Sharing confidential information among parties involved in family, couples, or group counseling.
5. Sharing confidential information about a client with the client's insurance providers.

Social workers who face these circumstances often need guidance concerning the proper handling of confidential information and the limitations of the client's right to confidentiality.

Self-Determination and Paternalism

Among the most venerated values in the profession is social workers' deep-seated respect for the client's right to self-determination. As the NASW's *Code of Ethics* (1996) states, "Social workers respect and promote the right of clients to self-determination and assist clients in their efforts to identify and clarify their goals" (standard 1.02).

However, experienced social workers know that extraordinary instances can arise that may require interfering with a client's right to self-determination (Biestek, 1957; Buchanan, 1978; Carter, 1977; McDermott, 1975; Perlman, 1965; Stalley, 1975). Examples include clients who threaten to seriously harm a third party or commit suicide. Especially since the well-known California Supreme Court decision in *Tarasoff v. Board of Regents of the University of California* (1976), for instance, there has been considerable consensus among social workers about their duty to take steps to protect from harm third parties who have been seriously threatened by their clients, even if this means interfering with the client's right to self-determination. In addition, social workers recognize their comparable duty to take steps to protect suicidal clients. As the NASW's *Code of Ethics* goes on to say in the standard concerning self-determination, "Social workers may limit clients' right to self-determination when, in the social workers' professional judgment, clients' actions or potential actions pose a serious, foreseeable, and imminent risk to themselves or others" (standard 1.02). Social workers are less clear about their duty to interfere with a client's right to self-determination when clients plan to engage in, or are engaged in, threatening or self-destructive behavior that is harmful but not life threatening or not likely to result in serious bodily injury to third parties. Examples include a client who chooses to be homeless in poor weather conditions and a client who refuses psychotropic medication that would likely improve the quality of his life. The overriding question, of course, concerns the extent to which people have a right to engage in behavior that is injurious to themselves and, conversely, the extent of social workers' obligation to act paternalistically in order to protect people from their own self-destructive tendencies.

Paternalism involves interfering with a client's wishes, intentions, or actions "for his or her own good." Paternalism can take the form of interfering with or restraining self-destructive clients for their own good, requiring them to receive services or assistance against their wishes, withholding information from them, or providing them with misinformation (a form of lying).

Social workers disagree about the condition under which various forms of paternalism are justifiable. Some believe that competent, informed, and thoughtful clients have a right to engage in self-destructive actions or behaviors, including taking serious risks, while others are more inclined to take steps against clients' wishes in order to protect them from harming themselves (Abramson, 1985; Dworkin, 1971; McDermott, 1975; Reamer, 1983).

Boundary Issues

Although the term "boundary issues" is relatively new to social work (and other helping professions), social workers have always understood the need to maintain clear boundaries in their relationships with clients. Boundary violations, which typically involve inappropriate "dual" or "multiple" relationships with clients, can cause great harm.

Dual or multiple relationships occur when social workers have a relationship with clients in more than one arena, whether sexual, social, professional, or business. Some dual and multiple relationships are not inappropriate or unethical. Examples include social workers who happen to encounter their clients at the dentist they share in common or whose children coincidentally attend the same summer camp as their clients' children. In such instances, social workers are usually able to manage encounters with clients outside of the clinical setting without a great deal of difficulty.

At the other extreme, unethical dual or multiple relationships involve some kind of exploitation, manipulation, or deception that is, or is likely to be, harmful to the client (Jayaratne, Croxton, & Mattison, 1997; Kagle & Giebelhausen, 1994). Examples include social workers who become sexually involved with their clients, borrow money from clients, invite clients to provide child care for the social workers' children, or invest in clients' business ventures. In these instances, social workers take advantage of their clients to further their own interests.

Some dual or multiple relationships raise boundary issues that are unclear, falling in an ethics "gray area." Examples include the following:

1. A clinical social worker's client was struggling with issues related to unemployment. The client had been having considerable difficulty locating an attractive job. One day the client informed the social worker that he finally "landed the job of my dreams." Unbeknownst to the client, the client's new job was in a company owned by the social worker's husband. The social worker was unsure about how to address this issue.

2. A social worker in private practice lived in a rural community. She was actively involved in a local soccer league. When the social worker went to the first league meeting of the season, she discovered that one of her clients had recently become a league official. Neither the social worker nor the client had known of the other's interest in soccer. The social worker was unsure about whether to continue participating in the league.

3. A social worker at a family service agency provided counseling to a client who had a serious substance abuse problem. The social worker and client had a very solid professional relationship. After working together for months, the client handed the social worker an invitation to attend the client's graduation from a local community college. The client told the social worker that it was very important to her to have the social worker

in the audience at the graduation, in light of the social worker's importance in the client's recovery. The social worker understood why the client wanted her to attend the graduation but was unsure about accepting the invitation to the social event, which would also be attended by a number of the client's friends and relatives.

Experienced social workers know that when boundary issues are unclear, they must be exceedingly prudent and obtain competent consultation and supervision. According to the NASW's *Code of Ethics*, "Social workers should not engage in dual or multiple relationships with clients or former clients in which there is a risk of exploitation or harm to the client. In instances when dual or multiple relationships are unavoidable, social workers should take steps to protect clients and are responsible for setting clear, appropriate, and culturally sensitive boundaries" (standard 1.06[c]).

Divided Loyalties and Conflicts of Interest

Some boundary issues involve situations where social workers feel caught between their obligation to their clients and to some other party, such as their employers, public agencies, or the courts. In these situations social workers may be unsure about to whom they owe their primary duty. Ordinarily social workers' primary commitment is to their clients, but circumstances sometimes arise that require social workers to choose between their client's and some other party's interests. As the NASW's *Code of Ethics* states, "Social workers are cognizant of their dual responsibility to clients and to the broader society. They seek to resolve conflicts between clients' interests and the broader society's interests in a socially responsible manner consistent with the values, ethical principles, and ethical standards of the profession" (p. 6).

Divided loyalties can be especially challenging in certain work settings. For example, social workers who are parole officers sometimes feel caught between their duty to respect clients' (that is, parolees') right to confidentiality and their obligation to report to parole boards or law enforcement officials confidential information about their clients' problems or misconduct. Social workers in military settings may feel caught between their clients' (that is, soldiers') rights and their duty to disclose to superior officers compelling information related to military security or safety. Social workers retained by employee assistance programs may feel caught between their clients' interest and their duty to disclose, for example, a client's serious drug-related impairment that poses a threat to other employees who are supervised by the client.

Professional and Personal Values

Some ethical dilemmas involve conflicts between social workers' personal and professional values (Reamer, 2001a). In these instances, social workers find that their own values clash with traditional social work values or the official positions of social work agencies or organizations (Levy, 1976). Examples include social workers who personally oppose abortion but work in settings that support the client's right to choose abortion, social workers who disagree with political endorsements made by social work organizations, and social workers who oppose political stands taken by social work organizations.

Social workers may also find that their personal values conflict with those of their clients (Hardman, 1975). This can occur when, for example, clients admit that they have lied to their spouses or partners, deceived their employers about their qualifications, failed to report income on their tax returns, or obtained welfare benefits fraudulently. In these situations, social workers must carefully examine the nature of their own values and the potential impact of their values on the way they serve clients and help clients struggle with moral issues in their own lives (Goldstein, 1998).

Whistle Blowing

Social workers, like all professionals, occasionally encounter wrongdoing engaged in by colleagues. This may involve colleagues engaged in unethical or illegal conduct, for example, colleagues who are sexually involved with clients, submit fraudulent clinical reports to insurance companies to enhance reimbursement, falsify credentials or qualifications, or use coercive or harmful treatment techniques.

Decisions about whether to report colleagues' misconduct—for example, to professional associations or licensing bodies—can be very difficult. Professional colleagues often feel loyal to one another and are reluctant to "blow the whistle" in a way that might end a colleague's career. Such situations can quickly become stressful for the whistle-blowers and jeopardize their own careers. At the same time, social workers typically feel a strong sense of duty and obligation to the profession and general public. It is difficult for social workers to ignore a colleague's misconduct that is causing harm to clients and other parties (Barry, 1986; Bullis, 1995; McCann & Cutler, 1979; Reamer & Siegel, 1992; Westin, 1981). Thus, the major challenge is for social workers to weigh their obligation to clients, the profession, and the general public against their duty to colleagues who are or may be involved in some kind of wrongdoing.

Managed Care

Managed care policies and procedures, designed to promote fiscal responsibility and constrain health care costs, have created a number of ethical issues for clinical social workers. Administrative policies such as capitation, case rates, utilization review, diagnosis-related groups, and prospective reimbursement have forced social workers to make difficult ethical, as well as clinical, decisions about the kind of clientele they will serve, the services they will provide, and the circumstances under which they will terminate services. Social workers operating in managed care environments sometimes encounter ethical choices about serving clients whose insurance benefits have been exhausted; providing inadequate or insufficient services to clients whose problems require more intervention than managed care authorities are willing to authorize; limiting their services only to clients who can pay for services out of pocket; exposing clients to privacy and confidentiality risks as a result of sharing information with managed care officials; and exaggerating clients' clinical symptoms, diagnoses, and prognoses to increase the likelihood that managed care officials will authorize services (American Medical Association, 1995; Corcoran & Winslade, 1994; Corcoran & Vandiver, 1996; Reamer, 1997b, 1998d; Ross & Croze, 1997; Schreter, Sharfstein, & Schreter, 1994; Schamess & Lightburn, 1998; Strom-Gottfried & Corcoran, 1998).

In addition there are ethical decisions about allocating agency and program resources. These include decisions about which programs will be eliminated or cut back when funds are not available for all of them and the criteria that will be used to allocate resources among programs and clients (Caughey & Sabin, 1995; Schamess & Lightburn, 1998; Reamer, 1998d).

ETHICAL DECISION MAKING

The applied and professional ethics field has produced a number of decision-making frameworks or protocols to guide practitioners who must make ethical decisions in the midst of an ethical dilemma. These frameworks, which often take the form of an outline of decision-making steps, encourage social workers to draw on a number of resources and tools when they encounter ethical dilemmas (Joseph, 1985; Loewenberg & Dolgoff, 1996; Reamer, 1995a). Typically these discussions identify a series of steps social workers can follow and issues that they can consider as they attempt to resolve difficult ethical dilemmas. What follows is one example (Reamer, 1999):

1. Identify the ethical issues, including the social work values and duties that conflict.
2. Identify the individuals, groups, and organizations that are likely to be affected by the ethical decision.
3. Tentatively identify all possible courses of action and the participants involved in each, along with the possible benefits and risks for each.
4. Thoroughly examine the reason in favor of and opposed to each possible course of action, considering relevant
    a. Ethical theories, principles, and guidelines
    b. Codes of ethics
    c. Legal principles

   d. Social work practice theory and principles
   e. Personal values (including religious, political, cultural, and ethnic values), particularly those that conflict with one's own.

5. Consult with colleagues and appropriate experts (such as agency staff, supervisors, agency administrators, attorneys, and ethics scholars).

6. Make the decision and document the decision-making process.

7. Monitor, evaluate, and document the decision.

As this outline indicates, one of the key features of this decision-making framework is the application of standard or classic ethical theory and moral philosophy (item 4a). Beginning at least with Socrates, Plato, and Aristotle, moral philosophers have developed various ethical theories, principles, and guidelines concerning matters of right and wrong, moral duty and obligation, social justice, and other key ethical concepts (Frankena, 1973; Hancock, 1974). Briefly, relevant ethical theories focus on what is known as *meta-ethics* (abstract discussions of the formulation, derivation, justification, and validity of moral theories) and *normative ethics* (the application of existing ethical theories, principles, and guidelines to actual ethical dilemmas). As one would expect, social workers tend to find normative ethics more relevant than meta-ethics.

   Theories of normative ethics are typically divided into two main schools of thought: *deontological* and *teleological* (Frankena, 1973; Reamer, 1990). Deontological theories (from the Greek *deontos*, "of the obligatory") assert that certain actions are inherently right or wrong, or right or wrong as a matter of fundamental principle. This perspective is most commonly associated with the eighteenth-century German philosopher Immanuel Kant. From a strictly deontological perspective, for example, social workers should never violate a law, regulation, or agency policy, no matter what the circumstances might be; should always tell the truth, even if telling the truth might be harmful; and should always honor their promises, even if doing so might have detrimental consequences. According to deontology, then, it would be unethical for a social worker to violate a mandatory reporting law concerning elder abuse even if the social worker believes that doing so would be in her client's best interest (for example, to preserve the therapeutic relationship). Similarly, from this point of view it would be unethical to exaggerate a client's clinical diagnosis in order to help the client qualify for insurance benefits, even if doing so would enable the client to obtain much needed services.

   In contrast, according to teleological (from the Greek *teleios*, "brought to its end or purpose") or consequentialist theories, ethical decisions should be based on social workers' assessment of which action will produce the most favorable outcome or consequences—an ethical cost-benefit analysis. According to the most prominent teleological school of thought, utilitarianism, ethical choices should be based on estimates of what will result in the greatest good for the greatest number of people ("positive" utilitarianism) or what will minimize harm ("negative" utilitarianism). From a utilitarian perspective, for example, it may be justifiable to force reluctant clients to take psychotropic medication against their wishes, "for their own good," even if doing so would violate the clients' fundamental legal and moral rights. Similarly, from this point of view, it may be legitimate to deceive insurance companies with exaggerated diagnoses if doing so would help vulnerable clients obtain the services they need.

There is much spirited debate about the strengths and limitations of various theories of normative ethics (Gorovitz, 1971; Smart & Williams, 1973). However, examining ethical dilemmas from these competing perspectives can help social workers understand, investigate, and thoroughly address the ethical dilemmas they face. In the end, this disciplined and systematic analysis may enhance the quality of the ethical decisions practitioners make. This process is similar to social workers considering different clinical theories and schools of thought (e.g., psychodynamic, behavioral, cognitive, solution-focused, task-centered) that recognize that there may be constructive disagreement about which perspective is the most compelling and valid in any given situation. Critically examining clients' needs using different theoretical frameworks and points of view may strengthen the effects of intervention.

Contemporary social workers can also draw on the substantial literature on social work ethics and, more broadly, applied and professional ethics. Most of this literature—which focuses on ethical issues in the profession, ethical decision making, ethical standards, and ethical misconduct—is of fairly recent origin (the majority of these works having been published since the early 1980s); many practicing social workers concluded their formal professional education before this literature was published.

In addition, social workers who encounter ethical dilemmas may find it useful to contact professional ethics consultants, agency-based ethics committees, and institutional review boards. Ethics consultation is commonly found in health care settings and is expanding to other settings, such as community mental health centers and family service agencies. In these settings, formally educated ethicists (usually moral philosophers who have experience working with professionals or professionals who have obtained a formal ethics education) give advice on ethics-related issues. These consultants can help social workers identify key ethical issues, analyze ethical dilemmas, and make difficult ethical decisions. They can acquaint social workers with relevant ethics concepts, literature, and other practical resources (Conrad, 1989; Fletcher, 1986; Fletcher, Quist, & Jonsen, 1989; La Puma & Schiedermayer, 1991; Reamer, 1995c; Skeel & Self, 1989). Social workers may also draw on the ethics expertise of NASW committees on inquiry (the panels that review and adjudicate ethics complaints) and state licensing boards. Some NASW chapters also provide consultation through an "ethics hot line."

Ethics committees, which exist in many health care and human service settings, often include social workers as members. The concept of ethics committees (often called "institutional ethics committees" or IECs) emerged in 1976, when the New Jersey Supreme Court ruled that Karen Ann Quinlan's family and physician should consult an ethics committee in deciding whether to remove her from life-support technology (although a number of hospitals have had something like an ethics committee since at least the 1920s). Ethics committees usually include representatives from various disciplines found in health care and human service settings, such as physicians, nurses, allied health professionals, mental health professionals, agency administrators, and clergy.

Most ethics committees spend much of their time providing case consultation and nonbinding advice. Committees are available to agency staff, clients, and perhaps family members for consultation about challenging ethical dilemmas. Relevant issues may include a client's right to refuse treatment, termination of services, the use of aggressive treatment, informed consent procedures, or release of confidential information (Cohen, 1988; Cranford & Doudera, 1984; Reamer, 1987b; Summers, 1989; Teel, 1975).

Many ethics committees also sponsor in-service or continuing education on ethical issues (for example, training on confidentiality, boundary issues, ethical decision making, and ethics risk management) and critique, revise, or draft ethics-related agency policy. Education may take the form of informal workshops, formal conferences, or what have become known as "ethics grand rounds."

Clinical social workers employed in settings that sponsor research (typically, health care organizations and educational institutions) may be involved in institutional review boards (IRBs). IRBs (sometimes known as human subjects protection committees) became popular in the 1970s as a result of increasing national interest in ethical issues in research and evaluation (Levine, 1991). As a result of strict federal regulations, all organizations and agencies that receive federal funds for research are required to have an IRB review the ethical aspects of proposals for research involving human subjects.

One of the most important resources for social workers who encounter ethical issues is the 1996 *Code of Ethics*. This is only the third code in NASW's history and reflects significant changes over time in social approaches to ethical issues.

The first code, which went into effect in 1960, included fourteen proclamations concerning social workers' ethical obligations (for example, every social worker's duty to give precedence to professional responsibility over personal interest; respect clients' privacy; give appropriate professional service in public emergencies; and contribute knowledge, skills, and support to human welfare programs). The second code, which went into effect in 1979, was far more ambitious. It included six sections of briefly stated principles (nearly eighty) related to social workers' conduct and comportment and their ethical responsibilities to clients, colleagues, employers and employing organizations, the social work profession, and society. Over time, however, particularly in light of the dramatic changes taking place in the applied and professional ethics field following the ratification of the 1979 code, NASW leaders recognized that a new code was needed.

The NASW *Code of Ethics* Revision Committee was appointed in 1994 and spent two years drafting a new code. This committee, which was chaired by the author and included a professional ethicist and social workers from a variety of practice and educational settings, drafted a code that includes four sections and is far more detailed and comprehensive than the two prior codes (Reamer, 1998a). The first section, entitled "Preamble," summarizes social work's mission and core values. For the first time in NASW's history, the association has adopted and published in the code a formally sanctioned mission statement and an explicit summary of the profession's core values. This mission statement and core values focus on social work's enduring commitment to enhancing human well-being and helping meet basic human needs; empowering clients; serving people who are vulnerable and oppressed; addressing individual well-being in a social context; promoting social justice and social change; and strengthening sensitivity to cultural and ethnic diversity.

This mission statement is critically important for clinical social workers. It implies that clinical social workers are obligated to be concerned about people who live in poverty and who are otherwise oppressed. Although the mission statement does not suggest that social workers should be exclusively concerned about low-income and oppressed people, it does suggest that these populations should be a priority to the greatest extent possible (while at the same time recognizing that affluent and other more privileged clients also have a very legitimate claim on social workers' expertise and resources). The mission statement also states that all social workers should be involved in social change and advocacy, addressing public policy issues that affect individual clients. Thus, where appropriate, clinical social workers should devote a reasonable amount of effort to such activities as legislative lobbying, letter-writing campaigns, and social protest to address important public policy and social justice issues (Richan, 1996).

The second section of the code provides an overview of its main functions, including an identification of the profession's core values; summarizing broad ethical principles that reflect social work's core values and specific ethical standards for the profession; helping social workers identify ethical issues and dilemmas; providing the public with ethical standards it can use to hold the profession accountable; socializing practitioners new to the field; and articulating standards that the profession itself can use to enforce ethical standards among its members. This section also highlights resources social workers can use when they face ethical issues and decisions.

The third section, "Ethical Principles," presents six broad principles that inform social work practice, one for each of the six core values cited in the code's preamble (service, social justice, dignity and worth of the person, importance of human relationships, integrity, and competence). A brief annotation for each principle is included.

The final and most detailed section, "Ethical Standards," includes 155 specific ethical standards to guide social workers' conduct and provide a basis for adjudication of ethics complaints filed against social workers. The standards are placed into six categories concerning social workers' ethical responsibilities to clients, to colleagues, in practice settings, as professionals, to the profession, and to the broader society. The 1996 code addresses a large number of issues that were not mentioned in the 1960 and 1979 codes, including limitations on a client's right to self-determination (an example would be if a client threatens harm to him- or herself or others), confidentiality issues involving electronic media (such as computers, facsimile machines, and cellular telephones), storage and disposal of client records, case recording and documentation, sexual contact with former clients, sexual relationships with clients' relatives and close personal acquaintances, counseling of former sexual partners, physical contact with clients, dual and multiple relationships with supervisees, sexual harassment, use of derogatory language, bartering arrangements with clients, cultural competence, labor-management disputes, and evaluation of practice. Many of the standards concern clinical issues, however, a number also focus on the obligation of all social workers to engage in activities designed to promote social change and challenge social injustice.

In general, the code's standards concern three kinds of issues (Reamer, 1994). The first includes mistakes social workers might make that have ethical implications, such as disclosing confidential information in public settings (e.g., restaurants or elevators) or inadvertently omitting important information on an informed consent or release of information form. The second category focuses on circumstances involving difficult ethical decisions, for example, related to ambiguous professional-client boundaries, release of information without client consent to protect third parties, labor-management disputes, social worker impairment, protection of research participants, termination of services, or allocating scarce resources. The final category concerns issues pertaining to social worker misconduct and unethical behavior, such as sexual indiscretions, financial exploitation of clients, or fraudulent or deceptive business practices.

MANAGING ETHICAL RISKS

Social workers have become more interested in ethical issues in part because ethics complaints and lawsuits filed against them for alleged ethical negligence or misconduct have increased (Berliner, 1989; Bernstein, 1981; Houston-Vega, Nuehring, & Daguio, 1997; Kurzman, 1995; Reamer, 1994, 1998a). NASW members may have ethics complaints filed against them for alleged violations of the association's code of ethics. Licensed social workers may have complaints filed against them for alleged ethical infractions. In addition, social workers may have malpractice and negligence lawsuits filed against them.

Complaints filed against social workers—whether in the form of ethics complaints or lawsuits—typically allege some significant departure from the profession's *standards of care*. This key legal concept refers to the way an ordinary, reasonable, and prudent professional with similar training would act under the same or similar circumstances (Austin, Moline, & Williams, 1990; Cohen & Mariano, 1982; Gifis, 1991; Hogan, 1979; Madden, 1998; Meyer, Landis, & Hays, 1988; Reamer, 1994; Schultz, 1982). Departures from social work's standards of care may result from a practitioner's active violation of a client's rights (in legal terms, acts of commission, i.e., misfeasance or malfeasance) or a practitioner's failure to perform certain duties (acts of omission or nonfeasance).

Some ethics complaints and lawsuits result from the social worker's mistakes and oversights. Some examples include social workers who disclose confidential information inadvertently during a hallway conversation that is overheard by a third party or who fax confidential material to the wrong location. Others stem from difficult, deliberate ethical decisions, for example, when social workers disclose confidential information without a client's consent in order to protect a third party from serious harm or when social workers terminate services to uncooperative or noncompliant clients. In addition, some complaints result from social workers' alleged misconduct or unethical behavior, such as sexual contact with clients or fraudulent or otherwise illegal activity.

When legal complaints are brought against social workers, plaintiffs (the parties bringing the lawsuit) must produce the following evidence:

1. At the time of the alleged negligence, the social worker owed a duty of care to the client (that is, the social worker was providing professional services to the client).
2. The practitioner breached the duty or was derelict in the duty (that is, the social worker failed to perform the duty based on prevailing standards of care).
3. The client suffered some harm or injury (examples include emotional anguish or injury to reputation).
4. The harm or injury was directly and proximately caused by the professional's breach or dereliction of duty (often known as "proximate cause" or "cause in fact").

For example, if a complainant alleges that a social worker was negligent (and unethical) because he disclosed confidential information inappropriately without the client's consent, the complainant would need to show that 1) the social worker owed a broad duty of care to the client by virtue of providing her with professional services; 2) the social worker breached that duty by disclosing confidential information without the client's consent, contrary to prevailing law, regulations, or standards in the profession; 3) the client was injured (for example, the information was used to terminate the client's parental rights or to terminate the client from a treatment program); and 4) the injury was the direct and proximate result of the unauthorized disclosure (as opposed to earlier trauma, for instance).

In some cases, prevailing standards of care are relatively easy to establish through citations of the profession's literature, relevant codes of ethics, or expert testimony. Examples include standards concerning sexual relationships with current clients, fraudulent billing, and a client's right to refuse certain kinds of treatment. However, in other cases there is disagreement or confusion about standards of care. Examples include the appropriateness of social (nonsexual) relationships with clients following termination of the professional-client relationship, the limits on a client's right to engage in self-destructive behavior, termination of services to clients who are unable to pay outstanding fees, and disclosure of confidential information without a client's consent to protect third parties who have not even been verbally threatened by the client.

A significant portion of ethics complaints and lawsuits involve social workers who are impaired in some manner (Reamer, 1992a). Impairment occurs when social workers' personal problems, psychosocial distress, substance abuse, or mental health difficulties interfere with their practice effectiveness (Bissell, Fewell, & Jones, 1980; Lamb, Presser, Pfost, Baum, Jackson, & Jarvis, 1987). For example, many cases in which there is evidence of boundary violations involve social workers who are leading troubled lives, manifested in the form of substance abuse, fragile marriages, employment problems, or financial difficulties. In one published prevalence study that included social workers, Deutsch (1985) found that more than half of her sample of social workers, psychologists, and master's-level counselors reported significant problems with depression. Nearly four-fifths (82 percent) reported problems with relationships, approximately one-tenth (11 percent) reported substance abuse problems, and 2 percent reported suicide attempts. Bissell and Haberman (1984) found that 24 percent of a sample of 50 alcoholic social workers that they surveyed reported overt suicide attempts, a rate higher than that reported by the dentists, attorneys, and physicians in their sample.

Several key studies highlight the disturbing problem of sexual exploitation of clients by clinicians. Pope (1988) reviewed a series of empirical studies and concluded that about 8 percent of male therapists and about 2 percent of female therapists acknowledged having had social contact with clients. Pope reported that one study (Gechtman & Bouhoutsos, 1985) found that 3.8 percent of male social workers admitted to sexual contact with clients.

Social work's first national acknowledgment of the problem of impaired practitioners came in 1979, when the NASW released a public policy statement on alcoholism and alcohol-related problems (NASW, 1987). By 1980, a small nationwide support group for chemically dependent practitioners, Social Workers Helping Social Workers, had formed, although this group struggled to generate significant membership (NASW, 1987). In 1982, NASW established the Occupational Social Work Task Force, which was charged with developing a strategy to address the problem of impairment, and in 1984 the NASW Delegate Assembly issued a resolution on impairment. The most recent significant profession-wide effort was in 1987, when NASW published the Impaired Social Worker Program Resource Book, prepared by the NASW Commission on Employment and Economic Support, to help practitioners design programs for impaired social workers.

With the exception of these efforts, and attempts by several NASW chapters to address this issue, social workers have paid relatively little attention to the phenomenon of practitioner impairment. Social work's literature includes very few publications on impairment, and the subject receives inconsistent attention in social work education. Social workers know relatively little about the prevalence of impaired practitioners or effective strategies for dealing with the problem.

CONCLUDING OBSERVATIONS

The social work profession has made major strides in its understanding of ethical issues. What began as a preoccupation with the morality of the profession's earliest clients (i.e., the poor) has evolved into a mature grasp of complex ethical dilemmas and relevant decision-making tools. Social workers' current use of ethical theory, codes of ethics, ethics consultation, agency-based ethics committees, institutional review boards, and applied and professional ethics literature is impressive, especially when contrasted with the profession's approach to ethics earlier in its development.

To build on these encouraging developments, we must take assertive steps to ensure that both new and experienced clinical social workers receive in-depth ethics-related education and training (Black, Hartley, Whelley, & Kirk-Sharp, 1989; Reamer & Abramson, 1982; Reamer, 2001b). Social work education programs and social work practice settings (such as community mental health centers, residential treatment programs, family service agencies, health care facilities, correctional programs, schools, substance abuse treatment programs, employee assistance programs, programs for senior citizens, and child welfare programs) must offer formal education and in-service training on the subject. In addition, professional associations and groups (such as the NASW and its state chapters, the Council on Social Work Education, the American Association of State Social Work Boards, and special interest groups related to group treatment, child welfare, mental health, substance abuse, oncology, disabilities, eating disorders, and so on) should sponsor continuing education workshops, seminars, and conferences devoted to social work ethics.

Professional and continuing education on ethics should address a wide range of topics. Potential issues include overviews of ethical issues and dilemmas in the profession generally or specialty areas within it, ethical decision-making frameworks, the relevance of ethical and moral theory to practice, the NASW's *Code of Ethics* (and other relevant codes), institutional ethics committees, institutional review boards, and ethics risk management (relevant malpractice and liability issues, common problems leading to ethics complaints, and so on). Specific risk management topics include (Barker & Branson, 1993; Besharov, 1985; Besharov & Besharov, 1987; Dickson, 1998; Houston-Vega et al., 1997; Madden, 1998; Reamer, 1994, 1998a):

1. Confidentiality and privacy—ethical risks related to the handling of confidential information pertaining to protection of third parties; mandatory reporting statutes concerning abuse and neglect of children, the elderly, and people with disabilities; alcohol and substance abuse treatment; sharing information with outside agencies and professionals, such as social service organizations and colleagues, news media, law enforcement officials, and collection agencies; sharing information with organizations; families, couples, and groups counseling; peer consultation or supervision; deceased clients; and minors. This training should also address inadvertent disclosures, for example, verbal disclosures in agency waiting rooms and hallways, elevators, restaurants, on cellular telephones, or answering machines and visual disclosures resulting from a failure to protect information on a social worker's desk or computer screen or faxed communications.

2. High-risk interventions—using interventions that are ethically questionable (for example, massage therapy or "body work" during a psychotherapy session or past-life regression techniques) or using interventions without adequate training or education.

3. Informed consent—the nature of standard informed consent procedures (for example, explaining the content of informed consent forms to clients and providing them with an opportunity to ask questions about the form as well as avoiding problems related to omitting an expiration date, having clients sign a consent form before the blank spaces are filled in or failing to obtain the services of an interpreter when a client does not speak or understand the primary language used in the social service setting).

4. Defamation of character—problems related to libeling or slandering clients based on untrue written or verbal statements made by a social worker that are injurious to clients.

5. Boundary violations—standards concerning boundaries related to, for example, sexual or social contact, gifts, sharing of meals, business dealings, religious activities, or barter.

6. Supervision—guidelines concerning proper supervision (based on the legal theory of *respondeat superior* or vicarious liability, according to which a

supervisor can, in principle, be found liable for the acts or omissions of supervisees, particularly if there is evidence of flawed supervision).

7. Documentation and recording—the need for careful case records to enhance client assessment, case coordination, treatment planning, service delivery, supervision, and accountability (for example, to insurers, utilization review staff, courts, and so on).

8. Consultation—the importance of consulting with qualified colleagues when necessary to meet a client's needs.

9. Referral—the importance of referring clients to qualified colleagues when necessary to meet a client's needs (for example, when clients are not making sufficient progress in treatment or a colleague's specialized expertise is needed to address a client's problem).

10. Fraud—the importance of accurate billing and documentation.

11. Termination of services—guidelines to ensure ethical termination of services when clients are uncooperative, are not making reasonable progress, or are unable to pay for services (especially when insurance benefits have run out and managed care officials are unwilling to authorize additional services).

In addition, clinical social workers should identify opportunities in their work settings to address ethical issues. Examples include appointing a task force or ethics committee that would be asked to identify ethical issues in the setting that require attention (for example, updating the agency's confidentiality or informed consent policies and procedure, writing new policies concerning boundary issues and dual/multiple relationships with clients, examining ethical aspects of procedures used to conduct agency-based research and evaluation, developing procedures for addressing worker impairment) or developing protocols for case consultation when ethical dilemmas arise.

Social workers also need to anticipate new and emerging ethical issues. It is hard to imagine what new ethical challenges may arise in the future; just imagine how hard it would have been for social workers in the late 1970s to forecast the ethical issues we now encounter related to HIV/AIDS and privacy issues involving Internet communications. In that era, no one had yet heard of HIV/AIDS or the Internet. Even a few years ago we would have been hard pressed to imagine some of the ethical issues clinical social workers now face with respect to managed care.

Finally, and most importantly, social workers must pay attention to their overall occupational mission, especially with respect to the clientele they serve. Especially in recent years, social workers have debated the extent to which practitioners have a moral obligation to serve low-income, disadvantaged, and economically vulnerable clients (Austin, 1997; Billups, 1992; Gil, 1998; Reamer, 1992a, 1997c; Specht & Courtney, 1994). Constraints imposed by managed care and other funding shortages have led some social workers to focus their practice on relatively affluent clients who can afford to pay fees out of pocket, thus bypassing insurers' and third-party payers' restrictions. If practiced widely, this response would lead to the virtual abandonment of social work's historic mission and what may be its most defining feature. Certainly social workers must be committed to serving all people, including those who are relatively affluent and privileged; however, social workers must simultaneously embrace their long-standing, unique commitment to the most vulnerable members of our society—a commitment that distinguishes social work from other clinically oriented mental health professions. Social workers must continually heed the forceful and compelling language added to the NASW *Code of Ethics* in 1996: "The primary mission of the social work profession is to enhance human well-being and help meet the basic human needs of all people, *with particular attention to the needs and empowerment of people who are vulnerable, oppressed, and living in poverty*" (p. 1, emphasis added). This also entails clinical social workers' abiding responsibility to be alert to and address issues of social injustice. In the end, it is this enduring concern that sets clinical social work apart from the other clinically oriented professions.

PART TWO

Applying the
Foundation of Change

CHAPTER 7

Shared Power in Social Work: A Native American Perspective of Change

Christine T. Lowery

Mark A. Mattaini

In this chapter, Lowery and Mattaini expand the discussion of social work practice perspectives and provide a Native American, sociocultural perspective in order to establish helping relationships. The concept of power is highlighted as a factor to consider in shaping relationships between client and practitioner as contributing partners in the assessment, planning, and delivery of treatment. Lowery and Mattaini convey the importance of different definitions of social work practice based on a Native American perspective on the role of power in the helping relationship. The authors explore the nature and extent of the role of adversarial power and review various types of adversarial power and social work practice. They describe the limitations of adversarial power styles of social work practice. The reader is given an analysis of the various models of shared power available for consideration to social workers as they develop a basis for planning change. The chapter includes useful examples of shared power-based practice methods across a number of fields of practice such as substance abuse, children and family practice, and so on. The chapter provides the practice principles needed by the emerging practitioner seeking ways to adopt nontraditional approaches to practice. The chapter concludes with a discussion of the Native American influence in the context of shared power and community social work practice.

This chapter emerged from a dialogue between a Pueblo woman and a white man regarding different perceptions of power, our different experiences with power, and the potential use of power in social work. As in any dialogue, our stances sometimes converge, sometimes overlap, and sometimes diverge. Our desire to ask thoughtful questions and listen to the answers is our common link; our commitment to social work is our strength. As the dialogue evolved, we discovered substantial coherence and resonance between traditional Native American thought and contemporary behavioral science, which suggested to us that they shared an important core.

While the meaning of empowerment is rooted linguistically and practically in the exercise of power, among both social workers and clients the concept of power is often troubling (Gitterman, 1989). The reasons for the struggle are deeply rooted in a western European view of power as limited and adversarial, a view that to some extent is maintained even among empowerment and feminist thinkers in social work. By contrast, a Native American understanding of shared power, potentially unlimited within the corporeal-spiritual boundaries of respect, offers a qualitatively different perspective for understanding and practicing social work. In a review of indigenous justice systems from the Ojibway in Ontario to the Salish in Washington State, Ross (1996), a Canadian attorney, repeatedly found that the emphasis was on teaching individuals from birth how to live together in ways that maintained the "integrity of spiritual principles and value" (p. 255), a proactive rather than reactive sense of justice. This view is strong in Pueblo thought (the first author's people), for Pueblo people have found ways to live together cooperatively, spiritually bounded in place and under circumstances of limited resources, for over 10,000 years.

THE WEB

One of the authors (CTL) once did an exercise with a group of young Indian women who played on a basketball team in an all-Indian school. This exercise, familiar to many social group workers, consists of tossing a ball of string back and forth, to and from every member of the group, and literally constructing a web. Each group member can see how she is connected to all other members of her team; when one group member moved, who else in the group might feel the tug, the change in the tension of the web?

Generally speaking, Native American philosophy acknowledges those visible and invisible connections that we share as human beings with each other and with all other life forces in our world. How we think about and behave toward one another as human beings frames our ability to contribute to that web, to that interconnectedness, in a positive or negative way. At Native American cultural gatherings where opening prayers are spoken, one may hear this phrase spoken in English, "We pray we will do things in a good way, with a good spirit, so that everyone may benefit." The words prepare the heart for appreciation "in a good way." And whether we call this social, moral, or natural ecology (Bellah, Madsen, Sullivan, Swidler, & Tipton, 1985), on a human level it is the same: it is the values, respect, gratitude, contribution, and adherence to spiritual laws that teach us how to treat one another.

How we are all connected or interrelated is not only an environmental condition. From a Native American perspective, it is a condition of the spirit, and knowledge of these connections contributes to our power and maintains a healthy spirit. As Vine Deloria (1995) notes, "The major difference between American Indian views and the physical world and Western science lies in the premise accepted by Indians and rejected by scientists: the world in which we live is alive" (p. 55). However, modern science is moving closer to Native American thought. Deloria continues, "Indians came to understand that all things were related . . . gradually, scientists have moved from philosophical physics to apply the concept of relatedness to biological phenomena and environments. Now many scientists believe that all things are related, and many articles, primarily coming from people in physics, now state flatly that all things really are related" (p. 57). A particularly strong example is the work of Fritjof Capra (1996), a theoretical physicist who has recently turned to ecology. Capra indicates that in contemporary scientific thought, "The material universe is seen as a dynamic web of interrelated events" (p. 39) and "all members of an ecological community are interconnected in a vast and intricate network of relationships, the web of life" (p. 298). When Indians speak in the traditional way of "all my relations" they refer to everyone and everything (Ulali, 1994; Silko, 1996); "man and woman, plant and animal, water and stone, all share the earth as equal partners—even as family" (*The Way of the Spirit*, 1997).

Empowerment is rooted in and results from the sharing of power within this matrix of "interrelatedness." Empowerment and shared power are realized in our power and in the power of others combined. An empowered person learns, recognizes, and uses the repertoires needed to participate authentically in sharing power. An empowered person can transfer this learning to other situations and model behaviors that can teach others. Inherent in empowerment and shared power is the understanding that, "Not only do I have power, but I can see you in your power and you can see me in mine." This understanding alone breeds a deep respect for one another. There is no hierarchy here. The responsibility for this work lies between people, and everyone will bear his or her own responsibility.

THINKING ABOUT POWER

Social work practice, if it is to be done in "a good way," requires a clear view of the nature of power. From a Pueblo perspective, power is a gift. There are many kinds of power: the power to sing, the power to teach, the power to heal, the power to pray, the power to bring people together in a good way. In social work there are many examples: the power to see through to people's hearts, the power to create and expand resources, the power to supervise in a way that encourages growth, the power to advocate for clients, the power to mobilize others for positive change. Because there are many kinds of power, power is not limited—in fact, its exercise in a good way leads to an overall increase in collective power.

Resources may be limited, but power is not materialistic. Power is not something one can "have" in a static sense, rather power is the expression of what one is, through what one does. At root, power is action, it is process, it is a verb. Recognizing one's own power as a gift is humbling and moves one away from one's ego and toward quiet contribution and appreciation of the power of others.

Our power, if we develop it, is limited only by our efforts to strengthen and share our gifts. Even when two of us demonstrate similar kinds of power, we each have our unique ways of contributing it. These contributions serve to strengthen you in your power and me in mine. This eliminates the need to compete with one another, to exploit one another, or to coerce one another, all of which are facets of adversarial as opposed to shared power. In traditional Tewa Pueblo society, there was diversity that included many roles, many powers, and many ways to contribute to the overall unity of society, a society in transactional continuity with the rest of the physical and spiritual world (Ortiz, 1969).

Contrast the sharing of power with a more traditional social work view like Hasenfeld's power-dependence perspective (1987), which seeks to achieve a "power balance between workers and clients" (p. 476). From that perspective, "A has power over B when A has the potential to obtain favorable outcomes at B's expense. Moreover, the power of A over B indicates the *dependence* of B on A" (p. 473, emphasis added). Within this view, rooted in traditional sociological thought, power is seen, by definition, as coercive and potentially exploitative. An increase in power for one person or group requires a corresponding decrease in power for another. If one gains, another must lose—a kind of mechanistic, hydraulic, zero-sum model.

Similarly, some modern feminist and empowerment thinkers in social work who speak of "shared power" mean something different than we do here. For example, Cohen (1998) discussed power imbalances between clients and social workers, concluding, "To reduce these power disparities, we will have to confront—and be prepared to give up—our power in relationship to our clients while simultaneously seeking to increase our power, through collective organizing and action, in relationship to our agency bureaucracies" (p. 441). Power, in other words, is limited and adversarial; for the client to gain power, the worker must "give up" power. Other feminist writers, however, redefine power as unlimited and facilitative, a view closer to that discussed here (e.g., Van Den Bergh & Cooper, 1995).

In Pueblo thought, there is no need for anyone to give up power, because it is not limited. The power of others can be frightening if we cannot see or understand our own power. The power of others can be threatening if one thinks he or she has none. However, if one understands one's own power as a gift that is actualized and strengthened, if used on behalf of us all, the very nature of the social work relationship and of practice changes. Authentic empowerment requires entirely new strategies that do not redistribute power or realign positions of power, but rather distribute opportunities to contribute and share responsibility. A commitment to practice that relies on shared power while refusing to participate in adversarial processes is far more radical than approaches grounded in disruption or conflict strategies. Those approaches (often labeled "radical") in fact support the use of the strategies that characterize the dominant—even the word tells the story—culture, which supports and reinforces oppression. The oppressed do not gain real power by competing with other groups and overcoming them or by achieving a balance of adversarial power. The question that social work must help both the oppressed and the oppressor to ask themselves is, "What responsibilities do we carry? How can we, collectively, make the best use of the power you bring to the table and the power we bring to the table? What are the opportunities we have to contribute?"

Is this realistic? Interestingly, thousands of years of experience (Silko, 1996) and contemporary behavioral science converge here (Mattaini & Lowery, 2000). Both indicate that constructional, shared power is resilient and potentially creative, while coercive, adversarial power by its very nature cannot be constructive. This understanding is not common in social work, and as a result, although many social workers are comfortable using the term "empowerment," they often struggle with the power that underlies it.

ADVERSARIAL POWER

Contemporary US culture and institutions rely heavily on egocentric, coercive, and competitive practices in many areas, and power is commonly understood in those terms. These practices constitute a major portion of the sociocultural matrix that shapes individuals, and to a large extent, society. Not only does dominant society rely on adversarial power to maintain social order, social welfare institutions and social work practice are often deeply rooted in this stance as well. In recent years, behavioral science has clearly elaborated the cost of coercion, competition, and exploitation, the processes underlying adversarial power (Sidman, 1989, 1993), but those analyses have only minimally affected the operation of social institutions. Social workers, however individually honorable, can be absorbed, often without being aware of it, into adversarial systems and cultures that fail to support shared power. Those systems damage rather than strengthen the web, and the individuals involved are also damaged in the process and, in turn, cause harm to others, particularly clients. Even recognizing the possibility of nonadversarial alternatives, however, is often difficult for people who have been raised in US society (Sidman, 1989).

Competition

Competition involves action to obtain good outcomes for oneself while constraining others from doing so. While such competitive practices produce demonstrably poorer aggregate outcomes for any complex system (Axelrod, 1984; Nowak, May, & Sigmund, 1995), they are deeply rooted in US society. Competition in business, sports, and personal relationships is commonly viewed as natural and productive. It is common to hear the argument that competition "brings out the best" in a person, but there is strong experimental evidence that games and sports that involve high levels of personal competition produce higher levels of aggression and interfere with performance in other areas of life (Bay-Hinitz, Peterson, & Quilitch, 1994; Sharp, Brown, & Crider, 1995; Biglan, 1995, 1996). Cooperative activities produce the opposite effects, and the results persist over time (Bay-Hinitz et al., 1994; Sharp et al., 1995). Cooperation need not preclude recognition and encouragement for doing one's best—"competing with oneself"—but that is a different phenomenon.

Is such competition as common in social work as in other institutions in the United States? Colleagues, students, and our own observations suggest that competition among workers for position and prestige, among students for grades or recognition, and among biological and foster parents for affection from the child and approval from the agency are deeply embedded in the system, although they can only damage the web, ultimately leading to poorer client (and social worker) outcomes. Unfortunately, this competitive dynamic can be nearly invisible from the perspective of the dominant culture, and it is difficult to acknowledge that we ourselves may participate in such patterns, although we may readily recognize the associated arrogance in others. Authentic acknowledgment of what we are and do—including those thoughts, actions, and feelings that may be potentially damaging—is essential to sharing power, as is a willingness to learn and be taught.

Coercion

Coercion is "our use of punishment and the threat of punishment to get others to act as we would like, and . . . our practice of rewarding people just by letting them escape from our punishments and threats" (Sidman, 1989, p. 1). Punishment produces problematic side effects, including depression, hopelessness, stress, illness, escape, and aggression (toward the punisher or often toward other, more accessible, targets; Sidman, 1989). Unfortunately, coercive strategies are common in parenting (Patterson, 1982), in intimate relationships (Pence & Paymar, 1993), and in social institutions, including human service settings. In substance abuse programs, clients are often terminated for drug use, disruptive children are commonly removed from foster homes, and staff supervision often relies on saying the same thing that was said on prior occasions, but doing so "longer, louder and meaner" (Daniels, 1994, p. 17). In each of these cases, those within the system are often unable to conceive of alternatives. In child welfare practice, relying primarily on the threat of loss of child custody to motivate parents to take mandated steps requires constant scanning for violations, and the behavior produced commonly lasts only as long as surveillance and a credible threat are maintained.

At a macro level, Schaef (1987) and Strick (1996) deal systematically with addictive processes in society and a coercive legal system, respectively. Schaef discusses the addictive society whose major premise is control or "the illusion of control" (p. 112), and Strick argues for restructuring of our adversarial legal system whose primary dynamic is punishment. Common to both discussions is the societal incongruence of our ethics and our behavior, our inability to be authentic, and our inability to understand power. Dualism (Schaef), or the either-or framework (Strick), enforces conformity, structures limits (only two choices), and eliminates the power of alternatives and new combinations.

Exploitation

Exploitation through apparently positive means is another common form of adversarial power (Biglan, 1995). Exploitation occurs by arranging conditions in which people are encouraged to act in ways that will ultimately be damaging to themselves and others by arranging short-term positive consequences for those actions, while concealing the long-term costs. For example, this approach is often used to lure urban youth into drug use and sales at an early age; the promise of immediate relief, pleasure, or cash is hard to resist for those with few other options. Is such exploitation present in social work and human services? Sexual involvement with clients or students, making commitments to clients or supervisees knowing that they may not be kept, supporting social policies that encourage the poor to take positions paying less than a living wage, or overdiagnosing clients to receive third-party payments (Kirk & Kutchins, 1988) are some examples of exploitation that have recently been discussed in considerable depth (McGowan & Mattison, 1998; Reamer, 1995a, 1995b), all of which are inconsistent with professional ethics and yet appear to be common.

Limitations of Adversarial Power

Reliance on adversarial power (coercion, competition, and exploitation) in social work occurs often enough that many clients' image of "social workers" is less positive than it needs to be to achieve optimal outcomes. Fulfilling or optimal alternatives do not emerge from constraint or punishment, which do not teach anyone how to construct a path that may lead to a good outcome, but only which paths to avoid. Structures based on coercion are inherently weak and are constantly at risk of collapse, because those constrained naturally will do as little as possible and only for as long as they have to, and they will escape or rebel at any opportunity. It is not surprising that many in society, including many social work clients, have become deeply suspicious of contemporary social institutions, often including social work itself. For the reasons elaborated above, the exercise of adversarial power cannot contribute to positive long-term outcomes in which all are included. The challenge to social workers, and social work students, is to examine their own practice environments and identify areas in which there may be unnecessary reliance on adversarial processes when shared power alternatives may be more constructive.

SHARED POWER

If power is to be constructive, an alternative, distinctive other paradigm is required. Social work need not, however, begin from scratch, for we understand relationships and contexts. Shared power is relational. Human beings are social animals, and constant reciprocal influence is built into who we are. The sharing of power involves recognition that power is potentially unlimited and constructive, rather than a path to personal aggrandizement. Shared power gives power life and contributes to an overall increase in the power of the group. Shared power mirrors good social work.

Shared power focuses on shared responsibility according to the strengths, talents—gifts—that each actor brings to the process. Responsibility requires the best use of the gifts we are given. We all carry full responsibility for contribution to human welfare. In the social work relationship, shared power does not mean "equality" of responsibility, however. Each actor carries different powers, and all of those are required; none is more or less important. Comparison and hierarchy are useless, for as one Ojibway elder from Canada explained, when all that is in the forest is needed, how can one be worth more than another? (Ross, 1996).

For example, we as social workers are held responsible for professional ethics because of the education in which we participate. Clients have responsibility for making changes in their lives. Social workers assist by mirroring awareness, offering options for exploration, reflecting change, and helping to construct opportunities for the person to take responsibility and contribute. In a substance abuse example, we might ask, "How does your drinking affect the well-being of your family? How does it affect your children? How can we make this different?" Instead, social workers sometimes make judgmental statements (e.g., "You need to stop drinking"), which set up an adversarial dynamic. Such a confrontation ignores the impact of a history of abuse and disrupted relationships. Such a confrontation bypasses opportunities for collective problem solving and mutual obligations of worker, client, and family systems to create healthier experiences. Sometimes, as social workers, we are dancing on the periphery of our own self-importance. Sometimes, we do not get to the best use of strengths and gifts, for our clients or ourselves.

The sharing of power allows everyone to contribute what they can to the social work process: time, material resources, experience, knowledge, expertise. The sharing of power establishes reciprocity in the social work relationship that goes beyond the personal strength perspective. While skill levels may differ, recognizing the gifts that we carry as human beings sets the stage for a different level of work. Sharing power requires awareness of where one's own power lies, authentic recognition of one's potential for causing damage, and a commitment to seeing and honoring the power of others. Such awareness permits access to our own genuine power and the power of those around us, namely, colleagues and clients. Shared power requires an ongoing commitment to seeing and challenging in oneself the egocentrism and ethnocentrism so effectively shaped by Euro-American culture. Shared power enables social work to move further along the continuum of respect and appreciation for diversity as well, because both people and peoples carry different powers and have different contributions that they can make to the collective.

Shared power requires explicit attention to every personal and professional action (there can be no real distinction because everything is connected) that may contribute or damage. This perspective involves seeing oneself as one of many contributors to the whole, rather than as someone important who makes a difference individually. This means practicing to contribute and construct on behalf of the collective, rather than managing one's image. The essence of authenticity is the release of self, not in sacrifice for the good of others, but in recognition of one's "connectedness" and the responsibilities that go with it. Shared power allows one to choose good paths because the decision making is contextual and relational, supports others in their choices, as opposed to simply punishing them for making poor ones, and lends real strength to effective advocacy and the construction of deeply useful helping relationships because one's own ego is not tied up in action taken. Positive outcomes are not guaranteed, but this is web building. A nexus of experiences in learning and relationship building is established, which creates points of strength that can be developed in future situations.

A commitment to sharing power in practice is also potentially freeing, since the social worker need not carry the entire responsibility for overall outcomes. One can then be more relaxed about the work, with the recognition that the social worker's role is to use his or her own power to contribute and to provide support for others involved in the case—clients, professionals, and collateral persons—as they recognize and contribute their own power to the work. Practice experience suggests, for example, that people want to provide food for their families and education for their children (especially if they have been extensively exposed to a community-oriented perspective) and want to resolve obstacles in their connections to their social world. The challenge, however, is to do so in an adversarial society where opportunities to be heard and to share power are limited or punished. The material that follows provides examples of social work practice with families and in substance abuse programs. These examples clarify how practice grounded in a shared power perspective differs from approaches that rely on adversarial power.

Practice rooted in shared power requires continual development in awareness and understanding. The examples that follow reflect various points on a developmental continuum of shared power. For example, self-awareness on the part of the worker is an essential beginning; providing additional options and resources is a further step; actively reaching for mutual recognition of and respect for the power of each contributor is more advanced still. The examples discussed here need to be further developed through application, reflecting a commitment to move practice ever further along the continuum.

Social Work with Families

State-of-the-art practice in child welfare cases calls for an arrangement in which everyone involved in the case has a strong voice, is heard, and shares responsibility—child, biological parents, foster parents, and social worker (Minuchin, 1995; Zlotnick, 1997). In cases where reunification is the goal, collaborative case planning is one way that all share power and responsibility for the process and outcome while building critical relationships. This does not minimize the social worker's responsibility to protect children, rather it expands the responsibility as well as the power to be shared with others involved in the case in order to create a process of potential growth and responsibility for all members. Shared power moves discussion away from blaming and models responsibility. It gives voice to the biological parents. State-of-the-art practice requires that, for example, parents have a strong role in the preparation of reports, have complete access to case records, and be viewed as partners in the work (Minuchin, 1995).

In collaborative case planning, participants can acknowledge where responsibility has been addressed or not and what needs to be done. The social worker (and the foster parents) is not omitted from this evaluation, and the foster parents and biological parents can address issues of social workers' responsibility as well. Because of their position in an adversarial, hierarchical system, biological parents are not consistently heard, nor are they consistently held responsible. And it is only recently that foster parents have founded organizations to collectively speak their concerns.

Shared power in child welfare involves encouraging and expecting (and allowing) everyone to contribute from their own power, namely, time, resources, knowledge, and skills. For example, some foster parents can share the power of their own lessons learned while recovering from substance abuse with biological parents who are addicts. Foster parents may draw power from a deep concern and respect for children, years of experience gained from child rearing, and a historical understanding of their community and culture. Biological parents' power may emerge from their intimate knowledge of the needs and preferences of each child, contributing from a concerned voice in planning for visiting and case resolution. Children, too, can often voice what feels right and what does not, and doing so helps them in the developmental task of creating their own power. The social worker's power may come from knowledge of child development and related practice approaches options for working with families having difficulties in child rearing (e.g., Greene, Norman, Searle, Daniels, & Lubeck, 1995; Howing, Wodarski, Gaudin, & Kurtz, 1989; Mattaini, McGowan, & Williams, 1996) and skills for encouraging constructive engagement among all parties.

In genuinely sharing power, hierarchical perspectives need to be actively abandoned. Systemic structures sometimes do not permit that everyone be heard, and individuals "in power" can misuse their positions to maintain their own belief systems rather than actively solving problems for the benefit of the collective. The challenge in such cases is to genuinely seek different voices and perspectives and incorporate them, rather than duplicating the adversarial arrangements that characterize the legal system. The goal in child welfare cases is not necessarily reunification, and effective family practice does not rely on punitive power. Rather, it is an issue of asking everyone, "What is required to provide for this child, and how can we all work to achieve that?" For parents, core questions include, "What do you need to provide better care for your child?" or "Are you at a point where this is possible?" Whether or not the goal is reunification, planning involves helping the parent and child to access what they need in a genuinely collaborative way.

Other emerging approaches to practice with families also rely heavily on shared power, and the evidence suggests that the better the sharing of power is operationalized, the better the results will be (Henggeler, Schoenwald, Borduin, Rowland, & Cunningham, 1998; Webster-Stratton, 1997). Multifamily groups, for example, are increasingly used with many client populations, including situations involving child maltreatment, battering, and adoption, among others (Meezan & O'Keefe, 1998). The presence and power of other families is a major dynamic in these groups. For example, McFarlane (1991), a pioneer in multifamily groups with families that include members struggling with schizophrenia, explicitly spells out the need to share responsibility among the families and professionals, noting that the group can even neutralize messages of blame that commonly come from professionals.

Identification of strengths, a focus on shared responsibility, and a primary focus on empowerment (including respecting families' choices in terms of treatment goals, assuming competencies, and collaborating to enhance connections with natural systems) are all among the core practice principles of multisystemic therapy, which is demonstrably more effective with families that include children and youth shaped in an antisocial climate than are standard interventions (Henggeler et al., 1998) and appears to be effective in cases of child maltreatment as well. These are consistent with the "Family Support Principles" of the National Association of Social Workers (cited by Zlotnick, 1997), including a call for family-centered, community-based services defined in terms of the family's strengths and definition of the problems, involving the family as a partner in the service-planning process, which requires program flexibility to fit the case (rather than offering services to families as defined by narrow categories of need determined by the agency or national policy), and attention to meaning and perceptions of problems and solutions inherent in cultural and ethnic interpretations of a family's dilemma.

Substance Abuse

Practically all social workers work with persons and families in which substance abuse is a serious issue, whether recognized or not. A shared power perspective suggests why a number of recent innovations in substance abuse treatment may be more effective than traditional approaches that rely heavily on coercive, confrontational strategies. Some reflect more advanced positions on the continuum of shared power than others, and some can be used in ways that minimize or maximize the sharing of power.

Family members are inevitably involved in the matrix of events that occur in substance abuse. Family members are often told that there is nothing they can do, that they have little to contribute to resolution of the problem, or even that as codependents they carry responsibility for the problem. These approaches do not respect the possible contributions that family members can make, do not explore their power. One alternative is some form of "intervention" (Johnson, 1973) in which family members actively confront the abuser and work toward engagement in treatment. In these approaches, family members often contribute in significant ways in the development of the intervention, in what can be an authentic sharing of power. At least as important, however, is that the intervention be conducted in a way that reserves to the substance abuser a voice in planning, opportunities to contribute to the process, and a share in responsibility for the outcome.

Three effective programs, in which significant others contribute toward moving the alcoholic toward treatment, demonstrate several points on the continuum from adversarial to shared power. One program, Pressures to Change, is designed to move through several graduated levels of action on the part of the nondrinking partner, and at each level the "pressure" is increased (Barber & Gilbertson, 1996, 1997). While not all of the levels employ adversarial strategies, the name of the procedure clarifies its coercive roots, and in fact the developers experienced substantial resistance from families to the more coercive levels of confrontation in the program. In unilateral family therapy (Thomas, Santa, Bronson, & Oyserman, 1987; Thomas & Yoshioka, 1989), the significant other is trained in a number of skill areas, culminating in either a "programmed confrontation," in which specific negative consequences of refusing to engage in treatment are clarified, or a "programmed request," in which the significant other and the social worker plan for how to make a potentially effective request for entering treatment. Further still along the shared power continuum is the reinforcement training approach (Sisson & Azrin, 1986). In this approach, a family member (usually the spouse) learns skills for 1) reducing the risk of physical abuse to him- or herself (primarily through making a safety plan), 2) encouraging sobriety, 3) encouraging engagement in treatment, and 4) assisting in treatment once the drinking partner enters. Clients are offered a range of skills (providing options) and assisted in developing their own individualized approach. They learn not how to "confront" their spouses, but when and how to effectively suggest treatment while supporting sobriety in very honest and authentic ways. Once the drinking spouse agrees to treatment (which nearly all do), he or she enters a program in which he or she participates actively in constructing a more effective life for him- or herself.

This approach, and certain other contemporary approaches in substance abuse treatment, like motivational interviewing (Miller & Rollnick, 1991), the community reinforcement approach (Meyers & Smith, 1996), and guided self-change treatment (Sobell & Sobell, 1993), are radically different from traditional substance abuse treatment in ways that may not be immediately apparent. None gives clients the message that they have no control over their lives, and all (if well implemented) offer clients opportunities to elaborate and experiment with what they believe will be of value to themselves, to contribute from their own strengths and power, and to share responsibility for the directions taken. Practicing such approaches requires more than individual workers having the awareness and commitment required for sharing power. Agency structures and policies also need to be firmly grounded in the sharing of and access to power, rather than in coercively forcing one program designed by the staff on every client, regardless of personal and cultural gifts and experiences. Within this matrix, client contributions to program design and operation are expected and honored.

In an interview conducted by the first author, one senior counselor in an on-reservation Native American residential alcohol and drug treatment center expressed a longing for shared power beyond teamwork, more discussion of cases, and shared knowledge among the treatment staff. (Ironically, the women counselors wanted more shared power, and the male supervisor and program director recognized that positive reinforcement of the gifts the counselors and women in treatment brought into the treatment program was one of the most powerful tools they had.) And the counselors recognized that helping women find their talents and gifts was power.

PRACTICE PRINCIPLES

Shared power involves the cocreation of an improved reality. A pathologizing or adversarial stance, in contrast, can at best reduce what is undesirable, usually ineffectively. One question that consistently arises in discussions with students and practitioners is how to operationalize the sharing of power in real world practice. There is no simple formula, of course; that would be inconsistent with an approach grounded in identifying and combining individual gifts and the unique collective cocreations that result. Several practice principles, however, are useful starting points:

1. The first step is the explicit identification of what powers, gifts, skills, and talents each party has to contribute to the practice encounter. Respectful

and explicit recognition and reinforcement of positive actions others take is among the most powerful steps one can take.

2. Workers committed to shared power make a continuous effort to identify the situations and ways they still rely on adversarial stances and to explore alternatives.

3. Breaking through authenticity is an essential repertoire that is often not supported by an adversarial culture. Repeatedly asking oneself, "Is this honest? Really honest?" is essential to shared power.

4. The social worker committed to shared power honestly labels adversarial processes for what they are ("speak truth to power"—nonpunitively) and declines to participate in them.

5. Sharing power is more difficult, but even more important, in settings characterized by high levels of diversity, in which it may be more challenging to honor and respect what others have to contribute.

6. Thinking and speaking at all times in terms of shared responsibility for achieving good outcomes frees the social workers and others involved from what may otherwise be experienced as a difficult burden.

7. Giving up the need to "make a difference," and instead recognizing that one acts not to save or fix someone else, but rather to contribute to the web of which one is oneself a part, can ease the transition from ego to collective.

It is difficult to maintain a commitment to shared power without support. Individual social workers need to participate in the cocreation and maintenance of empowerment cultures grounded in shared power within agencies and service networks (Lowery & Mattaini, in press). Two or three people who make a mutual commitment to the coconstruction of an empowerment culture can be surprisingly powerful, particularly if they are willing to look at themselves together in an authentic way. Sharing power can begin with the individual, but it is ultimately a collective effort.

CONCLUSION

Far from being an abstract ideal, the sharing of power is consistent with how the world is, whether viewed from the perspective of behavioral science or a Native American worldview. It is both practical and realistic. But establishing and maintaining it within social work requires a radical and painful reorientation. This requires an ongoing commitment to actively recognize and give up the coercive, competitive, and exploitative ways of viewing the world and clients that have often extensively shaped us as human beings/social workers in this society. Perhaps the most difficult stance to shift from is that of "expert." It is difficult to acknowledge that there are other systems of knowledge that more broadly explain the world than do some of our theories.

Because we do not understand the concepts or the language of these, or because we are not willing to acknowledge the capacities of others, particularly when we perceive their capacities as greater than ours, we are unwilling to explore these areas.

While the NASW's *Code of Ethics* (1996) states that "social workers elevate service to others above self-interest," doing so requires a level of self-awareness that is usually lacking in most people. The next step, recognizing that service to others is the best way to care for oneself because of one's essential connections in the web, is even less common. In Navajo (*Diné*) philosophy, First Man (essentially, the creator) recognized that his contributions for the benefit of all served him as well, and at the same time, these contributions made the best use of his medicine power (Farella, 1984).

Achieving the necessary awareness requires genuine feedback from others, since we are well defended against observing those patterns in ourselves. We also need to be willing to listen and respond honestly when those we trust say, "Your ego is too big," or "How is what you are doing making a contribution?" The first author "held up the mirror" frequently during the course of the dialogue that shaped this paper. The second author struggled with the challenges reflected back to him. Acknowledging patterns of egocentric adversarial behavior, authentically acknowledging the damage we can do and that we actually do, is an enormous personal and professional challenge. This is inevitably uncomfortable and often very painful. This process of awareness and exploration needs to be deeply interwoven into social work education if it is to become firmly embedded in practice.

Some individuals, both non–Native American and some with Native American blood, have tried to use traditional Native American power and spirituality for themselves, for economic gain or to enhance personal status in obvious or subtle ways. This egocentric stance is taken by persons who do not understand that real power by definition must be shared and is not about the individual. Lakota medicine people, for example, recognize that power is a gift that comes from outside of themselves and that they have a responsibility to use it well, on behalf of others (Crow Dog & Erdoes, 1995). The contrast between the two groups is profound.

Traditional sharing of power among Native American nations was sabotaged and subverted in the process of colonization (Lowery, 1999). The US Constitution, which borrowed heavily from the Iroquois Great Law of Peace, a model of shared power in which women played a critical role, is an important example of a general phenomenon (Jacobs, 1991). Governmental laws, regulations, and informal coercive actions attempted to graft sexist, adversarial practices onto cultures in which they were quite foreign. This example of adversarial power, like all others, was not only destructive, but also ultimately weak—the power of the constructive alternative continues to reemerge. Consider our legal system and one alternative:

> The most sophisticated legal mechanisms and benign procedural remedies cannot surmount an ethic that makes them artillery. Nor can the most constructive laws imaginable rise above a destructive legal method that applies those laws to actual problems; a method structured to produce neither new questions nor new answers, but only victors and vanquished. Psychic violence cannot lead beyond violence. (Strick, 1996, p. 204)

It must all go; we must start all over, Strick (1996) concludes. A contextual view is taken in the proposal for an effective legal system "conceived as an instrument for society's health and welfare" (p. 205). The new legal model proposed exudes shared power and is seen as "multi-referrant rather than bipolar, relativistic rather than resolute, preventive, ameliorative, information seeking, discussional, constructive" (p. 209). The new model must be expanded to engage the "participative experience and responsibility of every citizen, and enlist the support, involvement and ingenuity of local communities" (p. 209).

Such models were constructed in long ago indigenous communities. Sacred justice or restorative justice teaches adherence to spiritual law and heals and restores the spirit by rebuilding relationships within a community setting. Today, indigenous justice models are being revived and adapted in communities from Teslin, a Tlingit community in the Yukon, and the Ojibway-Cree community of Sandy Lake First Nation in remote Ontario, Canada, to the Navajo Nation (Arizona/New Mexico), formerly known for its Western-style court system, to Maori communities in New Zealand (Ross, 1996). Data from New Zealand using restorative justice practices have noted a drop in admissions to youth-offender custody facilities from 2,712 in 1998 to 923 in the period from 1992 to 1993, resulting in the closure of half of all such facilities (Ross, 1996). Prosecuted cases among older youth (ages 17 to 19) have declined by 27 percent from 1987 to 1992, "producing young adults less likely to be prosecuted in adults courts" (Ross, 1996, p. 23). This alternative clearly is powerful.

Adversarial, coercive power is by nature limited and weak. Shared power has no such limitations and has the potential to take social work practice to qualitatively different levels. We believe the sharing of power is the heart and soul of practicing social work "in a good way."

CHAPTER 8

Treating Depression in a Postmodern World: A Feminist Perspective

Nan Van Den Bergh

In this chapter, Van Den Bergh discusses the feminist approach to working with people who are depressed. Van Den Bergh also shows structure in her three-stage intervention, including restorying, restructuring, and recovering. In all of the stages, the emphasis is on active participation as a technique to reduce the client's depression. In addition, Van Den Bergh highlights the importance of the societal antecedents that facilitate depression in women and the usefulness of feminist treatment for both men and women social workers and for both men and women clients.

INTRODUCTION

The intent of this chapter is to explore the potential value of employing a feminist perspective when intervening with clients affected by depressive disorders, in particular, with women. Undertaking this endeavor seems warranted given the facts that 1) depressive symptoms are common among persons seeking mental health services, 2) social workers provide the majority of mental health services in the United States, and 3) the majority of social work clients are female.

What Is the Definition of Depression?

Within the larger rubric of mood disorders, which include depressive, manic, and mixed affective disorders, of primary concern in this chapter is the depressive disorder, characterized by one or more major depressive episodes, for example, at least two weeks of depressed mood or loss of interest accompanied by at least four additional symptoms of depression. To meet the criteria of a major depressive episode, five or more of the following symptoms need to be present during the same two-week period. Furthermore, at least one of the symptoms must be either depressed mood or loss of interest/pleasure, and those symptoms must represent a change from the individual's previous functioning: 1) depressed mood; 2) markedly diminished interest or pleasure; 3) significant weight/appetite changes, either losing or gaining; 4) insomnia or hypersomnia; 5) psychomotor agitation or retardation; 6) fatigue or loss of energy; 7) feelings of worthlessness; 8) diminished ability to think or concentrate or indecisiveness; and 9) recurrent thoughts of death (American Psychiatric Association [APA], 1994, p. 327).

By comparison, a dysthymic disorder is characterized by at least two years of depressed mood, in which the person is depressed for more days than not, accompanied by additional depressive symptoms that do not meet the criteria for a major depressive episode. Two or more of the following symptoms must be present while the person is experiencing a depressed mood: 1) poor appetite or overeating, 2) insomnia or hypersomnia, 3) low energy or fatigue, 4) low self-esteem, 5) poor concentration or difficulty making decisions, and 6) feelings of hopelessness. Pursuant to those symptoms, to qualify for a diagnosis of dysthymia, the following criteria must be met: 1) the person was never without the symptoms for more than two months at a time and 2) no major depressive episode was present during the first two years of the disturbance. Should this second criterion not be fulfilled, the individual may better qualify for the diagnosis of chronic major depressive disorder (APA, 1994, p. 349).

Extent and Degree of Depression

Since antiquity, depression has been recognized as a painful affective state associated with physical, psychological, and social distress (O'Neil, 1984). Based on contemporary epidemiological research, depression is one of the nation's leading mental health problems. A recent National Institute of Mental Health (NIMH)–sponsored endeavor to ascertain mental disorder prevalence in the United States, the National Comorbidity Survey (NCS), was the first mental health epidemiological research project to administer a structured psychiatric interview to a national probability sample of over 8,000 respondents, ages 15 to 54 years, in the noninstitutionalized civilian population of the forty-eight contiguous states (Kessler et al., 1994). In terms of general mental health trends, the NCS showed that psychiatric disorders were more prevalent than was suggested by prior research. Close to half of all respondents reported a lifetime history of at least one DSM-III-R disorder; one-fifth had experienced an affective disorder, one-fourth an anxiety disorder, and one-fourth had a history of a substance abuse disorder. In terms of twelve-month prevalence data, 30 percent of the sample had experienced a mental health problem, with 17 percent reporting an anxiety disorder, 11 percent a depressive disorder, and 11 percent a substance abuse disorder (Kessler et al., 1994). Analysis of these data by gender indicated that women were much

TABLE 8-1   Comparative Difference by Gender in Depression Prevalence

Affective Disorder	Male Depression Prevalence		Female Depression Prevalence	
	Lifetime	Twelve months	Lifetime	Twelve months
Major depression	12.7	7.7	21.3	12.9
Dysthymia	4.8	2.1	8.0	3.0

NOTE: Values are percentages.

more likely to experience affective disorders (with the exception of mania, for which there was no gender difference) and anxiety disorders than men, whereas men were more likely to have substance abuse problems and antisocial personality disorders. Gender differences are tabulated in Table 8-1 (Kessler et al., 1994, p. 12). As can be seen for both lifetime and twelve-month prevalence rates, women were almost twice as likely as men to experience a depressive disorder. Additionally, the NCS found that women had higher prevalence rates than men for experiencing three or more co-occurring mental disorders (i.e., affective, anxiety, substance abuse, etc.). Consequently, women in the United States appear to be more challenged than men to maintain a state of mental wellness, and additional research seeking explanations for gender differentials is definitely warranted.

Other demographic variables addressed by this survey, which warrant mention based on their potential interactive effect in predicting depression in women, were age, race, income, and ethnicity. Although the data are not broken down by the specific affective disorder, it is interesting to note that according to the twelve-month prevalence data, young people, ages 15 to 24, were significantly more likely, compared with other age groups, to experience an affective disorder, as were Hispanics (compared with non-Hispanic whites and African-Americans), people earning less than $19,000 per annum, and people with less than twelve years of education. Looking at lifetime affective disorder prevalence rates and significant group differences, people with lower incomes were more affected, and African-Americans were significantly less depression impacted than Hispanics and non-Hispanic whites (Kessler et al., 1994).

An interesting theme that emerged from this research was that for both lifetime and twelve-month prevalence rates, there was a consistent tendency for socioeconomic status to be more powerfully related to anxiety disorders than to affective disorders. That is to say, having increased financial resources seemed to have a more protective effect against the experience of worries and fears than of sadness. Consequently, it may be possible to conjecture that since women are more likely to be poor than men (Van Den Bergh, 1991), an improved economic condition, in and of itself, would not necessarily protect women from the risk of experiencing an affective disorder.

RESEARCH ON WOMEN AND DEPRESSION

Because women have been found to be at greater risk for developing a depressive disorder, substantial literature has been published on this theme. In the following section, a review of literature on women and depression with specific emphasis on reporting findings of studies funded under the aegis of the NIMH will be shared. NIMH-funded studies could be conceptualized as being divided between "nature" and "nurture" themes. Pursuant to the nature theme, research investigating the impact of biological factors, such as endocrinology and neurochemistry, has been funded by the NIMH, research that includes the role of genetics in the increased susceptibility to depressive symptoms. The nurture research has looked at the role of demographic factors, including age, race, socioeconomic status, and occupational role; sociocultural factors such as victimization; psychosocial factors such as social support and attachment/bonding as well as the role of personality dynamics in predicting depression rates in women.

Genetic Factors in Female Depression

A rigorous research design utilizing female-female twin pairs and longitudinal data collection has yielded some interesting findings concerning the possible biological explanations for an increased female depression ratio. In one study, where 680 randomly selected female twin pairs were interviewed regarding experiences with depressive symptoms, researchers found that the best-fitting structural equation model accounting for 50.1 percent of the variance in liability to major depression had the following predictors, in descending order: 1) stressful life events, 2) genetic factors, 3) previous history of major depression, and 4) neuroticism. These researchers suggested that female depression needs to be seen as a multifactorial disorder, with at least four interacting risk factors, including traumatic experiences, genetic factors, temperament, and interpersonal relations (Kendler, Kessler, Neale, Heath, & Eaves, 1993a). In a further elaboration of this study, the same researchers suggested that the role of genetics may be best understood as altering sensitivity to depression-inducing effects of stressful life events (Kendler et al., 1995).

In part because epidemiological research has suggested significant comorbidity, or co-occurrence, between substance abuse and affective disorders, researchers have attempted to ascertain those associational dynamics within female populations. Through the analysis of female twin pair data, researchers found that comorbidity between major depression and alcoholism in women is substantial, with significant correlations ranging from +.4 to +.6 (Kendler et al., 1993b). That level of dual diagnosis was deemed to result largely from genetic factors that influenced susceptibility to depressive symptoms or substance abuse; however, environmental risk factors also contributed to the co-occurrence rate. It is noteworthy that environmental factors played a more significant role in predicting major depression than in predicting alcoholism.

The theme from these genetic studies suggests that there is nothing biologically endemic to the condition of being female, in and of itself, which explains a greater depression rate in women. Genetic factors play a substantial, but not overwhelming, role in predicting the onset of depressive symptoms. It appears that the best explanation for the role of genetics in female depression is that one could inherit a heightened neurologic susceptibility to experiencing depressive symptoms when exposed to stressful life events.

Demographic Factors in Female Depression

Given the differential impact of gender in predicting depression, the role of other demographic factors interacting with gender and influencing the rate of female depression warrants investigation.

Age. While being younger, in general, seems related to greater depression for both genders, the depression incidence for young females is greater than for young males (Leon, Klerman, & Wickramaratne, 1993; Newman, Engel, & Jensen, 1991). Some research has suggested that gender differences in vulnerability to depression may be present prior to adolescence and could be associated with the impact of gender stereotypes on the construction of gender identity (Ruble, Greulich, Pomerantz, & Gochberg, 1993). Potential substantiation for that assumption is suggested by other research, which demonstrates that the nearly twofold increase in major depression in women compared with men peaks between adolescence and early adulthood (Leon et al., 1993). In a similar vein, it has been found that female adolescents, compared with males, reported more depressive symptoms associated with self-consciousness, negative body image, negative self-esteem, and identification with feminine rather than masculine cultural stereotypes (Allgood-Merten, Lewinsohn, & Hops, 1990). Other research has suggested that young women may experience a loss of hope and a sense of helplessness in managing day-to-day responsibilities by virtue of subscription to gender role stereotypes. Experiencing sexism and engaging in gender-based social roles that are stressful, or those that are not easily managed, may leave young women vulnerable to the onset of an affective disorder. The negative outcomes that could accrue from gender role confusion or ambivalence is also suggested through research findings based on analysis of age cohort data, which found that female vulnerability to depression was highest in the 1960s and 1970s, a period when traditional conceptions of gender roles were being questioned by the burgeoning feminist movement (Leon et al., 1993).

The studies noted above suggest that, attitudinally and behaviorally, conforming to gender role stereotypes may contribute to girls and young women having a more fragile self-image and, potentially, a sense of having less efficacy and mastery, which may make them more vulnerable to depressive symptoms.

However, research has suggested that accrued life experience may mediate the potential vulnerability to depression experienced by younger women, such that it may dissipate over the course of the life cycle. For example, depressive symptoms in a five-year study of women between the ages of 51 and 92 decreased with age; however, study subjects did experience feelings of enervation with age increases (Newman et al., 1991). These data suggest that with accrued life experiences, women may develop a sense of self separate from gender role stereotypes, which may allow them to view their life as having been worthwhile and productive. Age, then, may be associated with depressive symptoms as it corresponds to the identity development process one experiences over the course of the life cycle. Obviously, younger persons may be more vulnerable to the influence of stereotypes of how one is supposed to be; with life experience and maturation, a person is more likely to develop a sense of self based on one's lived reality. Using strength and empowerment concepts, it would seem safe to assume that the endemic process of maturation gives individuals more experiences whereby they can come to know their strengths and competencies, thereby potentially mediating the negative mental health impact that comes from conformity to female gender roles. Consequently, although a woman may have grown up conforming to gender role stereotypes, after being in the working world or having negotiated interpersonal relationships and attempts at family life, she may have a greater sense of her competencies and strengths.

Race.   Although the NCS, noted previously, found that African-Americans, in general, were less likely to be depressed than whites or non-Hispanic whites, other research has found that African-American women have a depression rate 42 percent higher than white women (Greene, 1994). The potential negative interaction effect between race and gender identity with regard to depression was suggested by one study of African-American gay men and women (Greene, 1994). Of these subjects, the women had depression scores similar to those for HIV-positive gay men; both groups ranked higher for depression than samples of nongay African-Americans and gay white men (Cochran & Mays, 1994). In other research focused on low-income African-American women, including women who had experienced mental disorders and controls without symptomology, clinically depressed subjects were more likely to have lower self-esteem and have a more external locus of control, that is, they perceived the forces of control as being outside of themselves (Goodman, Cooley, Sewell, & Leavitt, 1994). Low self-esteem could result from introjecting negative beliefs about oneself, as a result of being within a socially marginalized group. For example, research has found an association between internalized racism and depression (as well as a risk for alcoholism) within a sample of African-American women (Taylor & Jackson,

1990, 1991). The above studies do suggest the potential of an interaction effect between the negative experiences one could have based on gender and race prejudice/discrimination and increased susceptibility to depression.

Social class.   Social class factors, as measured by education and income, have also been found to be relevant in predicting depression for women. In particular, it appears that having less education and being poor may place women at greater risk. For example, research has shown that the groups of women for whom depression rates exceed 40 percent include those who are young mothers, urban, and poor (Brown & Harris, 1978; Belle, 1982; Weissman & Klerman, 1987). Research has also shown that rural women who are young, unemployed, and poorly educated also have depression rates greater than 40 percent (Hauenstein & Boyd, 1994).

The potential dampening effect of poverty and low education on mental health has also been observed in studies of women and employment. In a prospective study of the correlation between job loss and psychological distress among blue collar women, of those women who were laid off, having fewer financial resources was subsequently associated with greater depressive symptoms (Dew, Bromet, & Penkower, 1992).

Within a longitudinal study investigating the impact of employment status on depression symptoms, women who were initially unemployed with low levels of education and depressive symptoms, when subsequently employed, did not experience significant symptom relief (Bromberger & Matthews, 1994). This may be explained by their employment in lower-paying, low-status jobs, potentially contributing to a sense of blocked opportunity, which could be depressing.

Cross-cultural studies have also suggested the important role of social class factors, since high depressive symptoms were reported in one out of every three women living in poor residential areas in Puerto Rico (Jimenez, Alegria, Pena, & Vera, 1997). Factors associated with high depressive symptomology for these Puerto Rican women included being a female head of household and having high economic stress.

Patterns from the research studies noted above suggest that the impact of low education and income, shown to be predictive of affective disorders in the general population, seem to be strong predictors of depression potential for women. Due to the fact that the majority of the poor in the United States are women and children, there is a strong suggestion of an association between the feminization of poverty and a high depression prevalence rate for women.

Work role.   Research has been undertaken on the impact of work roles in predicting depression rates in women by comparing homemakers with full-time married employed women and employed with unemployed women, as well as comparing employed women's occupational groups and their differential depression rates.

Because the majority of women ages 18 to 64 are employed (Kemp, 1994), including those who have children under the age of 18, research comparing depression rates between women employed full time versus homemakers seems almost anachronistic. Results in this area have been equivocal. While some research has found that homemakers are more vulnerable to depressive symptoms than working women (Golding, 1990), other research has found that employed wives and homemakers have similar levels of depressive symptoms (Lennon, 1994). This study did find that having control over one's work was a depression buffer for homemakers, while less routinization of work mitigated depression for employed women.

Extrapolating from these studies could explain why secretaries may be more vulnerable to depression, as an occupational group, since they tend to experience low control and high routinization in their work environment. Research into the differential rates of depression among female workers, based on their job classification, which utilized a random sample of approximately 3,500 full-time employed women, found that secretaries were significantly more likely to be depressed than any other group (Garrison & Eaton, 1992). The explanations offered by the researchers for a higher secretarial depression rate included the following: 1) selection effect, that is, depressed women may be more likely to become secretaries; 2) greater non–work role stress experienced by secretaries than other employed women; and 3) the possibility that secretarial job conditions of high demand and low status result in dissatisfaction and stress leading to depression. The job conditions hypothesis seems compelling since secretaries, as an occupational group, because of high job routinization and low job control, may fall victim to learned helplessness, which could make them vulnerable to depression.

Other research related to work status and depression in women has examined role deprivation as a contributing factor. For example, in a three-year longitudinal study investigating the effect of employment status on depressive symptoms in middle-aged women, those women who were unemployed at baseline reported higher levels of depressive symptoms than employed women (Bromberger & Matthews, 1994). Three years later, depression levels tended to decrease for women who were initially unemployed and who subsequently got a job. However, within that group, those who retained depressive symptoms were women reporting low levels of education, social support, or marital satisfaction.

Operating from the opposite employment scenario but finding some similar predictors of depression, a prospective study of the effects of job loss on psychological distress in a cohort of blue collar women found that women who had been laid off had significantly more depressive symptoms (Bromberger & Matthews, 1994). Among those laid off, women who reported poor levels of support from their husband or partner and those experiencing more financial difficulties had higher depression levels.

Research examining work role and depression has suggested that role loss or deprivation seems to have some validity in predicting depression in women.

In addition, that research has suggested that role devaluation in terms of the type of work that women do and the conditions for that work may also play a contributing role. Women can be placed into roles within the family and the workplace that are undervalued as well as demanding. Having such a status could lead one to experience a sense of learned helplessness, since regardless of the effort expended in undertaking one's role responsibilities, the results may not be appreciated.

Sociocultural Predictors of Women's Depression

Victimization.   As a sociocultural variable, female victimization (including both incest and adult sexual assault) has been associated with depression and the dual diagnosis of depression and substance abuse. It is possible that 20 percent of the US female population has experienced child sexual assault, 12 percent before the age of 14 and 16 percent before the age of 18 (Bass & Davis, 1988). An association has been shown to exist between sexual victimization and depressive symptoms. In one study of rural women who reported depressive symptoms, which were ascertained from self-report questionnaires administered when visiting with their primary care physicians, a positive association was found between depression and the experience of child sexual abuse (Van Hook, 1996). Childhood sexual victimization has been uncovered as a theme in research with current or recovering female alcoholics and addicts, who also report other psychiatric symptoms in addition to substance abuse. For example, in a study of 146 primarily African-American and Latina females who were pregnant or parenting and recruited from both drug treatment and nontreatment sites (i.e., homeless shelters or jails), 51 percent reported having been victims of at least one forced sexual encounter, and 46 percent of women who had been victimized were 16 years old or younger at the time of the assault (Paone & Chavkin, 1992). The researchers hypothesized that their female respondents had abused drugs, in part, to self-medicate the depression and anxiety experienced from the victimization they had experienced. In undertaking a retrospective review of National Institute of Alcohol Abuse and Addictions research, Wilsnack (1993) reported that experiences of childhood sexual abuse seem to be emerging as important antecedents of elevated female lifetime depressive episodes, problem drinking, and lifetime multiple drug abuse.

The theme of violence against women and the negative impact of that on female mental health has also been explored by Miller (1993), who reports that results from the National Women's Study (a national telephone survey of 4,008 female respondents over the age of 18) indicated that 13 percent of adult women in the United States have been victims of at least one rape; the majority of those sexual assaults occurred before the age of 18. Additional data from that study indicated that rape victims were more likely to have reported nonmedical use of prescription drugs (15 percent vs. 3 percent), marijuana (52 percent vs. 16 percent), cocaine (16 percent vs. 3 percent), and other hard drugs (12 percent vs. 1 percent). Research with college women found that 27 percent had experienced rape or attempted rape since age 14. The fact that women self-medicate with alcohol and/or drugs in order to alleviate internalized stress states (with depressive or anxious symptoms) resulting from being victimized is posited as the theoretical link between victimization and mental health/substance abuse problems for women. Therefore, although female substance abuse is not the primary subject of this chapter, the high comorbidity rates reported for women having more than one mental health disorder (affective disorder, substance abuse problem, anxiety) suggests that the victimization of girls and women is a definite risk factor for that higher dual diagnosis rate.

Psychosocial Predictors to Women's Depression

Social support.   As was suggested in the work role research, social support is a factor that can buffer the impact of negative life events and potentially reduce risk for depression (O'Neil, 1984; Aneshensel & Stone, 1982). This assumption appears to have some cross-cultural validity. For example, within a random sample of approximately 1,000 Puerto Rican women ages 18 to 64, having few contacts with friends as well as a poor perception of family support was correlated with an increased level of depressive symptoms (Jimenez et al., 1997).

The impact of social support as a buffer to stresses that could be experienced by older women has also been investigated. In one study of 271 community-dwelling elderly women, low perceived family support, regardless of perceived support from friends and level of connectedness to a social network, was associated with poorer psychological well-being (Thompson & Heller, 1990). The social support quality versus quantity theme was also borne out in research assessing potential depressive symptoms for female caregivers of frail family members. Within this study (Rivera, Rose, Futterman, Lovett, & Gallagher-Thompson, 1991), women more likely to be depressed, despite having equivalent access to social support resources as nondepressed caregivers, had a higher incidence of negative interactions with others.

Wetzel (1994) suggests that it may be appropriate to conceptualize social support as an important factor in assessing "goodness of fit" between an individual and her social environment, hence, it is predictive of one's social and occupational functioning. She indicates that research reveals that lack of supportiveness in the family and at work, as well as a lack of control in both environments, increases women's vulnerability to depression.

Attachment/bonding.   Related to the concept of social support, attachment has been studied as a factor potentially contributing to mental health. Attachment, or the quality of one's bonding experiences with others, has been investigated in terms of the impact of the early loss of a significant other on the potential to be depressed or anxious. Earlier research investigating the relationship between attachment loss and the experience of depression has been somewhat equivocal (O'Neil, 1984), which is reassuring since it suggests that early loss does not inevitably lead to depression. Hence, individuals (including children) may have a remarkable ability to handle major loss. In some more recent attachment/mental health research, a study comparing female nonpsychiatric controls with women having major depression found that severely depressed subjects reported little attachment to their mother, at any age, and less attachment to their peers during development than nonpsychiatric controls (Rosenfarb, Becker, & Khan, 1994). Another study that attempted to assess the relationship between childhood parental loss and subsequent adult experience with depressive or anxiety symptoms and that utilized female twin pairs indicated that an increased risk for major depression and generalized anxiety disorder occurred for subjects experiencing parental separation but not parental death. Interestingly, panic disorder was associated with parental death and maternal, but not paternal, separation. The overall outcome of this female twin study indicated that between 1.5 percent and 5.1 percent of the variance in affective and anxiety disorders could be accounted for by childhood parental loss (Kendler, Neale, Kessler, Heath, & Eaves, 1992). Consequently, it may be appropriate to assume that attachment, as a psychosocial construct, has a rather low predictive ability in explaining depressive disorders in women.

Personality and Psychodynamic Predictors to Women's Depression

Traditional psychoanalytic literature has suggested that psychodynamic factors such as personality characteristics are believed to play a contributory role in all affective disorders. The importance of personality type in predicting depression, is on a continuum ranging from less impact with conditions, such as bipolar disorder, (believed to have a more biologic etiology), to dysthymic disorder, where one's temperament is believed to be more prone to major depression or "neurotic" recurrent depression (dysthymia). Personality types believed to be more depression prone include: 1) oral dependent personalities that constantly need recognition, approval, admiration, and demonstrations of love; 2) obsessive, conscience-ridden personalities with bottled-up aggressive and self-destructive tendencies; and 3) cyclothymic personalities who vacillate between subclinical experiences with mania and depression (O'Neil, 1984).

Traditional psychoanalytic perceptions of depression also suggest that there is an impaired sense of well-being associated with experiencing stressful life events where loss is frequent. Feelings of helplessness and hopelessness can ensue, and the depressed person may wish to give up. Additionally, anger and aggression, along with guilt and self-blame, can also be factors in clinical depression that can result in feelings of being an unworthy and unlovable person.

Those psychodynamic formulations seem to make sense in predicting female depression, particularly when considering some of the prior research regarding demographic and sociocultural predictors. It would appear that traditional gender role socialization, experiences with racism and sexism, a greater likelihood of being poor, occupational segregation into low-paying and low-status jobs, as well as experiences with childhood and adult victimization, could all create conditions whereby feelings of loss and anger might manifest themselves as depression. It may be that the intractable nature of those life stressors could contribute to a pervasive sense of powerlessness, whereby the development of a depression-prone personality could be a logical outcome.

Despite the fact that belief in certain psychodynamic predictors of depression has had more heuristic value for guiding treatment than empirical verification, NIMH has sponsored research investigating the role of personality factors in predicting women's depression. By the use of a longitudinal twin study design exploring the relationship between personality and major depression, findings indicated that neuroticism was associated with risk for experiencing a depressive disorder (Kendler et al., 1993c). In an elaboration of that research, when neuroticism was placed within a structural equation model for women's depression, it was ranked below the stronger predictors of stressful life events and genetic predisposition (Kendler et al., 1993c).

Although consideration of personality type may have some impact in predicting depression in women; Jimenez (1997) suggests caution in the use of personality-type diagnostic categories when addressing issues of women's mental health. She believes that psychiatric conceptions of what constitutes a mental disorder in women have served to try to control women's behavior. For example, a prevailing psychopathology applied to women from Victorian times up until the last twenty years was hysteria, described as demanding and sexually manipulative behavior which exploited the traditional feminine role. Hysteria and depression frequently co-occurred. It was renamed histrionic personality disorder in DSM-III (APA, 1980) at the same time that borderline and dependent personality disorders were introduced. Both of those personality-type diagnoses, which can co-occur with depression, are overwhelmingly applied to women (Widiger & Weissman, 1991).

Criteria for borderline personality disorder include a pattern of unstable and intense interpersonal relationships, impulsiveness, inappropriately intense anger, and identity disturbance. In a study measuring clinicians' gender weighting of diagnostic criteria for borderline personality disorder, all the criteria for this diagnosis were judged to be feminine, except excessive anger. The findings of that study suggest that women who become as angry as men may be perceived as mentally disordered (Sprock, Blashfield, & Smith, 1990).

As the polar opposite of a borderline personality, dependent personality disorder embodies the qualities associated with a traditionally feminine gender role such as inability to make decisions without advice and reassurance, difficulty disagreeing with others because of fear of loss of support, and difficulty initiating projects due to a lack of self-confidence. A study of gender bias found that dependent personality disorder was rated as the most feminine of all the personality disorders (Sprock et al., 1990).

Borderline and dependent personality classifications may serve to pathologize women for both conforming to gender role expectations and for acting out against them. They seem to narrow the degrees of freedom for what constitutes appropriate female behavior, in addition to the potential harm created by stigmatizing women seeking help for dangerous metamessages about gender role and social norms; to that extent, their existence may exert some level of social control. In a perverse way, those personality classifications may add to the environmental risk factors for women and depression.

Consequently, despite traditional psychoanalytic concepts regarding the role of personality type in depression risk and some empirical evidence, when considering the impact of temperament in predicting women's depression, it is necessary to simultaneously consider the environmental factors implicated in the development of personality type. Clearly, limiting and discriminating life experiences could easily lead one to feel both helpless and angry.

FEMINIST PERSPECTIVES AND THEIR IMPLICATIONS FOR PRACTICE

Feminist Theories and Principles—An Overview

It is important to understand that there is no one universal feminist framework that can be used to inform practice; rather there are multiple perspectives (Wetzel, 1986; Bricker-Jenkins & Hooyman, 1984, 1986; Van Den Bergh & Cooper, 1986a, 1986b; Van Den Bergh, 1995; Saulnier, 1996). However, what does tie the varying feminist perspectives together is that they derive from a focus and analysis about the conditions of women's lives, which have engendered inequality and injustice. Feminist frameworks are extensive, spanning formulations developed from the early years of the feminist movement to the contemporary concerns of ecofeminism and global feminism. A thorough delineation of multiple feminist frameworks and how they can be employed within social work practice has been developed by Saulnier (1996); below is a brief summary of those feminist theories:

1. *Liberal feminism* is concerned with equal opportunity in employment and reproductive freedom.
2. *Radical feminism* is concerned with eliminating the patriarchal structure in the family and in social/economic systems.

3. *Socialist feminism* operates under the belief that women's oppression is derivative of economic class exploitation.

4. *Lesbian feminism* names heterosexism as the key oppressive system for women.

5. *Cultural feminism* discerns profound trait differences between women and men; female traits such as nurturing are considered superior to male traits.

6. *Ecofeminism* explores the similarities, overlaps, and interactions between the oppression of women and the exploitation of the environment.

7. *Womanism* looks at the interlocking oppressions of racism, sexism, and classism.

8. *Postmodern feminism* deconstructs global assumptions about women and attempts to reconstruct truths based on examining perceptions and standpoints of marginalized populations.

9. *Global feminism* examines cross-cultural oppressive practices affecting women and girls, including exploitation as cheap labor and enslavement within an international sex industry.

Despite the diversity within the theoretical formulations noted above, there are several common conceptual themes that can be gleaned from them, including 1) interconnectedness, 2) empowerment, 3) restructure/rename/reorder, and 4) valuing women's experiences. Each of those principles has some utility as a way to begin thinking about working with female clients who are depressed.

For example, by using an interconnectedness lens, it is possible to see that there can be a relationship between societal political/economic realities and one's sense of social class as a predictor, in that women who are poor are significantly more likely to express depressive symptoms than those with greater financial resources. Hence, it may be helpful to assist a client in seeing that her depression may, in part, be due to the endemic stresses associated with meager financial resources. Additionally, when working with women of color, it may be helpful to engage in a dialogue with them about the potential implications of experiencing racism and sexism as contributing to the circumstances leading them to seek help for their depressive symptoms.

Empowerment serves as both a process and a goal. In working with clients, it is important to work with their strengths, helping them to gain clarity on competencies, which they may have overlooked. This would seem to be particularly important with young women, who are at significant risk for depression and who may not have a sense of their capabilities. Another idea emanating from the female depression research that could be applicable to this empowerment principle would be assisting clients in identifying interpersonal and structural supports that they could use, particularly in time of stress. Helping clients to see their own competencies as well as opportunities to experience mutual aid and peer support can be a powerful antidote to depression.

All of the research related to the potentially detrimental effects of internalizing conventional gender role stereotypes underscores the need to assist clients in restructuring and renaming any negative self-concepts they may have internalized about being female. Dealing with a client's thought processes is an integral component of much psychodynamic work with depressed clients (Van Den Bergh, 1992). Hence, this principle underscores the importance of investigating the extent to which a client's depression may be related to the introjection of gender role stereotypes that are limiting or otherwise detrimental to her sense of efficacy and empowerment. Validating a client's own perception of what it means to be a wife, mother, partner, daughter, and so on can be an empowering experience, allowing someone to switch a self-perception of inadequacy into efficacy.

Utilizing the principle of valuing women's experiences would entail working with a client to utilize her own life experience as the basis for determining "truths" in the sense of what is important to her, what she values, the goals she has, and so on. This principle underscores the need to see that in every life experience, even those that are painful, something may have been gained or acquired. This is particularly important when working with clients who have experienced victimization. By no means is the goal to minimize the negative event, but to help uncover some strength or competency that may have developed by virtue of having had to cope with that life stress. For example, one's possible difficulty in trusting others, based on having been victimized, could be reframed as a healthy self-vigilance and caution, in order to determine over the course of time who is worthy of trust.

Feminist Direct Practice Approaches—A Critique

Considerable literature has been published defining how to do feminist therapy and what constitutes feminist social work. Much of this was articulated in a prior chapter addressing feminist approaches to treating depression, covered in a former edition of this book. The reader is referred there for a more elaborated discussion on the development of feminist practice principles (Van Den Bergh, 1992). In the section that follows, mention of feminist therapy methods will be made, along with critiques of them.

Feminist therapy has been defined as the incorporation of feminist values into a given psychotherapeutic process, be it cognitive behavioral, object relations, self-psychology, and so on. Consequently, feminist practice has not been focused on the utilization of particular methods, although group interventions were initially favored as valuable for establishing a sense of commonality as well as mutual aid and peer support for women experiencing a common problem, such as depression (Haussman & Halseth, 1983).

Perhaps the most defining characteristics of a feminist therapy approach include 1) employing a "political analysis" to whatever challenge may bring a client for services (the personal is political); 2) assuming that gender has played a key role in the development of the problem; 3) reconceptualizing power within the therapeutic relationship; and 4) supporting client individualization. Of those precepts, the most criticized, particularly in terms of its applicability to women of color, is the notion that the therapeutic relationship should be one of equals. In terms of how that principle becomes extrapolated to practice, Lundy (1993) noted that during the initial contact with a client, the worker should be explicit that 1) their relationship is collaborative and 2) the client is the expert, not the worker. Self-disclosure on the part of the therapist is also seen as a way of equalizing any power imbalance that may exist between the worker and client.

Critique of that relationship-equality theme has been offered by a group of feminist social workers employed by public mental health systems. They have noted that the notion of equality between the practitioner and client is a myth, particularly in public mental health services. Those practitioners saw the therapeutic relationship as the historical embodiment of differential power-knowledge relationships between the "haves" and "have-nots," which have a disciplinary quality of maintaining the status quo (Rossiter, de Boer, Narayan, Razack, Scollay, & Willette, 1998). Similarly, Baines (1997) refutes that the "equal" relationship precept is something that clients want, explaining that oftentimes women who are poor want the worker to use her "privilege" in order to leverage landlords, or others, to be responsive to her needs. Furthermore, the self-disclosure feminist value could actually highlight the differences between a worker and her client, if the latter perceives status differentials between them, thereby revictimizing poor women and women of color by reemphasizing the difficult to attain middle-class standard.

As an additional critique of those feminist therapy principles, when working with women of color, it is important to see that gender may not be the most potent contributing factor to the duress causing them to seek services (Lewis & Kissman, 1989). Rather, it is important to explore with a client her perception as to how gender is relevant within whatever scenario has caused her to seek services and to discern what meaning gender has within her cultural context (Brown, 1995). For women of color, race and gender oppression cannot be separated into distinct entities. Consequently, their "personal is political" analysis must include reflections on the multivariate, interlocking stressors that may contribute to their sense of subjective distress.

Furthermore, a focus on individuation does not correspond with the interdependent realities of many women who rely on extended family and other support networks for purposes of maximizing resources within oppressive environments. Additionally, focusing on the development of autonomy does not give credence to the deep meaning many women gain from being part of an ethnic or cultural community, which gives them a sense of history, legacy, and individual pride (Baines, 1997).

Themes that seem to run through the above critique of feminist practice principles are those of diversity and multiplicity. The notion of multiple realities and the need to be aware of them as sources of strength has evolved, in part, from the influence of postmodernism on feminist practice. In the next section, themes associated with a postmodern feminist perspective will be explored in terms of their relevance in guiding an intervention approach with depressed clients.

POSTMODERN FEMINIST PRINCIPLES AND PRACTICE APPROACHES

Postmodernism is a philosophical perspective about the creation of knowledge, and it has been exerting an impact on social work practice and research. Two premises of a postmodern approach have particular relevance for social work and for feminist practice. First, postmodernism espouses the theory that the development of knowledge is controlled by those who wield societal power; therefore, scientific truth may not be representative of what marginalized populations consider to be truth. Second, there is no one standard way of determining truth; rather, there are multiple realities that are dependent on the standpoint of the perceiver. To some extent, all of the activist social movements have been postmodern in the sense that they question what is "true," "right," and "normal" for those subjugated within society, such as ethnic minorities, women, gays/lesbians, those differently abled, and so on.

A paradox exists in applying postmodern precepts to feminism, since to some extent postmodernism would suggest that it is futile to define a feminist practice approach. This is because 1) there is no one feminism and 2) there is no one unitary experience of being female. An interesting literature has developed surrounding the meld of postmodern feminist theory and social work practice (see, for example, Sands & Nuccio, 1992; Gross, 1998a, 1998b; East, 1998; Laird, 1995a). Despite the ostensible contradiction of generating a postmodern feminist perspective; there have been efforts to define how those two constructs can coexist in a way to inform a particular approach to practice. For example, Laird (1995a) suggests that through a postmodern feminist treatment approach client problems can be seen as linguistically created stories and problem-saturated narratives that are drawn from dominant societal discourse replete with beliefs that are pejorative to women, ethnic minorities, the poor, and so on. Consequently, one can see client interventions as political acts that encourage clients to challenge the status quo in their thinking and to make changes in their personal lives, which serve to restructure conventional ways of doing things (Laird, 1995b). By reviewing the literature that seeks to define a postmodern feminist practice approach, several themes seem to be particularly relevant as guideposts for thinking about how to work with depressed clients.

Deconstruction

A postmodern strategy for determining truth is to deconstruct narrative, or text, in order to determine its underlying assumptions. As a process it allows for recognizing biases and, having done so, potentially reconstructing a narrative to include perspectives previously marginalized. Questions that could be used in the process of deconstruction might include 1) What are the assumptions? 2) What are the biases? 3) Who is saying this truth? 4) What is left out? and 5) What is your truth?

For example, let us consider the situation of a single mother who presents with depressed symptoms and indicates she is seeking help because of concern that she is not doing a good job parenting her 11-year-old son. In the course of exploring the challenge with her, she indicates concern about her son's development into puberty and fears he will become a "momma's boy" because there is no man in the family. Using a postmodern feminist perspective, it seems plausible that the client has internalized negative valuations about women as "less than" and consequently worries her son may become defective without the influence of a male parent. It is also likely that she has internalized some sexist and heterosexist assumptions that "mommas' boys" may become gay men. Consequently, by deconstructing the dominant societal discourse within this client's narrative around gender issues, it is then possible to reconstruct a new story focusing on both her strengths and those of her son in order to help her feel comfortable about both her parenting experiences and her son's predictable adolescent development.

Similarly, a woman who is an adult incest survivor may present with depressed symptoms concerning a sense of powerlessness regarding establishing a life separate from an abusive partner. Deconstructing being an incest survivor might mean helping her to see that sexist assumptions are, in part, responsible for beliefs holding women responsible for, and therefore deserving of, their victimization. By exposing that potentially internalizing assumption, it is then possible to assist the client in reconstructing a sense of her strengths and competencies based on her actual lived experiences. For example, helping the client to focus on the competencies she has demonstrated through advocating for her children with teachers, her willingness to seek additional training or education, and the actions she has taken to defend her children against her partner's anger would all allow the client to "restory" her personal narrative as a victor, not a victim.

The above examples seek to demonstrate how engaging in a deconstruction process with clients could assist them in questioning core beliefs potentially interfering with their sense of self and contributing to feelings of helplessness or hopelessness. By then embarking on a reconstruction process emphasizing their strengths and competencies acquired through accrued life experiences, a postmodern feminist approach to helping depressed clients would be employed.

Multiple Discourses

This postmodern precept exhorts that there are multiple truths and types of knowledge, which have given rise to the concept of a feminist standpoint and are complementary to the notion of cultural competence.

Standpoint perspectives are a kind of enlightened consciousness about 1) an individual's location in the social structure and 2) how that location impacts one's learned experience (Swigonski, 1993, 1994). Consequently, one's standpoint emerges from a critical consciousness about how gender, color, age, social class, sexual orientation, and so on interact to affect one's quality of life.

As a complement to a standpoint perspective, practitioners who have written on feminist culturally sensitive or competent treatment indicate that for women of color, race and gender oppression cannot be separated into distinct entities and that subjective experiences of distress (depression or anxiety) emanate from multivariate interlocking stressors (Lewis & Kissman, 1989; Greene, 1994; Suarez, Lewis, & Clark, 1995; Brown, 1995; Freeman, 1994). Consequently, a culturally literate and antiracist feminist therapist must have an understanding of the role of multiple identities and oppressions in the client's perception of self and her surroundings, as well as a willingness to acquire familiarity with a client's cultural/ethnic heritage and the role of "isms" (racism, sexism, etc.) in affecting the client's quality of life. In other words, a practitioner must have an understanding of the client's standpoint as it pertains to her depression and the potential role of stressors associated with poverty, racism, and sexism in contributing to her subjective distress.

For example, in working from a feminist culturally sensitive standpoint with clients from Hispanic and Latino backgrounds, Comas-Diaz (1988) indicates that practitioners must first understand that in traditional Hispanic cultures there is not necessarily a differentiation between physical and emotional concerns; therefore, strong emotions are believed to cause physical illness. Consequently, Hispanic/Latina women could report somatic complaints as a means of expressing their needs and thereby obtaining support from others. Additionally, it may be important to determine the potential impact of cultural gender roles on the client's challenge, such as concepts of *marianismo* (female powerlessness) and *hembrismo* (female powerfulness), as potentially important in contributing to whatever conflict a client may be having. Additionally, a practitioner should discern the extent to which a client's level of acculturation may be contributing to her distress. On the one hand, a client could be culturally amphibious (i.e., equally able to live in Hispanic as well as in US culture), or, on the other hand, she may be culturally schizophrenic (some degree of acculturation with confusion created by conflicting values), which could create both anxiety and loss.

For example, a highly educated professional Latina could experience depression and anxiety in attempting to reconcile her desire not to marry and start a family with her family of origin's belief that it is most important for her to be a wife and mother. A culturally sensitive feminist practitioner would assist the client in acknowledging this cultural clash and to work with her to arrive at some synthesis of personal needs and cultural loyalty.

Freeman (1994) suggests, in working with African-American women, that assisting clients with an enhanced sense of their Afrocentric competencies can be a self-healing process, which may be necessary for clients who have lost a sense of hope and belief in themselves through racism and sexism. She defines the process of building Afrocentric competence as composed of three entities: 1) helping clients to clarify their ethnic self-concept as African-American women, 2) assisting them in developing an ethnic self-esteem by pursuing perceptions of themselves and their ethnic groups, and 3) aiding clients in identifying and developing ethnic competencies in terms of the abilities and resources they could utilize for individual and community survival. Examples of cultural competencies that African-American women could possess or develop include 1) using oral traditions for passing on beliefs and traditions, 2) negotiating equal status between themselves and men, 3) restorying self-worth to generate alternative positive interpretations of potentially negative events, and 4) applying gender and cultural centrality when making life decisions, that is, emphasizing the importance of kinship, family, and clan.

Synthesizing these culturally sensitive standpoints means that when working with women of color it is important to engage in a cultural deconstruction that examines the potential role of the multiple stressors of race, class, and gender realities in contributing to the client's subjective distress. However, it is equally important to underscore gender, ethnic, and class strengths with which the client already identifies in order to reconstruct a personal perspective and environmental context that is empowering. For example, in working with a woman who is a member of an ethnic minority and who is experiencing frustration and disappointment in her role supervising a work unit primarily composed of majority-culture males, it would be important to validate her experiences of racism and sexism while also taking inventory of the gender and cultural strengths she demonstrated in her management role. Also, it would be extremely appropriate to provide her with information about community groups of other professional women of color, with whom she could seek mutual aid and peer support.

Subjectivity

Intimately connected with the themes of deconstruction and multiple discourse, the postmodern theme of subjectivity suggests that an individual's sense of self is not static; rather, it changes contextually through dialogue and interaction with others. Persons exploited and marginalized can develop a subjective sense of self whereby their inherent strengths and capabilities can become clouded by having internalized racism, sexism, classism, and so on, leading to states of despair, shame, and hopelessness. The antidote to experiencing self-denigration is what hooks (1989) calls self-recovery, a process of reuniting fragments of one's identity and recovering aspects of individual and collective history that can be used in the service of personal empowerment. Searching out one's gender's cultural history can allow for knowing the voices from the past (hooks, 1989).

All of the civil rights activist movements and the women's movement have focused on researching and discovering contributions of marginalized populations to society, as well as highlighting heroines and heroes to be emulated as role models. Hence, the postmodern subjectivity premise delineates that one can be continuously self-empowering by being engaged in a developmental process of identity construction. The feminist component of this postmodern subjectivity principle is that personal change is the starting point for structural change.

The significance of this theme in working with women who are depressed is that it encourages collaboration with them to develop a dynamic sense of what it means for them to be women. Since research on women and depression has suggested that depression may lessen over the course of the life cycle, it suggests the merit of encouraging women to see that they do not have to define themselves by a culturally dictated script; therefore, there is no one way that they are supposed to be. For example, it is curious that in Asian cultures, there are fewer reported symptoms related to becoming menopausal than is the case for women in the United States. Age is a more venerated life stage in Asian culture, whereas in the United States a premium is placed on youthfulness. For women who are menopausal and may be experiencing that transition as a crisis, it would be important to help them reflect on their own strengths and competencies, while underscoring that in many cultures, entering midlife is honored as a state of wisdom and freedom.

Just as it is necessary to acknowledge that clients' sense of self and truth are subjective, fluid, and contextually based, it is also important to acknowledge that engaging in practice, be it clinical, organizational, or research oriented, is an intersubjective process. Both the practitioner and the client are affected by the exchange of feelings and ideas; knowledge is cocreated within the treatment process through dialogue and collaboration. Consequently, as a practitioner it is important to ask the following questions:

1. How is this work making a difference within the client and within myself?
2. What is the impact of our dialogue/collaboration on what we seek to know?
3. What are we coming to mutually understand?

TOWARD A POSTMODERN FEMINIST APPROACH WITH DEPRESSED CLIENTS

Considering the themes of deconstruction, multiple discourse, and subjectivity leads toward suggesting the following as precepts that could inform one's practice approach:

1. Restory
2. Restructure
3. Recover

These "3Rs" might be employed with clients who are depressed, in particular with women, in the following way: First, it would be important for the practitioner to be listening for any culturally associated belief systems that a client may expose in her description of the presenting problems that could be limiting or devaluing. By using deconstruction questions, one goal might be for the client to challenge erroneous, outdated, or prejudicial assumptions, similar to what would occur within a cognitive therapy approach aimed at uncovering cognitive distortions. Additionally, the practitioners would need to listen for personal and cultural strengths as well as competencies and bring them from the margin of the client's consciousness to center view. In determining a path to the solution, a client would be encouraged to restory her personal narrative to define goals that are based on her perception of what she wants, not what may be others' goals or what may be considered the "right" thing for her to do based on cultural stereotypes. An assessment of personal, interpersonal, cultural, and environmental strengths would be undertaken; when appropriate, information and resources could be offered as augmentative to extant competencies and opportunities.

Working within a collaborative relationship, an assumption would exist that both the client and practitioner possess expert knowledge that could be utilized to achieve the therapeutic goals. The client would serve as the expert in formulating a standpoint regarding her perceptions of the factors that contribute to her depression, as well as resources within herself and the environment that might be utilized in assisting her in feeling better. The practitioner would be seen as having expertise in facilitating the client's empowerment process and in possibly offering suggestions regarding the appropriateness of a psychopharmacologic evaluation or in providing other information and referral resources. Explicit within the working relationship would be the assumption that undertaking change is necessary in order for the client to feel better and that such action might challenge the status quo within her immediate environment as well as in the broader sociocultural context.

Another explicit understanding regarding the client's change process would be that there is not a single, static standard toward which she should strive. Rather, a client would be encouraged to see her healing process as a "work in progress," and, as such, permission would be afforded to engage in a dynamic, evolving and developmental endeavor of self-definition and self-recovery. To that extent, an evaluation of practice focus would be on progress, not perfection, and the "right" way to be might be defined as that which, contextually, offers her a sense of meaning, purpose, and empowerment. Inherent within this belief would be the acknowledgment that a client's sense of self is subject to change based on differing life experiences and needs. Therefore, one could be encouraged to embrace life's developmental changes and crises as opportunities to acquire even more understanding about the breadth of one's abilities, interests, and priorities. To be both patient and compassionate with oneself would be an important tenet of the self-recovery process.

The essence, then, of a postmodern feminist approach to practice would be to assist each client in uncovering her uniqueness, her connectedness, and her strengths, in order to give voice to her truths and passion to her pursuits.

CHAPTER 9

Behavior Analysis and Therapy for Persons with Phobias

Bruce Thyer

In this chapter, Thyer discusses anxiety disorders and shows how to use exposure therapy with persons who are experiencing a specific phobia. This chapter reflects many of the components of a structured intervention, beginning with the need for an accurate assessment. Thyer shows how to make assessments based on 1) observable behavior, 2) client self-report, and 3) physiological measures through the use of well-defined problems. Each of these assessments is considered in terms of its utility in evaluating change in the person with the phobia over the course of treatment. Moreover, the assessments make it possible to isolate what caused the person to experience anxiety, which facilitates fitting the specific form of treatment to the client's problem. Thyer's discussion of exposure therapy also demonstrates client preparation, well-explicated components of the intervention (including homework), and how to evaluate the client's change.

INTRODUCTION

This chapter will review the current state of evidence-based psychosocial treatments for clients who suffer from one of two disorders, specific phobias or social phobias. Omitted from consideration will be topographically similar problems such as panic disorder, agoraphobia, posttraumatic stress disorder, obsessive compulsive disorder, and other conditions generally categorized as anxiety-related disorders.

At present, the most widely used nosological system for disorders of behavior, affect, or cognition is called the *Diagnostic and Statistic Manual of Mental Disorders* (DSM; American Psychiatric Association, 1994). Now in its fourth edition, the DSM attempts to distinguish various psychosocial problems experienced by individuals using supposedly specific criteria, the presence, absence, or magnitude of which can be reliably judged. It accomplishes this with varying degrees of success, depending on the disorder in question. Fortunately, the criteria for specific and social phobias are not difficult to discriminate. Most simply put, a "**specific phobia** is characterized by clinically significant anxiety provoked by exposure to a specific feared object or situation, often leading to avoidance behavior," and a "**social phobia** is characterized by clinically significant anxiety provoked by exposure to certain types of social or performance situations, often leading to avoidance behavior" (American Psychiatric Association, 1994, p. 393, boldface in original).

TABLE 9-1   Subtypes of Specific and Social Phobias

Phobia Subtypes	Selected Examples
Specific	
Animal type	Dogs, cats, insects, snakes, birds
Natural environment	Heights, water, thunderstorms
Blood-injection-injury	Sight of blood, seeing or receiving injections, invasive medical procedures, trauma-related sounds (e.g., sirens, cries of pain)
Situational	Flying, driving, bridges, closets, elevators
Other	Choking, fear of vomiting
Social	
Generalized	Fearful of most social situations

Specific phobias (SPPs) have various subtypes related to the nature of the anxiety-evoking stimulus (AES), and these are outlined in Table 9-1, along with some examples. Social phobias (SOPs) typically relate to situations wherein the individual is exposed to the scrutiny of others and she/he is afraid of acting in a manner that will provoke criticism or ridicule from others, leading to personal embarrassment or humiliation. Typical AESs for SOPs include public speaking, musical or theatrical performances, eating in public, using public lavatories (when other people are present), parties, and other social settings. SOPs have only one possible specifier, called "generalized," which is used to distinguish individuals with fairly specific social anxieties (undertaking a musical performance) from those with more pervasive AESs, situations often encountered in everyday life, such as conversations with attractive individuals or discussions with authority figures (hence the term generalized). The dividing line separating a discrete SOP from a generalized one is a matter of clinical judgment, as opposed to explicit quantitative criteria, but the DSM criteria in this case do seem to be fairly reliable (see Mannuzza, Scheier, Chapman, & Liebowitz, 1995).

It is important to note that for both SPPs and SOPs additional diagnostic criteria include the requirement that the individual recognize the unreasonable nature of his/her fears, that if the AES cannot be avoided then it is endured with intense distress, and that the problem creates problems in one's normal psychosocial functioning.

SPPs and SOPs can be quite handicapping. Fear in circumstances that pervade one's everyday life can render daily existence an absolute misery, leading to the possible development of other disorders, such as severe depression or alcohol abuse (see Thyer, Parrish, et al., 1986). Rarely, individuals with severe phobic disorders have been known to resort to suicide (Pegeron, Curtis, & Thyer, 1986). In no way should these conditions be considered trivial.

Interestingly, SPPs and SOPs are among the most common so-called mental disorders in the contemporary United States. According to the results of the national epidemiological catchment area study (Robins & Regier, 1991), which remains the most comprehensive community-based study of mental disorders ever undertaken, the one-month, one-year, and lifetime prevalence of phobic disorders are almost 7 percent, 10 percent, and 14 percent, respectively. This latter figure is roughly equivalent to the lifetime prevalence of alcohol abuse and almost double that of affective disorders. The phobic disorders are more common among black and Hispanic individuals compared with whites and more common among women compared with men.

I would like to point out that my use of the criteria found in the DSM does not imply that I endorse the view that the conditions contained therein are "things" or "real entities." Since I do not believe in the existence of the mind, I am very dubious about the whole concept of mental disorders. These constellations of associated signs and symptoms are more accurately construed as disorders of behavior, affect, or intellect, and very few of the conditions found in the DSM have been shown to be independent entities (e.g., mental retardation secondary to Down syndrome). Unless a compellingly clear biological etiology is established for a DSM-defined disorder, to view it as a thing apart from the behaviors that define it constitutes the logical errors of reification and circular reasoning.

PROBLEM IDENTIFICATION

The clinical interview conducted by a knowledgeable social worker, psychologist, or other mental health professional remains the mainstay of the diagnostic process. Because the criteria are generally easy to apply, it is usually not necessary to employ a comprehensive structured clinical interview such as the Structured Clinical Interview for the DSM-IV (SCID; First, Gibbon, Williams, & Spitzer, 1997). However, use of the SCID can be an excellent training tool for the novice clinician or for the experienced practitioner otherwise unfamiliar with the DSM criteria for the anxiety disorders.

A structured clinical interview that is specifically focused on the differential diagnosis of anxiety disorders is known as the Anxiety Disorders Interview Schedule (ADIS; DiNardo, Mora, Barlow, & Rapee, 1993). A child version of the ADIS is also available (Silverman & Nelles, 1988), and the ADIS is much less cumbersome (i.e., less boring for practitioner and client and takes less time) than the SCID, although at the expense of comprehensive coverage of *all* the potential diagnoses found in the DSM.

The SCID and the ADIS are also a systematic way to exclude potential differential diagnoses and may be particularly indicated for use with clients who present with a complex clinical picture or with multiple diagnoses. It is not uncommon for clients in the early stages of what will eventually emerge as panic disorder with agoraphobia (PDA) to present with circumscribed fears that resemble SPPs (e.g., driving, shopping, going to the barber, etc.). However, most apparent instances of SPP can be readily differentiated from PDA via a careful history taking related to the experience of spontaneous panic attacks. The compelling association between the evoked nature of phobic anxiety stands in marked contrast to the apparently unprovoked experience of panic, which does bear considerable subjective resemblance to phobic anxiety (Thyer & Himle, 1987).

Few biological disorders can be mistaken for SPP or SOP, and certainly the developmental status of the client needs to be taken into account. Irrational fears, sometimes quite marked, are common in childhood (and to a lesser extent in adolescence). For the most part, these are transient and only troubling to a minor extent. A formal diagnosis of SPP or SOP is not warranted unless the child's social, school, or occupational functioning is significantly impaired. To make a diagnosis of SOP with clients under the age of 18, the impairment has to have been present for at least six months.

ASSESSMENT AND MONITORING

Once the diagnosis of SPP or SOP has been made, and an agreement has been entered into with the client to undertake treatment, additional efforts should be made to assess problem severity and client functioning in a quantitative manner and to repeat these assessments on a number of occasions over the course of intervention. If these assessments can be repeated a few times prior to beginning treatment, it will be so much the better.

The clinician's assessment of client functioning related to a phobic disorder can only involve three approaches to gathering data: client self-reports, the observations of others or direct observations, and selected physiological indices of stress (Hudson & Thyer, 1987). Fortunately each of these areas is fairly well developed in terms of client-friendly and practical approaches to measurement, and a few of the more useful ones, to be viewed as adjuncts to the clinical interview, will be reviewed below.

SELF-REPORT ASSESSMENT METHODS

The value of both projective (e.g., Rorschach Test, Thematic Apperception Test, Sentence Completion Test, etc.) and generalized objective (e.g., MMPI, Brief Symptom Inventory) tests is quite low, and these measures are not recommended when initially assessing the presumptively phobic client or for monitoring the outcomes of treatment. In addition, overall structured measures of client stress and discomfort in life are not usually of use in treating the phobic individual, as opposed to some more preferable highly focused indicators. However, when an overall indicator of anxiety is desirable, the Clinical Anxiety Scale (CAS; Westhuis & Thyer, 1989) is a rapid assessment instrument (RAI) that is easy for clients to understand and for practitioners to score and interpret. Generally, individuals meeting the DSM criteria for an anxiety score greater than 30, and those who are not clinically anxious score less than 30. A copy of the CAS appears in Figure 9-1, and is meant to illustrate one example of a contemporary RAI that can be used in practice. By having the client complete the CAS several times before and during intervention, the practitioner has a credible quantitative indicator of overall anxiousness that can be used to supplement one's clinical judgments regarding response to treatment. Additional information on the CAS can be found in Fischer and Corcoran (1994, pp. 122–123).

However, of greater value are more specific RAIs that have been tailor made for specific subtypes of phobic disorders. A number of these RAIs are listed in Table 9-2. With the advent of such focused measures, the usefulness of more global indices of fearfulness has substantially diminished. It should be emphasized that the field is rapidly progressing, and new RAIs pertaining to SPPs and SOPs make their appearance almost monthly. The clinician of the new millennium can be expected to access comprehensive computerized journal and book databases (PsychINFO is currently the best such resource) regularly to obtain the latest information on assessment and treatment approaches, not just for the phobic disorders, but for all psychosocial problems.

Behavioral Observations

Structured behavioral observations of client reactions while undergoing exposure to AESs can be a very valuable method of clinical assessment. Given that avoidance behavior is one of the defining criteria for the diagnosis of SSP or SOP, attempting to evaluate a presumptively phobic individual without observing his or her behavior would seem to be an incomplete form of assessment. A corollary of this position is that behavioral observations should take place under conditions closely resembling those encountered by the client in real life, as opposed to artificially contrived circumstances arranged by the therapist. This is not always logically feasible or acceptable to the client, so analog behavioral assessments may be used instead.

A behavioral approach test (BAT) is one such structured method of assessing phobic behavior. For example, a client meeting the criteria for an SPP centered around a fear of dogs may be asked (with informed consent, of course) to confront a small dog tied to a secure leash about twenty feet away. From twenty feet, the client is asked to step closer and closer, until he or she absolutely refuses to draw nearer. At each distance (e.g., twenty feet, eighteen feet, fifteen feet, etc.) the social worker asks the client to self rate their subjective anxiety on a zero (no fear) to 100 scale (as fearful as one can imagine being) and record these subjective units of distress (SUDS) ratings for each increment of distance. More sophisticated BATs can also make use of simple heart-rate monitors, clip-on devices that attach to the client's finger and dis-

FIGURE 9-1   The Clinical Anxiety Scale

CLINICAL ANXIETY SCALE (CAS)

Name: _____   Today's Date: _____

This questionnaire is designed to measure how much anxiety you are currently feeling. It is not a test, so there are no wrong or right answers. Answer each item as carefully and as accurately as you can by placing a number beside each one as follows:

> 1 = Rarely or none of the time
> 2 = A little of the time
> 3 = Some of the time
> 4 = A good part of the time
> 5 = Most or all of the time

---

1. I feel calm. _____
2. I feel tense. _____
3. I feel suddenly scared for no reason. _____
4. I feel nervous. _____
5. I use tranquilizers or antidepressants to cope with my anxiety. _____
6. I feel confident about the future. _____
7. I am free from senseless or unpleasant thoughts. _____
8. I feel afraid to go out of my house alone. _____
9. I feel relaxed and in control of myself. _____
10. I have spells of terror or panic. _____
11. I feel afraid in open spaces or in the streets. _____
12. I feel afraid I will faint in public. _____
13. I am uncomfortable traveling on buses, subways, or trains. _____
14. I feel nervousness or shakiness inside. _____
15. I feel comfortable in crowds, such as shopping or at a movie. _____
16. I feel comfortable when I am left alone. _____
17. I feel afraid without good reason. _____
18. Due to my fears, I unreasonably avoid certain animals, objects, or situations. _____
19. I get upset easily or feel panicky unexpectedly. _____
20. My hands, arms, or legs shake and tremble. _____
21. Due to my fears, I avoid social situations whenever possible. _____
22. I experience sudden attacks of panic that catch me by surprise. _____
23. I feel generally anxious. _____
24. I am bothered by dizzy spells. _____
25. Due to my fears, I avoid being alone whenever possible. _____

NOTE: Copies of the CAS and scoring instructions are available from the Walmyr Publishing Company, POB 6229, Tallahassee, FL 32314-6229.

TABLE 9-2 Examples of Specialized RAIs Used in Treating Phobic Clients

Phobia	Citation to Specialized RAI
Specfic	
Driving	Ehlers, Hofman, Herda, & Roth (1994)
Flying	Howard, Shane, & Clark (1983)
Heights	Baker, Cohen, & Saunders (1973)
Spiders	Muris, Merckelbach, Holdrinet, & Sijsenaar (1998)
Dental treatment	Stouthard et al. (1995)
Social	
Performance anxiety questionnaire	Cox & Kenardy (1993)
Mathematics anxiety	Richardson & Suinn (1972)
Test anxiety	Spielberger (1977)
Social phobia	Safren, Turk, & Heimberg (1998)
	Leary & Kowalski (1993)
	Beidel, Turner, & Marns (1995)
	La Greca & Stone (1993)
	Davidson, DeVeaugh-Geiss, & Tupler (1997)

play his or her heart rate. These are inexpensive and readily available at sporting goods stores. Heart rate can be recorded concurrently with the client's subjective quantitative ratings (0 to 100) of fear. Obviously, a more phobic individual will not come as close to the dog, will report higher levels of fear, and have higher heart rates at each step along the way. As treatment progresses, this BAT can be repeated to ascertain in a quantitative manner if the client is improving and so augment one's clinical judgments and observations.

BATs for some AESs are relatively easy to contrive, whereas the arrangement of other AESs (e.g., thunderstorms, fear of vomiting) require considerable ingenuity on the part of the therapist. For example, audio or videotape recordings of difficult to recreate events (e.g., thunderstorms, sight of blood) may be a useful substitute. Of course, if such assessments are simply impractical, then treatment can proceed in their absence.

SOP-related AESs can be particularly difficult to contrive, however, a growing empirical literature addresses this issue, and some practical standardized behavioral assessment measures are being developed. For example, the therapist can arrange for the socially phobic client to have a conversation in the consulting room with the type of individual who would normally be avoided by the client (for example, an attractive member of the opposite sex in the case of a dysfunctionally shy individual). The author has accompanied some social phobics (again with informed consent) into real-life situations such as restaurants, bars, and lavatories for the purposes of surreptitiously (with respect to bystanders) observing their reactions in the circumstances that evoked severe fear.

The simulated social interaction test (Mersch, Breukers, & Emmelkamp, 1992) is one office-based SOP equivalent to a standardized BAT used in instances of SOPs. Asking public-speaking phobics to deliver brief talks in front of small audiences and videotaping their performance can be a very useful form of behavioral assessment, particularly as the tapes can be reviewed with the client and used to help point out his or her positive elements, and cue him or her into awareness of subtle indicators of fear. This can introduce the crucial element of skills building into treatment and involve coaching and specific training exercises to improve one's oral delivery. It can also be extremely validating as a part of the termination process for a successfully treated client to compare videotapes of his or her before and after public-speaking performance.

Physiological Measures

Almost all phobic clients display some type of excessive physiological arousal when they confront their unique AESs. This may involve elevations in heart rate, pulse, and blood pressure, perspiration, tremor, and problems with breathing, as well as more subtle responses, such as profound changes in hormone levels, all in preparation for the so-called fight or flight response. Particularly severe phobics may also experience such reactions not only when actually confronting their AES, but also when they are anticipating such confrontation (as in the public-speaking phobic who has to give a speech the following day or a test-phobic student facing an end-of-semester examination). Fairly constant anticipatory anxiety of this nature can be quite debilitating over time, perhaps to the bewilderment of the client's family and friends who can see nothing obviously wrong.

In routine clinical practice the therapist will rarely assess physiological responses of clients, except perhaps in specialized treatment clinics. One notable exception is the measurement of heart rate, readily conducted via wrist palpation or using the fingertip clip-on monitor mentioned above. Heart rate is a good general measure of physiological arousal, and a true measure of clinical success can be obtained not by simply having the client say that he or she feels much better, but by corroborating such self-reports with improvements in standardized RAIs relevant to their phobic disorder, by demonstrable reductions in avoidance behavior and other overt indicators of fear ascertained via approach tests or simulated interactions, and by the absence of heart-rate elevations during exposure to formerly feared situations. Such a clinical outcome is a truer appraisal of where the client is in his or her therapy than is assessment conducted via conversations in the consulting room alone.

BEHAVIOR ANALYSIS AND THERAPY

At present, the psychosocial treatment of choice for clients meeting the DSM criteria for SSPs or SOPs is the behavioral approach called exposure therapy (ET). A very large number (too many to recount in this chapter) of conventional and meta-analytic reviews of the literature have concluded that ET conducted in real-life settings produces clinically meaningful, rapid, and long-term positive improvements for most clients with SPP or SOP (e.g., Donohue, Van Hasselt, & Hersen, 1994; Feske & Chambless, 1995; Taylor, 1996; Ost, Mavissakalian, & Prien, 1998). Almost all so-called cognitive behavioral therapies include extensive elements of therapist-assisted or self-conducted real-life exposure to AESs, and there is little evidence that solely office-based verbal psychotherapy of any variety or theoretical orientation is effective in helping phobic clients. There is considerable evidence that treatment with psychotropic medications can exert a palliative influence for SOP, but the effects are transient, typically lasting only as long as the client remains on the medication regimen. However, "pharmacological treatments have not proven effective for specific phobias" (Roy-Byrne & Cowly, 1998, p. 328), and their use is best avoided.

There are a number of variations of conventional ET that have appeared in the practice literature in the past few years, and among the most widely reported is the technique labeled eye-movement desensitization and reprocessing. Initially advocated as a treatment for posttraumatic stress disorder, it has recently been tested with specific phobics. The results have been largely negative (Bates, McGlynn, Montgomery, & Mattke, 1966; Muris, Merckelbach, Holdrinet, & Sijsenaar, 1998), and at present the procedure cannot be considered as a first-choice treatment for SPPs or SOPs. Similar caveats exist for procedures involving hypnosis or so-called thought field therapy. Below I describe how to undertake a course of ET with phobic clients.

CLIENT PREPARATION

Initially, client education about the nature and treatment of phobic disorders takes place through one-to-one instruction in the consulting room. Clients are informed that the onset of the majority of phobic disorders is associated with one or more traumatic experiences with the animals, objects, or situations the person has come to fear. Simply put, a large proportion of dog phobics have had a frightening experience with dogs; perhaps they have been bitten or knocked down (see, for example, Thyer, 1981). Many driving phobics develop their fears following an automobile accident. Large-scale studies involving recall interviews with clinical phobics reveal that over half of these individuals report such a traumatic onset to their phobia (Ost & Hugdahl, 1981).

Although many phobics have had a direct traumatic experience with the AES that initiated the onset of their fears, another large proportion has had an indirect or vicarious traumatic experience. Examples include seeing a childhood companion being severely bitten by a dog, witnessing a car accident, or viewing a frightening movie involving snakes or insects. Role modeling on the part of parents or siblings may also play a part in the etiology of some phobias. If a child witnesses a significant other displaying fear of certain animals or objects or when in selected situations, it is not uncommon for that child to acquire similar phobic behavior and associated emotions.

The above data are consistent with the hypothesis that a large proportion of clinical phobias are etiologically related to the processes of respondent (i.e., Pavlovian) learning. This view is corroborated by experimental laboratory-based demonstrations of the induction of conditioned fearlike reactions in humans (Malloy & Levis, 1988).

Once a conditioned fear reaction is established, a second learning process may account for the well-known persistence of phobias, that is, their resistance to apparent spontaneous remission (at least among adults). A phobic who is inadvertently or intentionally exposed to his or her AES generally displays a fairly consistent constellation of signs and symptoms. Efforts to escape the situation almost always occur, as do elevations in heart rate, respiration, blood pressure, and certain hormones, and the individual experiences the subjective sense of severe fear. If these efforts to escape or avoid the AES are successful, the individual's avoidance behavior is negatively reinforced, one of the fundamental learning processes associated with operant conditioning. If being in the presence of a phobic stimulus generates aversive internal states (i.e., fear, anxiety, agitation, etc.), then any action that successfully ameliorates such states (i.e., helps the person calm down) is likely to be strengthened.

You should explain to your client that, like most phobics, he or she probably has an extensive history of coming into contact with the AES, becoming frightened, and then fleeing the situation as quickly as possible. Each act of successful flight or avoidance in effect terminates the aversive situation and hence strengthens avoidance and escape behaviors. Over time, phobic escape and avoidance become more and more likely. This process probably accounts for the persistence of phobias over time. Functional equivalents to overt escape from a phobic situation may include the use of sedative drugs such as alcohol or benzodiazepines, which may account for abuse of these agents by the clinically anxious (Thyer, Parrish, et al., 1986). The mechanism of positive reinforcement, in which there is a significant payoff for the display of phobic behavior for some individuals, may also be at work; this, either intentionally or inadvertently, may help to maintain dysfunctional fears. For example, a phobic family member may find that his or her excessive display of fear and the corresponding demands made upon the family are useful in gaining attention and solicitous concern.

You should emphasize to your client that there is no such thing as a "phobic personality," that the existence of a phobia in no way implies the presence of deep-seated psychological problems, and that "crazy" phobias are not precursors of insanity. You may want to read selected portions of the DSM to your clients to further illustrate that the problems they are experiencing are recognized and understood. A major point to be driven home throughout all these efforts at client preparation is that phobic clients are in no way responsible or to blame for their fears and that they or their families could have done little up to this point to help them overcome their phobias.

You may wish to recommend to phobic clients some of the self-help books on understanding and overcoming phobias. *Living with Fear* (Marks, 1978) is among the best. Virtually every phobic client can identify with one of the case studies in this book, which is empirically based yet packed with clinical anecdotes. Such books reinforce for clients the fact that that they are not alone in suffering from phobias and that help in the form of behavior analysis and treatment is extremely effective in alleviating most instances of pathological fear. It is best for clients to read such materials at home, where they may be assimilated at leisure, and to jot down any questions generated by their reading for discussion with the therapist.

Client preparation continues by bringing up the subject of treatment itself, which is addressed in the self-help books. The basic principle on which virtually all effective treatments for phobias are based is therapeutic exposure, or programmed confrontation. To the extent that the phobia truly is an irrational response and that there is little or no realistic element of danger involved in confronting the AES (which is by definition the case in phobias), ET is the treatment of first choice, both in terms of clinical effectiveness as demonstrated by hundreds of controlled experimental studies, and in terms of client acceptability.

ET involves arranging for clients to gradually confront aspects of their phobic stimuli in a controlled manner. This should be undertaken in real life as much as possible, as opposed to exposure in fantasy. Most clients have had a number of episodes of unavoidable confrontation with their AES through the years and may object that such experiences simply exacerbate the problem. Upon inquiry, however, it will almost inevitably be revealed that such exposure trials were of relatively brief duration and that when these episodes were terminated clients were still extremely fearful. Common examples might be the public-speaking phobic who can recall having to "tough out" a required public talk in a college class, or the flying phobic who was forced to endure a two-hour flight in order to attend a funeral. You should agree that brief periods of exposure or confrontation that terminate when the client is still agitated are not productive but clearly differentiate such experiences from the therapeutic procedure that you propose.

In ET you and the client plan a series of potentially frightening confrontations with the client's phobic animal, object, or situation, ranging from very mildly anxiety-provoking situations to those that the client believes would be absolutely terrifying. The client is asked to take one of the more frightening situations and project what would happen if he or she were somehow forced to confront that situation. Say, for example, that a client with a dog phobia states that being in a room with a German shepherd would be one of the most awful experiences he or she could imagine. The social worker–client dialog might go like this:

> Social Worker: All right, now tell me, what do you think would really happen if you were sitting in a room alone with a German shepherd seated three feet in front of you?
>
> Client: Oh my God! That would be awful. I would go crazy!
>
> Social Worker: Do you really mean that, truly insane? Or do you mean that you would be severely frightened?
>
> Client: Well, I suppose I wouldn't actually go crazy, but I think it would be the most terrifying thing I have ever done in my life.
>
> Social Worker: I agree, it would be terrifying, and you wouldn't go insane. But now tell me, what would you actually do? How would you feel?
>
> Client: Well, my subjective anxiety would be sky high, 90 or more on that scale you talked to me about. My heart would be going a mile a minute, I'd be sweating, and looking about frantically for a means of escape.
>
> Social Worker: Yes, that's probably a realistic description. Now tell me, suppose that the dog simply looked at you, didn't growl or bark or try to touch you. Imagine that you've been seated in this room for over an hour. Would you be as frightened after sixty minutes as you were in the very beginning?
>
> Client: Well, probably not, but I'd still be terrified and I'm not willing to do that!
>
> Social Worker: Of course not, and I'll not suggest that you do. I am simply trying to use an extreme case to illustrate how ET is likely to work. Would you agree that after two hours of this, as long as the dog just sat there, that your subjective anxiety would be lower than it was when you began, that your heart rate would be slower and your shaking would be diminished? How about after six hours, wouldn't you be getting a bit bored?
>
> Client: Yes, I'd be pretty sick of the whole thing by then, I imagine.
>
> Social Worker: Yes, and that is precisely the point. Virtually any frightening experience can be overcome if you confront it long enough to become bored, provided, of course, that the activity is not actually dangerous. That is how we will try to work together to gradually help you overcome your fear of dogs. Now I know you are not willing to enter a room containing a German shepherd, but how about one that has an eight-week-old beagle puppy on a leash tied to the opposite wall?

At some point the client will allow you to arrange a mildly anxiety-evoking confrontation with his or her phobic stimulus. You then move from the stage of client preparation to the actual conduct of ET.

EXPOSURE THERAPY

You should set up an appointment with the client at which you will recreate the appropriate anxiety-evoking situation. Then you will have to arrange the logistics. Small animals must be obtained from friends or a local pet shop or caught in the wild (e.g., bees and other insects). You must locate small lockable rooms for sessions with claustrophobic patients, an automobile for use with driving phobics, and high buildings for work with clients who are afraid of heights. If the client is afraid of certain objects, a selection of these stimuli must be gathered. With living creatures, arrangements must be made to restrain them appropriately to prevent clients from coming into more intimate contact than they are willing to experience at that stage of therapy. Secure leashes or animal cages may be needed, or glass jars or a terrarium for smaller animals. In some cases only a portion of a client's AES may be acceptable for initial stages of ET. One client seen by the author had a severe fear of birds. Early treatment sessions involved the use of a series of feathers, because initially she would not tolerate an entire bird and found the touch of feathers to be very anxiety evoking.

At the actual exposure session, you should greet the client in the consulting room or other appropriate location with the AES out of view or out of the room. You should deal with any last-minute questions and provide the client once more with the following reassurances:

1. There will be no tricks or surprises during the session. You will be responsible for ensuring, for example, that the animal does not escape and in general see that the client is not exposed to greater levels of contact than he or she agrees to.
2. The client's permission will be obtained at each stage of the process prior to making any changes.
3. The client may terminate the session at any point by simply making a firm request to stop.

The next step is to get the client's permission to begin the exposure to the AES, perhaps at a specified distance away from the client. As this is done, you should observe the client carefully and ask him or her to rate his or her subjective anxiety. Give reassurance as necessary that the AES is harmless, controlled, restrained, etc. Urge the client to look carefully at the AES, to refrain from averting his or her eyes or body, and to note various features of the AES that you point out. Generally, clients initially are highly anxious, but with the passage of time, often just a few minutes, begin to calm down. With support, facilitative suggestions, the judicious use of humor, or some coaxing, they can be persuaded to approach the AES (or let you bring it closer) and eventually touch it. Periodically the client should give you a rating of subjective anxiety, and you may wish to note the client's heart rate by palpation or through use of a cardiotachometer.

Variations on this process should be used, depending upon the client's AES. A person with height phobia may accompany you to the first landing of a lengthy stairwell and look down the central well until calm. At that point, you suggest moving to the second landing, repeating the process, and so forth until the highest level is reached. You may take a person with driving phobia to a deserted shopping mall's expansive, empty parking lot, seat him or her behind the wheel, and with you seated alongside, have him or her circumnavigate the lot. Continue this until the client is calm, at which point you may seek permission to move the practice scene to a nearby residential street, and from there to a quiet business district, etc.

With social phobics, most of whom are afraid of public speaking, the unique feature of their AES may require some creative arrangements on the part of the social worker. One series of programmed confrontation exercises that the author has developed involves having the client prepare a written speech of about three minutes in length that he or she delivers to the social worker in the privacy of the consulting room over and over until he or she is comfortable making the speech. At this point, permission is sought to admit a third person to the sessions (another person with a public-speaking phobia is ideal for this purpose), and the process is repeated. Secretaries, fellow social workers, other agency staff, or friends of the client may also be used. When the client becomes comfortable with an audience of two, subsequent sessions incorporate three, four, or more additional members of the audience. Video-taped practice with immediate feedback is also useful with clients who fear giving public talks, both to help them improve their manner of delivery and to demonstrate that although they may be feeling very shaky internally, most often an external observer cannot detect any signs of tremulousness.

A variation of this approach is to bring public-speaking phobics to a classroom environment (the author has used graduate classes for this purpose) and arrange for most of the class to remain in the hall or nearby lounge while the client begins making the speech to an initial audience of one or two unfamiliar students. As the client becomes more comfortable, the social worker obtains permission at intervals to bring in one or two more students, until the class reaches its maximum audience size. If the client becomes distressed, members of the audience may be asked to leave. In this manner, the AES (public-speaking situation) can in effect be titrated in a careful manner so as to never overwhelm the client, yet provide an appreciable challenge.

As noted earlier, a large body of empirical research has documented the value of ET in the treatment of SPPs and SOPs, the phobic avoidance associated with agoraphobia, panic disorder, certain cases of obsessive-compulsive disorder, and various features of posttraumatic stress disorder (Marks, 1987; Cooper & Clum, 1989; Clum, 1989; Steketee, 1987). Exposure-based techniques also seem quite helpful in ameliorating various pathological conditions dominated by private events, internal states that have been given labels such as "obsessions," hypochondriacal concerns, and morbid grief (see Himle & Thyer, 1989; Mawson, Marks, Ramm, & Stern, 1981). ET has been found to be appropriate with a number of special populations as well, including the mentally retarded (Matson, 1981), the elderly (Thyer, 1981), and the blind (Thyer & Stocks, 1986). The following brief case description and single-subject study will further illustrate the conduct of ET in the treatment of phobias.

CASE DESCRIPTION

Mrs. Wilkes (a pseudonym) was a fifty-six-year-old woman who was self-referred to the Anxiety Disorders Program of the Department of Psychiatry at the University of Michigan Medical Center, where the author was employed as a clinical social worker. Her presenting complaint was a severe fear of birds that resulted in significant phobic avoidance and a generalized distress in her life because of the apparent pervasiveness of birds. Mrs. Wilkes was unable to give any account of the onset of this fear, noting that she had been frightened of birds ever since she was a small child. In terms of daily life, when she left the house she would often have her husband depart first, stand by the car in the driveway and scan the yard for birds. If none were apparent, Mr. Wilkes would signal her to come out, at which time she would quickly scurry from the front door to the car, which her husband would open for her.

She was unable to visit friends' homes if she knew they owned a pet bird. She could not go into pet stores that sold birds, and was reluctant to shop at local supermarkets. This latter restriction had originated several years earlier when a live sparrow flew into the grocery store where she was shopping and fluttered about the ceiling. Upon inquiry, she stated that she could not buy fresh chicken, only frozen. This was because of her self-admitted irrational fear that the fresh, plucked, plastic-wrapped birds would somehow become reanimated and come after her. She knew this was unlikely with frozen chickens, however. The precipitant for her seeking treatment was her imminent departure with her husband on a long-looked-forward-to vacation in Jamaica. A few weeks earlier Mrs. Wilkes had heard a story from a friend who had stayed recently at the same resort hotel where the Wilkeses had reservations. Apparently the hotel had a large dining patio that had trees filled with parrots, cockatiels, and similar exotic birds that were so tame that they would fly down to the tables and peck tidbits from the diners' fingers. This story, unwittingly told by a friend who was ignorant of her bird phobia, filled Mrs. Wilkes with great distress and caused her to seek help before her departure.

Mrs. Wilkes had been happily married for over thirty years and had several grown children and an accommodating husband who was puzzled by his wife's irrational behavior but did not make a major issue of it. He was supportive of her efforts to obtain help. Mrs. Wilkes had no other past psychiatric history or behavioral disorder and was rather embarrassed about seeking treatment for her phobia. It is worth reiterating that although certain aspects of Mrs. Wilkes's fear of birds bordered on the psychotic (e.g., her fear that dead birds in the poultry case at the supermarket would come alive), she was not psychotic and would admit sheepishly that although she really knew that the dead chickens would not hurt her, she nevertheless could not control her fearful feelings. Mrs. Wilkes decidedly met the diagnostic criteria for specific phobia but for no other clinical condition or personality disorder.

Treatment planning.   The usual client preparation process was completed without incident, and although Mrs. Wilkes remained curious about the origins of her bird phobia, she accepted the author's contention that it was unlikely that we could arrive at a clear etiological understanding (both her parents were deceased), and that in any event treatment could be effective without knowing the origins of her fears. She read and discussed *Living with Fear* and its accompanying description of and rationale for a program of therapeutic exposure. She was amenable to this approach, especially when it was made clear to her that it was the one most likely to yield rapid and long-term improvements.

Stimulus mapping of her phobia failed to reveal any significant elements that had a bearing on treatment. She was equally afraid of large and small birds, and their color, gender, or variety made little difference. Birds in a cage were barely tolerable from a distance, if she was sure that they could not escape. She avoided eating chicken, game hens, or other poultry, and did not watch television programs or movies about birds or read stories about or look at pictures of them.

We constructed a hierarchy of potential AESs, which ranged from looking at a color picture of a bird to being in a locked room containing several live birds on the loose. She agreed to begin our first session with my bringing a caged pigeon to our next meeting. Friends who worked in a laboratory that used pigeons for research agreed to let me borrow a pigeon and a clear plastic cage for a few hours.

Evaluation and conduct of ET.   I elected to evaluate my sessions with Mrs. Wilkes by using systematic BATs conducted before and after each ET session. I would measure her approach behavior to the caged pigeon, along with her heart rate as she got progressively closer to the cage. By attaching a portable cardiotachometer to her finger, I could record her heart rate as she approached the bird. Thus, before each session I could assess how close she would come to the bird, her subjective anxiety, and one physiological response (heart rate) at various levels of approach. This process would be repeated after each session. By systematically assessing her phobia through the use of standardized BATs, it would be possible to evaluate the effects of our intervention program through the use of a special type of research design called the "repeated pretest-posttest single-subject experiment" (see Thyer & Curtis, 1983).

Mrs. Wilkes arrived for her appointment on time. I seated her comfortably in my office and tried to put her at ease with some preliminary conversation. I explained that I did, as promised, have a caged live pigeon in an adjoining room. I gave her the rationale for the use of BATs before and after each treatment session, explained the procedure, and obtained her consent. She waited in the hall while I placed the caged bird at the far end of my office, some eighteen feet from the door. I went to the hall, attached the cardiotachometer (a soft foam rubber clip) to her index finger, and asked her to give me a SUDS rating. It was a 95, and her heart rate was 110 beats per minute, mildly tachycardic. She agreed to accompany me back into the office and stood fifteen feet from the caged bird. Her SUDS went to 98 and her heart rate to 120. She agreed to come to within twelve feet, and we continued in this manner until she stopped six feet from the pigeon, saying that she had had enough. I praised her for her efforts, unclipped the cardiotach, and seated her about fifteen feet from the bird. I sat in front and to the side of her, between her chair and the bird, and quietly encouraged her to sit and look at the bird. Over the course of the next ninety minutes she remained with me in the room, interacting from a distance with the bird. As her SUDS scores declined, I asked her to inch her chair (which was on wheels) a bit closer to the caged bird. In this manner I eventually was able to get her to touch the outside of the plastic cage. At this "high point" of treatment I suggested that we stop, to which she agreed with evident relief. I reminded her that we needed to repeat the BAT once more, which we did. Both her SUDS scores and heart rate were lower during this second BAT, and her approach improved to where she could touch the cage. The data for the BATs conducted before and after the first treatment session are depicted in Figure 9-2. The data for the remaining series of four additional treatment sessions are depicted in Figures 9-3 through 9-6.

As may be seen in Figures 9-2 through 9-6, Mrs. Wilkes made consistent improvements at each treatment session. In these figures, the abbreviation OR stands for out of the room, IDT stands for indirect touch (i.e., touching the cage), and DT stands for directly touching the bird. She often could not start a new session at the point where she had left off at the previous session, but these mild regressions were quickly recovered. At the conclusion of the fifth session, she was comfortably holding the pigeon in her hand, was agreeable to allowing the bird to walk freely about the room and on the desk next to where she sat, would allow me to wave the flapping bird over and around her head, and even played catch with the bird, both tossing it to me and letting me toss it to her, accompanied, of course, by a great flutter of wings. She would permit the bird to be placed in her lap, on her head, and on her shoulder; both of us learned not to wear our best clothes during these sessions.

Mrs. Wilkes agreed to undertake certain extratherapeutic tasks, to be performed between sessions three through five. Examples included going for walks in her neighborhood; setting out bread crumbs and birdseed in her yard and stepping outside when birds were present; going grocery shopping in stores she had previously avoided, purchasing fresh chicken and preparing fresh chicken dinners for her husband (a treat he had not enjoyed in years!); visiting pet stores and asking to examine various birds, and feeding pigeons at the park. These tasks were accomplished successfully, albeit with some initial trepidation. Had there been significant problems, I would have accompanied her on some of these exercises.

FIGURE 9-2   Behavioral Treatment of a Bird-Phobic Woman: First Treatment
Session (90 minutes)

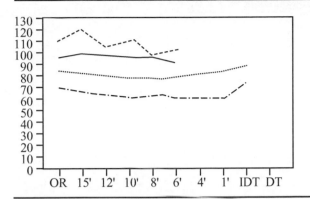

FIGURE 9-3   Behavioral Treatment of a Bird-Phobic Woman: Second Treatment
Session (90 minutes)

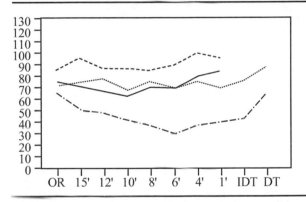

FIGURE 9-4   Behavioral Treatment of a Bird-Phobic Woman: Third Treatment
Session (90 minutes)

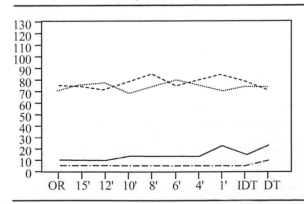

FIGURE 9-5 Behavioral Treatment of a Bird-Phobic Woman: Fourth Treatment
Session (120 minutes)

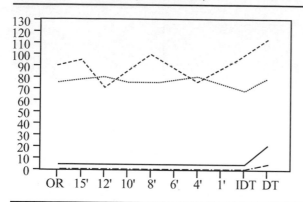

FIGURE 9-6 Behavioral Treatment of a Bird-Phobic Woman: FifthTreatment
Session (120 minutes)

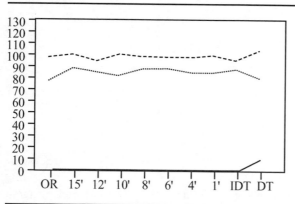

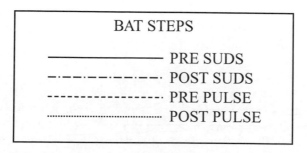

When Mrs. Wilkes was free of avoidance behavior in the consulting room, was undertaking ET homework exercises comfortably, and reported that she no longer feared birds or dreaded her vacation (the precipitant to her seeking treatment), therapy was discontinued. A few telephone contacts were made in the week or so prior to her departure on vacation to confirm that all was well. Two weeks after treatment concluded, I received a postcard from Jamaica from Mrs. Wilkes: "Having a wonderful time! Wish you were here!" The postcard had a picture of a tropical bird.

SUMMARY

Matching Interventions to Client Problems

The technique of ET is a valuable clinical skill that most human service professionals should acquire. Given that the anxiety disorders are the most prevalent so-called mental disorders, and that the treatment of choice for virtually all anxiety disorders defined in the DSM usually involves some elements of ET, it seems appropriate that clinicians working with patients who meet the criteria for simple or social phobia, obsessive-compulsive disorder, agoraphobia, panic disorder and its associated phobic avoidance behavior, and post-traumatic stress disorder should be familiar with this approach. Carefully designed studies have examined the levels of client acceptance and the dropout rates associated with offering clients a program of ET; client acceptance is higher and dropouts are equivalent to those of conventional dynamic psychotherapies.

Components and Sequencing of Exposure-Based Interventions

Once it has been determined that a given client meets the DSM criteria for one or more disorders for which ET is an indicated approach, the following processes go into the design and sequencing of this treatment procedure. First, careful stimulus mapping of the salient features of the client's AES is undertaken to determine the design and structuring of programmed confrontation exercises. Next, the client is aided in beginning this process of gradual exposure to AESs so that he or she is able to remain in the proximity of the AES until he or she is calm and can repeat this process over and over. Such exposure exercises may occur initially in the client's imagination, using simulated stimuli (e.g., rubber snakes as opposed to live ones), but real-life practice should eventually supplant such exercises.

In many cases clients can successfully undertake a program of self-conducted ET unaccompanied by an expensive therapist, guided instead by a self-help manual, a computer-assisted instructional program, or weekly visits with the behavior analyst (Ghosh & Marks, 1987). Self-conducted therapeutic tasks undertaken by the client outside of the consulting room, in the real-life environments where phobic behavior is most problematic, are essential to the process of behavior analysis and therapy and vital to ensuring that treatment gains are maintained and generalized. Such requests of clients by the behavior analyst have ample precedent in the literature of psychodynamic psychotherapy, intriguingly enough, although the theoretical rationales for such endeavors differ (e.g., Herzberg, 1941; Omer, 1985).

Client progress should be reviewed regularly with the social worker, either over the telephone or in the consulting room. If self-conducted treatment does not yield satisfactory results, therapist-assisted exposure exercises may produce the desired benefits. If local self-help or support groups for phobics are available, the client should be encouraged to explore these options as well (Thyer, 1987).

The use of single-system research designs to evaluate the efficacy of social work practice employing exposure therapies is especially helpful. Hudson and Thyer (1987), Thyer (1987), and Thyer and Curtis (1983) provide detailed descriptions and examples of such methods of practitioner-guided evaluative research.

CONCLUDING REMARKS

The origins of ET, although often purely empirical, may be clearly tied to the advances in contemporary social learning theory that form the experimental foundations of behavior analysis and therapy (Thyer, Baum, & Reid, 1988). I believe that it is increasingly important for social workers, psychiatrists, psychologists, and other human service professionals to receive thorough training in the modern formulations of respondent, operant, and observations learning principles (Thyer, 1992). Many psychosocial interventions derived from these learning theories have been rigorously tested through research studies and found to be effective. Moreover, many of these research therapies have been and are being evaluated in terms of their effectiveness when applied in more representative clinical and agency settings and are demonstrating equivalent efficacy (see Shadish et al., 1997; Wade, Treat, & Stuart, 1998; Westbrook & Hill, 1998).

Therefore, as the evidence-based foundations for intervention in the human services continue to accumulate, an ethical mandate begins to emerge suggesting that social workers should be trained in such interventions and should provide them to clients as first-choice treatment options, where such knowledge exists (Myers & Thyer, 1997). Social workers engaged in helping individuals suffering from SPPs or SOPs must acquire skills in behavior analysis and therapy in order to reliably assist these clients. The empirical evidence is very compelling in this regard and cannot be ignored by the ethical practitioner.

CHAPTER 10

Competency-Based Treatment of Marital Discord

Norman H. Cobb
Catheleen Jordan

In this chapter, Cobb and Jordan show how to help couples in dysfunctional relationships, focusing on promoting social competencies by developing functional social skills. One of the foundations of change they emphasize is defining a couple's problem by considering five areas of functioning: values, communication, negotiation and contracting, stress, and time management. Cobb and Jordan describe how to help couples with each of these problem areas to facilitate matching the client problem with specific clinical procedures. The components of the intervention are explained precisely, including a step-by-step protocol that uses active client participation and homework assignments.

Between 1980 and 1995, the rates of divorce and marriage (US Census Bureau, 1997) gradually declined in the United States, however, the 2.3 million marriages in 1995 were overshadowed by 1.2 million divorces or annulments. In the United States, almost half of marriages end in divorce (Gottman, 1994). In Europe, the divorce rate is growing, and in some countries, such as Sweden, Norway, Denmark, and Finland, the rate is nearing the US rate (Bodenmann, 1997). The census data also suggested that "two-parent families were more likely to break up if the father was unemployed, if both parents worked full-time, or if the family was poor rather than nonpoor" (Janzen & Harris, 1997, p. 344).

The statistics do not take into account the number of relationships that ended with no formal legal proceedings, nor do they reflect the number of couples who stay together although the relationship is characterized by their dissatisfaction. For example, Barker (1984) reported that about 50 percent of wives have been hit by their husbands, at least 41 percent of married men and 20 percent of married women have been involved in extramarital affairs, and 80 percent of couples have considered divorce at some point in their relationship. Frequently, in homes where spousal abuse is present, children are also abused (Stanley & Goddard, 1993), because the abusive acts are tied to power and intimidation (Erickson, 1992).

Although the true extent of dissatisfaction and dissolution is difficult to estimate (both formally and informally), marriage and couple counseling is an important field for intervention by social workers and other helping professionals. This chapter addresses dysfunction in intimate relationships and presents important interventions to build the skills and competencies of partners. The problem is discussed in terms of background, clinical manifestations, and assessment issues and how these aspects logically dictate the suggested intervention package. While the terms indicative of marital relationships are used extensively in this chapter, the concepts and issues are clearly relevant for all couples.

PROBLEM IDENTIFICATION

From a social learning, cognitive behavioral perspective, marriage relationships are seen as a product of the reciprocal interactions between marital partners in the context of their unique environment. Through the interaction of their personal values, beliefs, and expectations, the spouses create for themselves complex systems of individual and mutual behavior patterns. These strongly influence the satisfaction of the partners in the relationship and each partner's personal self-esteem or cognitive image.

Unfortunately, couples have varying degrees of skills with which to establish healthy systems of behavior. Although all couples could benefit from enhancing particular relationship skills, dysfunctional couples demonstrate significant deficits in these important skills. For example, many couples have rigid systems of verbalized or hidden rules, which might include: "Don't talk about our problems to others," "Always say nice things about the way my body looks," "Don't make a lot of noise when we're having sex." Many couples, particularly dysfunctional ones, lack the skills to discuss their value differences and communicate the desire to negotiate solutions.

BACKGROUND DISCUSSION

Several theoretical models contribute to an understanding of couples from the social learning–cognitive behavioral perspective. Behavior modification emphasizes that the partners' reinforced behavior increases and punished behavior decreases. The different levels of positive and punishing behaviors determine satisfaction or dissatisfaction. Dissatisfaction can result from a high rate of punishing behaviors or a low rate of positive reinforcers (Jacobson & Dallas, 1981).

Jacobson and Christensen (1996) reported findings from their pilot study indicating that behavioral exchange and communication training are significantly more effective when the therapist emphasizes "acceptance." The authors reported that 75 percent of couples receiving behavioral intervention, with a focus on acceptance, reported high levels of marital satisfaction, versus 50 percent of couples receiving behavioral intervention alone.

Starting from social learning theory, Bandura (1977a, 1977b, 1986) emphasized that people's behavior is reciprocally determined in the give and take of relationships. For example, when two people communicate, the initial message has significant impact on the listener. The message not only defines the topic, but it alters the way the receiver thinks and reacts to the other person. When the listener returns the dialogue, the new message affects the thoughts, feelings, and reactions of the first person. The reciprocal give and take effectively changes each person in the process. Consequently, both partners carry a significant burden of responsibility for their mate's positive and negative behavior. If conversations about home chores frequently evolve into criticism of the partner's attempts at housekeeping, the partner learns to avoid the task as well as the criticism.

Exchange theory demonstrates the reciprocal relationship between rewards and costs. Couples stay in relationships in which the rewards are greater than the costs (Thibaut & Kelly, 1959). Research indicates that distressed relationships are characterized by greater numbers of punishing (vs. rewarding) events and that negative exchanges are likely to occur in escalating chains of coercive behaviors (Filsinger & Thoma, 1988; Patterson, Chamberlain, & Reid, 1982). Therefore, distressed couples are even more sensitive to the harmful effects of negative behaviors and interactions (Huston & Vangelisti, 1991; Jacobson, 1984).

From a social competency perspective (Gambrill & Richey, 1985), basic skills are necessary for communication, sexual performance, employment, child rearing, and a host of other activities. While different clinicians and lay persons may argue over the list of "necessary" skills, all agree that the lack of certain skills often contributes to a couple's distress. Partners may lack basic communication skills, such as the ability to disclose feelings, demonstrate accurate empathy, communicate understanding, make requests, and negotiate conflicts (Gottman, 1979; Jacobson & Margolin, 1979). The skills approach in therapy allows couples and therapists to look beyond the idiosyncratic behaviors of individuals and focus on learning more effective and efficient tools for making changes in their relationships. For example, a couple may report frequent arguments about a wide variety of issues. They may discount the interactions as "charming banter" or they may allow the dissatisfaction to question the authenticity of their commitment. In actuality, they may not have the skills to clearly state their needs or negotiate mutually satisfying solutions. These possible skill deficits with their various clinical manifestations are more readily assessed when viewed from the theoretical perspectives of social learning, exchange, and social competency.

CLINICAL MANIFESTATIONS

Clinical manifestations are observed in at least one of six major areas of couples functioning: conflicting values, communication, negotiating and contracting, stress, coping skills, and managing time. In the area of values, distressed couples experience difficulty solving problems and correctly evaluating their relationship. Couples report differences between the early months of their relationship and their current situation. They frequently describe how similar they were in the beginning and how much the other one has changed. They were unaware of the basic differences between them that were previously obscured by the excitement of dating and the "honeymoon" period. Partners frequently become preoccupied with the conflicts or frustrations and discount the possibilities of the less obvious differences in values and perceptions. Consequently, recurring fights over the same issues are commonly a manifestation of value conflicts. The arguments may focus on the "correct" roles of males and females, differing attitudes about extended family members, disagreements about child discipline, disputes over intimacy, or personal uses of leisure time (Jordan, Cobb, & McCully, 1989).

Couples who interact poorly may be suffering from poor communication patterns in addition to differences in values, ideas, or needs. Poor communication is not a function of amount but rather an issue of quality. Some couples follow a totally honest, totally open communication style. As attractive as this may sound or even appear in treatment sessions, "totally open" may be a form of verbal brutality. Few relationships can survive long periods of unedited, poorly timed communication. Other couples do not listen to each other. They tend to hear only the first part of their partners' message because they start thinking of what to say in response.

Similarly, clients who are quite successful communicators at work are not automatically effective communicators at home. The expectations for communication at work and home are often very different. The superior-subordinate interaction style at work does not work well in close interpersonal relationships (Bartolome & Evans, 1980; Bartolome, 1983). When partners assume a subservient or a dominant role, they guarantee that one person's concerns will not be heard and the other person's opinions will not be sufficiently evaluated. In a variety of not so subtle ways, subservient partners criticize (or retaliate against) their partners for being bossy, opinionated, or overpowering. In turn, however, subservient partners may be treated as unimportant or insignificant. In some cases, individuals assume these communication styles to avoid fights or disagreements because of a mistaken belief that fighting is dysfunctional. However, much to their surprise, relationship problems are fueled by resentment, low self-efficacy, and even boredom.

While couples frequently communicate about specific problems, the critical and oftentimes overlooked issue is the couple's lack of skills to resolve recurrent problems. Furthermore, the problems that they do solve characteristically result in one partner being the winner and one partner being the loser. One partner's resentment over past fights or solutions may indicate a failure to negotiate and safeguard the needs of both parties.

Failure to negotiate agreements costs time, and, unfortunately, many partners blame themselves for being inadequate, "always tired," "overwhelmed," or unable to handle all the pressures. For example, wives may report dissatisfaction because they do more household and child-rearing tasks than their husbands. They often feel guilty (and resentful) about their fatigue and frustrations. The husbands, however, are not immune to these pressures, and a growing number of men report frustrations due to lack of time to accomplish family responsibilities. Couples may describe the loss of private and intimate time to be alone or with their partners.

The failure to manage time is only one of the numerous sources of stress for couples. Individuals report not measuring up to their idealized image of a parent, house manager, lover, friend, employee, and so forth. Partners report conflicting feelings about working outside the home, caring for extended family members or friends, or having insufficient time to be alone or pursue important ventures. They may report being overwhelmed by children who need time, partners who need support, houses that get dirty only hours (or minutes) after cleaning, or interpersonal problems and deadlines at work. Unfortunately, partners may not correctly identify their marital relationship as the source of stress.

Partners experiencing a great deal of stress may lash out at each other and focus attention on the other partner's more irritating characteristics. The stress can cause physical problems such as elevated blood pressure, sleeping problems, headaches, and other medical/mental problems. After reviewing the literature on stress and life in dual-career and dual-earner marriages, the authors believe stress to be inevitable for modern families who report a moderate to high level of activities such as work commitments, school programs, dance classes, meetings, schedule conflicts between family members, and so forth. Finally, individuals and couples experiencing predictable changes, such as marriage, childbirth, children beginning school, and so forth, experience significant stress (Andolfi, 1980). In essence, high levels of stress are common in contemporary society.

Effective coping skills are crucial components for effective marriages. Bodenmann (1997) reported that couples under considerable stress were unable to communicate effectively and ameliorate the negative impact of stress. Partners were unable to find common perspectives with which to solve their problems. Similarly, when both partners experience considerable stress from employment, child care, or so forth, one partner may be unable to temporarily take a supportive or corrective role in the relationship. As a result the relationship is harmed and the care taking or nurturing in the idealized marriage is absent. To make matters worse, ineffective coping skills result in the accentuation of the stress or problem.

ASSESSMENT AND MONITORING METHODS

Initial contacts with couples may yield vast amounts of data. For example, many distressed couples show the tension in their faces, as well as in gestures and angry interactions. The very power of their emotions may cover up the basic skill deficit that produces a complex scenario of frustrations and disappointments. Other couples may be quite skilled at hiding their frustrations. For example, dual-career couples may present confident exteriors to colleagues and clients when they know, all too well, that their business personae are not working at home.

The complexity of clients' problems and personal styles dictates that assessments of couples in marital distress occur from a multidimensional, systems perspective. Spouses are viewed as unique individuals interacting in complex relationships within nuclear families, extended families, and the community. Clinicians must identify the unique expectations that spouses have for themselves and their partners. For example, are their conflicts due to value differences, or to their deficits in communication skills or in negotiating conflicts? Is the couple having problems due to an inability to manage time schedules, or because of internal or external stress?

Assessment can be facilitated by the use of measurement instruments. There are two types used for slightly different purposes: global measures and rapid assessment instruments. The global instruments are designed to look at overall conceptions of marital and family functioning. These are usually lengthy questionnaires or interview schedules that are completed at the beginning of therapy. A popular example is the Stuart Clinical Aids (Sheafor, Horejsi, & Horejsi, 1997), which include the Marital Pre-Counseling Inventory, the Family Pre-Counseling Inventory, the Sexual Adjustment Inventory, and the Pre-Marital Counseling Inventory. The Stuart questionnaires are valuable as a starting point for looking at the couple in the context of their individual, couple, family, and external systems (work, extended family, etc.) issues. Questions focus on the areas of a couple's adjustment and satisfaction, parent-child relationships, personal life satisfaction, and so forth. These questionnaires can be mailed in to be computer scored. Practitioners can utilize the information to get an overview of couple and/or family functioning to aid in assessing, operationalizing, and prioritizing problems.

Other measures can be utilized to give a more specific view of the marital relationship itself. Fredman and Sherman (1987) reported instruments for measuring general marital satisfaction and adjustment including the Locke-Wallace Marital Adjustment Test, the Spanier Dyadic Adjustment Scale, and the Notarius and Vanzetti Marital Agendas Protocol, which is a fifteen-item questionnaire that has been used to standardize other marital adjustment instruments. The test measures global adjustment, areas of possible disagreement, conflict resolution, cohesion, and communication. Scores range from 2 to 158, with most nondistressed couples scoring above 100. Some of the questions may assume stereotypical roles for husbands and wives.

The Spanier Dyadic Adjustment Scale was designed to assess the relationship of either married couples or unmarried couples living together. The four subscales used in the test are dyadic satisfaction, dyadic cohesion, dyadic consensus, and affectionate expression. The scale is designed to be used in whole or part; the subscales are designed to stand alone. The test is short and easy to administer; and each of the subscales has high reliability and validity coefficients, with the exception of the affect subscale which, therefore, should be interpreted with caution.

The Notarius and Vanzetti Marital Agendas Protocol measures problems in the marital relationship in four sections. To complete the test, each spouse is asked to respond to a list of common issues couples face. They read the list four times to respond to the following four issues: 1) relationship problems they may be experiencing, 2) spousal agreement about the seriousness of the problems, 3) expectations about the chances for problem resolution, and 4) assignment of spousal blame for continuation of problems.

The Udry Marital Alternatives Scale allows the couple to evaluate their thoughts about whether they could do better if they were married to someone else or not married at all. Two main factors emerge from the test: the spouse replacement factor and the economic maintenance factor. Studies suggest that couples with higher scores on the test have a higher probability of divorcing or separating. This test is helpful for couples trying to decide whether to stay together and for those couples who have not evaluated what the alternative to marriage might be.

Fredman and Sherman (1987) also reported instruments for measuring communication and intimacy including the Larzelere and Houston Dyadic Trust Scale, the Bringle Self-Report Jealousy Scale Revised, and the Waring Intimacy Questionnaire. The Larzelere and Houston Dyadic Trust Scale is an eight-item test that measures belief in the partner's benevolence and honesty. The test correlates highly with other measures of love and self-disclosure, but not with generalized trust or social desirability.

The Bringle Self-Report Jealousy Scale Revised measures three types of factors: minor romantic, major romantic, and nonromantic. The test is a twenty-five–item questionnaire; scores range from 0 to 100, with higher scores indicating more jealousy. Respondents rate how pleased versus upset they would be if confronted with specific situations, such as "at a party, your spouse kisses someone you do not know."

The Waring Intimacy Questionnaire is designed to measure eight factors of marital intimacy: conflict resolution, affection, cohesion, sexuality, identity, compatibility, expressiveness, and autonomy. The test consists of forty items and can be used to look at a spouse's perception of marital intimacy while it reveals the discrepancy between the two spouses' answers.

Other instruments useful for assessing couples in the context of their family system include the Olson scales and the Beavers-Timberlawn scales (Fredman & Sherman, 1987). The most widely used of the Olson package of scales is the Family Adaptability and Cohesion Evaluation Scales III. This scale measures four types of dimensions of family adaptability: chaotic, flexible, structured, and rigid; and four types of dimensions of cohesion: disengaged, separated, connected, and enmeshed. The 111-item, self-report inventory is designed to be answered twice, first to assess the family as is, and secondly to assess the family as the member would like the family to be. The discrepancy between scores on the "perceived" version versus the "ideal" version allows practitioners to assess couples' marital satisfaction.

The Beavers-Timberlawn Family Evaluation Scale is a popular tool to observe the family as they interact. The practitioner asks the family to "discuss as a group what you would like to change about your family." This interaction is videotaped and coded by trained observers on the following five dimensions: structure of the family, mythology, goal-directed negotiation, autonomy, and family affect.

In contrast to these global measures, rapid assessment instruments (RAIs) are used for assessment but also have applicability in monitoring therapeutic progress. This monitoring can be conceptualized in a single-system design and can be used to gather baseline (pretreatment) scores over the course of the assessment period and later to compare baseline scores with those from the treatment phase of therapy.

Examples of the goals of RAIs and other assessment measures for specific problems include the following:

1. To assess value conflicts (reported in Fredman & Sherman, 1987): The Dunn, Dunn, and Price (1975) Productivity Environmental Preference Survey identifies potential sources of conflict. Areas measured include each spouse's preferences in functioning in the immediate environment, in emotionality, in sociological needs, and in physical needs. The Pendleton, Poloma, and Garland (1980) Dual-Career Family Scales are composed of six scales that measure working wives' views of marriage. The six scales measure marriage type (traditional vs. nontraditional), domestic responsibility, satisfaction, self-image, career salience, and career line. The Tetenbaum, Lighter, and Travis (1981) Attitudes toward Working Women Scales identify sources of conflict when wives work or have careers.

2. To assess communication problems (reported in Fredman & Sherman, 1987; Corcoran & Fischer, 2000a): The Bienvenu Marital Communication Inventory is a forty-eight–item questionnaire that measures relationship hostility, self-disclosure, regard, empathy, discussion, and conflict management. The Locke, Sabaught, and Thomes (Navran, 1967) Primary Communication Inventory is a twenty-five–item inventory that measures both verbal and nonverbal communication, as well as the individual's self-perception of their own communication ability and the spouse's perception of the individual's ability. The Beier-Sternberg Discord Questionnaire is a ten-item instrument that measures the couples' discord or conflict, as well as their degree of unhappiness related to the discord. The popular Clinical Measurement Package (CMP; Hudson, 1982) includes the Index of Marital Satisfaction, the Index of Sexual Satisfaction, the Index of Family Relations, the Index of Parental Attitudes and

Child's Attitude toward Father and Child's Attitude toward Mother. Each scale has a clinical cutting score. The CMP also has a new computerized version so that clients can quickly and easily fill out measures before each therapy session. The computer version also scores the instruments, interprets, and graphs the data.

3. To assess negotiation skills (reported in Corcoran & Fischer, 2000a): The Heppner Problem-Solving Inventory is a thirty-five–item questionnaire that measures the awareness of problem-solving abilities in the areas of getting along with friends, feeling depressed, choosing a career, and deciding whether or not to get a divorce. The twenty-item Infante and Wigley Verbal Aggressiveness Scale identifies each spouse's willingness to attack the self-concept of the other.

4. To assess stress and time management (reported in Corcoran & Fischer, 2000a): The MacDonald Irrational Values Scale is a nine-item scale that measures spouses' irrational beliefs; it is based on the Ellis-theory model. The forty-item Weissman Dysfunctional Attitude identifies attitudes and beliefs that may contribute to stress and is based on the Beck-theory model. The thirty-item MacKay and Cox Stress Arousal Checklist measures stress on two dimensions—stress and arousal. The first dimension measures feelings from pleasant to unpleasant; the second dimension measures the general sense of well-being.

INTERVENTION

Treatment of Choice

The treatment chosen for couples with marital problems is a skills-focused approach. The elements of the package are values clarification, communication training, negotiation and contracting skills training, time-management techniques, and stress-management techniques. The intervention package takes into account that negative and positive behaviors in marital relationships occur independently (Jacobson, Waldron, & Moore, 1980; Weiss, Hops, & Patterson, 1973). Simply stated, decreasing the negatives in the relationship does not directly increase the positive behaviors, and, consequently, certain positive behaviors need to be learned. The skills perspective emphasizes the acquisition of positive behavior patterns. Research and practice wisdom support their effectiveness.

Research Support

The systematic approach to skills training has a long history of successful utilization (Curran & Monti, 1982; Gambrill & Richey, 1985; Carkhuff, 1971; Pierce & Drasgow, 1969). A systematic approach to teaching key elements of communication was successful for distressed couples in group settings (Wells,

Figurel, & McNamee, 1975), with individual couples (D. F. Beck, 1976; Carter & Thomas, 1975), with dysfunctional families (Bright & Robin, 1981; Robin, 1982), and with adolescents and their parents (Ostensen, 1981). Markman and colleagues (Markman, 1979; Markman, Renick, Floyd, Stanley, & Clements, 1993) have documented the long-term effectiveness of communication training and conflict management for four to five years following treatment.

As in the Markman et al. (1993) study, communication training has been evaluated concurrently with other skills training. Baucom (1982; Baucom & Hoffman, 1986), for example, studied the effectiveness of communication training and contracting with distressed couples. Similarly, communication training was successfully used as a stress reduction method with couples (Ewart, Taylor, Kraemer, & Agras, 1984).

Contracting and negotiation skills training is a logical step in therapy after training in communication skills (Stuart, 1980). Research demonstrates the effectiveness of contracting skills as an effective tool for enhancing marital relationships (Azrin, Naster, & Jones, 1973; Jacobson, 1977; Jacobson & Martin, 1976; Weiss, Hops, & Patterson, 1973).

Contracting and negotiation skills help couples resolve marital conflicts and the trials of daily living, however, individual and marital stress must receive direct attention. Research on the success of stress-management techniques is quite encouraging for the practitioner-teacher (Cormier & Cormier, 1985). Various types of meditation helped clients reduce anxiety (Girodo, 1974) and drug usage (Shapiro & Zifferblatt, 1976). Relaxation training (King, 1980) reduced incidents of insomnia (Woolfolk, Carr-Kaffashan, McNulty, & Lehrer, 1976), alcohol consumption (Marlatt & Marques, 1977), and stress. For example, Denicola and Sandler (1980) successfully used stress management with parents who abuse their children. Charlesworth, Williams, and Baer (1984) combined progressive relaxation, autogenic training, stress hierarchy, imagery, systematic desensitization, cognitive restructuring, and assertiveness training to successfully reduce stress for white-collar workers.

Practice Wisdom Support

While few clinicians will be surprised by the fact that a couple's conflicts frequently stem from differences in values, the effectiveness literature for values clarification is largely devoid of researched strategies for helping clinicians. The marital therapy field has approximately relied on axioms such as couples fight about what "should" occur in married life (Stuart, 1980). Our practice wisdom emphasizes that the idealized picture of marriage contains numerous myths. Individuals consequently prepare themselves for marriage in order to fit these beliefs, however, an individual's values and myths infrequently match the spouse's beliefs.

Partners frequently are not fully aware of how their cherished myths and/or values conflict with their images of themselves, the values of their spouses, and the values of society. For example, working women may fear that value conflicts between their work and home life will threaten their femininity or male support (Schwartz & Waetjen, 1976). Similarly, males may feel threatened by normal home tasks that do not fit their definitions of what men should do. Partners need help clarifying discrepancies between their own images and the demands of modern home life. Many clinicians will not be surprised that Keith and Schafer (1998) found that working couples with traditional male and female values experience a higher threat to their mental health.

A strong personal identity is hard to maintain when couples are directly or indirectly questioning and confronting each others' beliefs about the relationship (Brittan, 1973). Many therapists emphasize that spouses with weaker senses of identity have more conflict with their partners (Barry, 1968). Sekaran (1986) emphasized the importance of a strong self-concept and self-identify to support working women who must continually tolerate ambiguity. The ambiguity comes from conflicts between their work world and home responsibilities. Conflict may result between partners when they fail to support each other as whole persons in each area.

Whereas values clarification enables couples to enhance their common understanding of each other's values, good communication serves as the vehicle to convey information about one's values and show appreciation for the values of the partner. The majority of couples place very high emphasis on communication as a major criterion for marital satisfaction (Jacobson & Moore, 1981). At the same time, clinicians know that communication problems signal distress in the couple's relationship (Gottman, 1979; Markman, 1979). Jacobson and Holtzworth-Munroe (1986) emphasized that regardless of whether poor communication is targeted as a causal factor of dysfunctional relationships or as a dominate component, the quality of communication is significantly related to the level of marital distress. Nonverbal elements of communication are also important. Mehrabian (1972) asserted that only 7 percent of the feeling message is "heard" in the words. The remaining message is delivered through the vocal tone and facial expression. This evidence underscores the reality that communication is exceedingly complex, far more than most couples (and many professionals) realize. Clinicians might benefit from reading Watzlawick, Beavin, and Jackson's (1967) description of the multidimensional nature of communication. While the metacommunication and content of messages can enhance interaction, they often obscure the complex meanings within the communication (Nierenberg & Galero, 1973).

In addition to the practice wisdom on the importance of communication, the therapeutic relationship requires that clients be willing to cooperate during clinical sessions and in the client's day-in and day-out activities. Jacobson and Gurman (1986) very clearly emphasized this requirement with their expectation that couples be willing to enter into collaborative sets. The agreed collaboration requires an explicit commitment to compromise and change.

Fortunately, an important goal of negotiation and contracting skills is the resolution of problems in such a way that both partners feel and believe that they gained from the resolution. For example, the research on household responsibilities clearly shows that women are still performing two and one-half more hours of home tasks than their male counterparts (Pleck, 1997). In all families, particularly in dual-career or dual-earner marriages, partners need to know how to negotiate and contract the division of labor in the home. Men frequently need encouragement to examine the consequences to their wives (and their marriage) of stressful and inequitable home and child-care responsibilities.

The very nature of the husband and wife's stressed lives distracts them from using the obvious stress and time-management skills. Many couples are unable to see the problem clearly, and they need an external agent, such as the therapist or other caregiver, to intervene and stop the cycle of increasing stress. Clinicians concur with McLaughlin, Cormier, and Cormier (1988), who studied dual-career women with children. They found a significant relationship between low levels of stress or distress and the high use of coping strategies and time management.

STRUCTURE OF INTERVENTION

The treatment package was first suggested by Jordan et al. (1989) for dual-career couples and is adapted for use with other marital couples in distress. The treatment package is first described, and then limitations are discussed.

Treatment Process: How to Do the Treatment

The five steps of the intervention package are goals and values clarification, communication training, negotiation and contracting skills training, time-management techniques, and stress-management techniques.

Goals and values clarification.   The first step in interviewing with distressed couples is to assist them in identifying the similarities and differences regarding their overall life and family goals. What did they expect the marriage to be like? How is it different? What do they like/dislike about their roles as spouse, parent, worker, in-law, friend, and so forth? What do they like/dislike about their spouses? The therapeutic aim at this stage is to help couples establish mutual and individual goals and values.

Therapists can use rather simple procedures to enable clients to share their goals and values. For example, clients may be asked to separately list on paper various pieces of information such as their preferences for the marriage, pro and con statements about their marital relationship, or positive and negative aspects of their roles as parents. Periodically during the listing of information, the therapist may ask each client to share two or three preliminary ideas. This minor interruption stimulates clients' thinking and helps them clarify the task. Following the completion of the lists, clients share ideas from their lists and discuss similarities and differences.

Helpful variations on this procedure include asking spouses to list their expectations for their partners and compare that list with their expectations for themselves. As an aside, some partners, such as first-time parents, have been quite surprised at differences or conflicts in expectations. Many couples are surprised that the inclusion of an infant in the family initiates a change in roles toward more traditional family and marital roles. Only when this reality is addressed do partners gain the awareness to initiate strategies to avoid rigid and unhealthy traditional roles. For example, careful planning may ensure that fathers have more involvement with their children and mothers avoid the onslaught of numerous overwhelming child-care tasks and expectations.

This task can accomplish more than the mere listing and sharing of similarities and differences. Values assumed for healthy relationships may be communicated to couples through the structure of the exercise. For example, wives and husbands may be instructed to separate their lists of work and home responsibilities. This strategy enables clients to separate the values of the work and home and acknowledge the difference between the settings. By separating the two roles, partners can see themselves as competent within each setting and perhaps avoid or reduce the tendency of one set of expectations infringing on the other.

Clients may also be asked to jointly list their goals for the family and their marriage. Couples may be encouraged to set goals in terms of future time periods, for example, goals for the next four months, the next two years or the next five years. The short-term and long-term consequences of each goal may then be explored.

The listing or comparison of goals and values frequently leads to important discussions and possible resolutions, because the therapeutic setting "gives permission" for discussion of sensitive issues or the presentation of topics that have never been addressed. Therapists should emphasize that couples will benefit even more if this task is repeated at home. Some issues for discussion are: In what ways do the couple agree/disagree on the traditional or nontraditional nature of their relationship? In what ways are spouses' lifestyles, hobbies, and interests compatible? Which are incompatible? What are the long-range plans for their family, and how are they taking steps to make those plans materialize? A matrix such as the one depicted in Figure 10-1 may help couples determine how each spouse rates the importance of work versus family life and how each perceives self in terms of traditional or nontraditional characteristics.

Communication training.   Communication skills training focuses on teaching couples both verbal and nonverbal elements of good communica-

FIGURE 10-1   Sex-Role Orientations and Central Life Interests

Sex-Role Orientations

	1 *HUS/WF* *Both* *Trad'l*	2 *HUS-* *Notrad'l* *WF-* *Trad'l*	3 *HUS-* *Trad'l* *WF-* *Nontrad'l*	4 *HUS/WF* *Both* *Nontrad'l*
1. HUS/WF Work				
2. HUS Fam WF Work				
3. HUS Work & Fam WF Work				
4. HUS Work WF Fam				
5. HUS/WF Fam				
6. HUS Work & Fam WF Fam				
7. HUS Work WF Work & Fam				
8. HUS Fam WF Work & Fam				
9. HUS/WF Work/Fam				

SOURCE: Adapted from Sekaran (1986).

tion. Rice (1999) noted four necessary elements that must be present before communication skills may be learned and integrated as part of a couple's healthy relationship. These are as follows:

1. A positive feeling between spouses who value and care for each other and are motivated to want to develop sympathetic understanding.
2. A willingness to disclose one's own attitudes, feelings, and ideas.

3. An ability to reveal attitudes, feelings, and ideas clearly and accurately.
4. A reciprocal relationship in which disclosure and feedback originate with both partners, who listen carefully and attentively to each other (p. 342).

Gambrill (1997, pp. 335–339) identified steps that may be followed by those requesting a behavior change from their partners:

1. Ask, "Does it really matter?"
2. Consider the other person's perspective.
3. Plan and practice what to say.
4. Choose the right time and place.
5. Start with positive feedback.
6. Be specific about what you want and why.
7. Personalize and own feedback.
8. Avoid negative comments.
9. Match your style of presentation to the message.
10. Offer specific suggestions for change.
11. Be willing to compromise.
12. Offer positive feedback.
13. Avoid sidetracks.
14. Persist.

Specific communication skills may be taught following the framework developed by Gottman, Notarius, Gonso, and Markman (1976) for couples communication. They taught couples how to listen and validate each other, how to level or communicate directly, and how to edit unproductive information. Couples learn to intervene in their own arguments, their faulty communication interactions, or their situations of possible misunderstanding. By teaching them how to call a halt to troublesome interaction, both partners can agree that stopping an interaction or asking for clarification and feedback is permitted (and extremely beneficial). Also, therapists may emphasize that by using this strategy partners demonstrate their caring and eagerness to understand.

The stop-action approach is easy to teach and use. The first step describes the "stop action" as a nonconfrontational request. For example, a spouse may ask a partner to set a time to talk about an issue or a conversation. The partner may say, "I am a little worried about our finances. I would like to set aside some time for us to talk about our money. When is a good time to talk so that we won't be interrupted by the kids or the television?" In the second stage of a stop action, a partner makes a direct request for feedback from the spouse. The request focuses attention on the possible impact of the message. To illustrate from the example above, the partner may ask, "Do you feel the need to talk about the money?" In the third stage the partner is taught to respond to the request by stating what he or she thinks the partner meant by the request. The other spouse should be instructed to listen for possible misunderstandings between the original request and the interpretation (or feedback) provided by the partner. Partners should keep in mind that differences between initial messages and perceived intent are common. Consequently, this commonality dictates the use of the stop-action steps.

The fourth step instructs partners to listen and respond to content and feeling in the original request. In the example above, the request asks for a time to solve problems and at the same time communicates a worry about the family finances. Partners commonly focus on either the request or feeling and in doing so fail to communicate clearly with their spouse. This failure frequently causes the worried partner to feel unsupported or not heard. This step instructs partners to ask for clarification if both the feeling and the request are not heard. The fifth step asks the listener to summarize or paraphrase what he or she thought the partner intended by the message. The sixth step is important because the message is validated even though the listener may not agree or sympathize with his or her partner's concerns. The listener might say, "I certainly understand that you are worried about the family finances. Also, it is frustrating to find the time to sit and talk about it." Finally, the partner should check to see if the impact of the message is in keeping with the intent. This evaluation allows partners to clarify any discrepancies that might still exist.

Leveling is recommended for the numerous couples who avoid conflicts with their spouses and do not discuss problems. The first clear indication of couples avoiding topics may appear in the goal and value clarification period of this intervention package. The leveling technique consists of five steps. In the beginning, partners are taught to express their feelings despite their fears that something catastrophic will result. Partners may have previously avoided crucial topics for fear that their spouses will not love them anymore or they will leave them.

Unfortunately, these fears have a component of truth that clinicians should not deny or discount. The irrational aspect of fears, however, can be rationally examined in a worst-case/best-case discussion. For example, clients may be asked what they think will be the worst possible and best possible consequences of discussing an important topic with their spouses. The subsequent discussion should also consider less extreme consequences. In the process, the clinician teaches the client to examine decisions in a cost and reward framework. The ultimate decision point for overcoming fears about communicating rests on the evaluation that the rewards outweigh the costs.

The second step in leveling requires that partners examine their own feelings to help them better express their ideas as well as their feelings. Unfortunately, and quite surprisingly to most clinicians, many clients do not know the appropriate words to express their feelings or they lack the experience of expressing feeling with words. This is especially true for men who received little encouragement as children to verbalize their feelings. Clients can benefit from using a feeling chart or similar list of feeling words to help them associate words with their emotions. Various feeling lists categorize descriptive words and help readers better discriminate between words associated with frustration versus anger, happiness versus self-satisfaction, and so forth. For example, a wife may communicate her emotions more effectively with her partner when she expresses her frustration over the child-care responsibilities with feeling words such as "despair," "overwhelmed," or "pulled in different ways" rather than with angry words such as "bitter," "hate," or "detest."

The third aspect of leveling encourages partners to write feelings on paper and give each other time to read and think about them before responding. This approach short-circuits the tendency of many partners to prematurely respond with inappropriate or defensive words that do not communicate caring or a willingness to hear and support the other partner. This method helps reduce the fear of communicating on threatening topics.

The fourth step clearly addresses the need for partners to be more assertive in asking for what they want. Couples frequently lack workable agreements about the difference between assertive and aggressive behavior. They worry or fear that what they define as "assertive" will actually be destructive or demanding. A frequently underlying theme, however, the belief that getting needs met is selfish or self-centered. Assertive partners are sometimes criticized for being too demanding while their mates believe they must avoid assertiveness and resort to devious methods to meet basic needs.

Clinicians should help couples define and differentiate between aggressive and assertive. Additionally, the couple should discuss the rights of persons to have their needs met in the midst of loving relationships. A result of this discussion is at least a covert permission to ask each other and other persons for certain needs to be met. The process of asking, however, does not come easily to many people. Couples should be encouraged to openly list their needs and share those needs with their spouses. Richard Stuart's Caring Days Model (1980, discussed later in this chapter) is effective for this task. Regardless of the approach a therapist may choose, the mere process of asking and the concomitant permission to ask is usually well received by both partners.

The final step in leveling provides couples with a needed mechanism and permission to inform their spouses about their readiness to hear or communicate. In everyday life many demands, frustrations, or even positive mental states dispose someone to react certain ways. Gottman et al. (1976) refer to this state of being or attitude as a "filter" that affects all incoming messages. For example, when working partners meet home from their jobs, they may need to warn their partners that they have had a horrible day or a splitting headache. This final leveling skill may consist of an agreement between partners that each has the right, even the responsibility, to prepare their spouse. While discussing this idea with clients, clinicians may emphasize the therapeutic or care-giving aspect of this skill. A component of this agreement should include a listing of ideas of how the other partner might respond to the warning. For example, if the partner who has spent all day caring for the children announces that they have been "terrible," the other spouse will know that a good response is to take over and watch the kids for the remainder of the evening.

Whereas leveling encourages partners to communicate, editing is recommended for those couples who overcommunicate about their problems. For example, they have angry fights over every issue, and, unfortunately, most of those arguments include all the problems at once. Characteristically, many couples start fighting or discussing a concern and fifteen minutes later the partners cannot remember what they originally discussed and usually failed to resolve.

In the simplest form, editing involves being polite to your spouse. In therapy, couples may benefit from a brief discussion comparing how partners interact with friends or business acquaintances compared with how they interact with each other. Not surprisingly, most couples find that they are less polite and thoughtful of their partners than they are of persons outside the family. For example they nag, interrupt, put each other down, or bring up old unresolved issues. Couples should be reminded that while the home setting or marital relationship permits more honesty or directness, much of what happens in the name of openness is more properly characterized as honest brutality and, consequently, is quite destructive.

The principles of editing include the following: 1) Make requests in terms of what you can, rather than cannot, do (i.e., "I can go shopping with you, but only for one hour." Edit out, "I have a million things to do, how can you waste your time like that!"). 2) Give sincere praise (i.e., "You were so thoughtful to buy me this tie for my birthday." Edit out, "Even though it is a God-awful shade of purple and you know I hate that color."). 3) Be considerate (i.e., instead of saying "Quit telling me how to drive," you edit this out and say nothing). 4) Listen and express interest in things important to your spouse (i.e., do not only talk about yourself, but also ask your spouse about his or her job, hobbies, day, etc.). 5) Do not interrupt your spouse; let him or her continue and finish the conversation. 6) Say something nice that your spouse will like to hear, rather than putting him or her down. 7) Accept responsibility for what mistakes you make, rather than making a self–put down. 8) Stay in the present; do not dig up past grievances to manipulate and divert a conversation with your spouse. 9) Do not think only of yourself; be empathetic and try to recognize and act upon the wishes of your spouse.

When couples agree that the principles to editing will help communication, they should be encouraged to use simple methods to remind themselves and each other about the need for editing. For example, individuals may be instructed to plan discussions with their mates. The plan should focus on one topic that is central to a particular problem. Tangential or alternative problems should be openly delayed and even scheduled for discussion at a later time. Additionally, couples may be encouraged to openly allow one or the other person to interject in the discussion, "We are getting off the subject. This new problem is important, however, can we set aside time to talk about it, like this evening after supper?" This approach affirms the importance of their partner's concerns but does not allow those concerns to interfere with the current issue. Similarly, couples need to be alerted to the simple technique of silently asking themselves if what they need or want to bring up in the discussion relates to the current issue or is merely tangential. Also, couples may need to inquire if the initial topic is the problem that really needs their attention or do they need to set it aside and change to the new topic? This technique allows for a clear and conscious break in the discussion and requires the concurrence of both partners. In short, editing may help couples communicate politely and rationally and avoid the seductive confusion of competing problems.

While these steps are very effective, Gottman (1993, 1994) has recently emphasized the need for partners to become aware of their physical arousal during communication. He contends that physical arousal interferes in partners' ability to respond effectively. Becoming aware of physical responses is particularly helpful for men, because with increased awareness, they are able to evaluate their anger-related cues. Deschner (1984), in her program to teach a cognitive behavioral method for anger control, delineated the physical responses associated with anger. She prescribed a time-out method to intervene in domestic violence.

The method contains the following steps: 1) The client recognizes the physiological and environmental signs that he or she is getting mad enough to be out of control. 2) The client communicates to the spouse that he or she (i.e., the client) needs to leave the situation and take a time-out. 3) The client thinks about the fight and focuses on what he or she did to contribute to the argument. 4) The client returns to communicate his or her "technical error" and discusses better solutions.

In another area of good communication skills, Gambrill and Richey (1985) made additional recommendations. Practitioners may give feedback about spouses' voice qualities that communicate unintended messages. For instance, talking too loudly or too softly can communicate that partners are either domineering or submissive, confident or sad. The tone in which they speak can indicate that they are depressed (flat, monotonous tone) or sophisticated (deep, resonant tone). People who vary the pitch of their voice are perceived as more dynamic and extroverted. Pace and clarity, that is fast or slow, can communicate boredom or anger. Similarly, a gregarious person may be viewed as socially competent unless he or she monopolizes the conversation by talking too long. Also, more successful communicators balance general statements versus more detailed statements, because too many general statements may label someone as superficial and too many details may bore others.

In the clinical setting, couples may benefit from the opportunity to give feedback to each other about the tone and clarity of voice. For example, they may practice speaking where their voice is clearly audible, not too loud or soft. The voice should be warm, the pitch and tone should reflect interest, and the tempo should be moderate, not too fast or slow. While the physical proximity will vary with the situation, spouses should indicate interest and warmth.

Clinicians should also help partners become aware of the length of time that each person speaks. In arguments or discussions where the amount of dialogue is dramatically unequal, one partner is probably controlling the flow of information and the definition of the problem. Unfortunately, the quieter member is losing the opportunity and possibly avoiding the responsibility to contribute information, personal feelings, or differences of opinion. Clinicians may want to teach clients appropriate and agreed-upon hand gestures that signal the desire to talk. For example, couples frequently agree that balanced dialogue is effective even though one partner tends to talk more than the other. Therefore, they can agree that holding up the hand with the index finger pointing up is an acceptable signal to change speakers.

Certainly, an equalization in the length of time partners speak facilitates self-disclosure and intimacy, but the listener also may facilitate communication through constructive feedback and active listening. Clinicians should model active listening and help the partner to role-play this skill. During this role play couples can also practice exchanging feedback. They frequently need help discriminating between constructive and destructive feedback. If partners have difficulty making this distinction, the clinician may ask partners to give feedback for a few minutes then reverse roles and encourage each partner to return appropriate and inappropriate feedback to its source. Practice sessions in the office or a controlled setting help clients anticipate and avoid errors associated with too little helpful feedback or too much critical feedback.

In addition to verbal communication, clinicians must also focus clients' training on the very powerful nonverbal communication. For example, clients are quite surprised when they learn that when communication is broken down into its parts, that is, content, facial expression, tone of voice, and so forth, the largest percentage of the effective or "heard" communication is actually nonverbal. Unfortunately, clients and clinicians downplay the importance of these skills and overlook the necessity to learn and practice nonverbal skills.

Elements of appropriate nonverbal communication include (Hepworth, Rooney, & Larsen, 1997) facial expressions, posture, voice, and physical proximity. Desirable facial expressions include eye contact, a warm expression, eyes at same level as spouse's, facial expressions that change appropriately in response to the partner's conversation, and a mouth that is relaxed or smiles when appropriate. Posture includes expressiveness of arms and hands with appropriate gestures and body relaxed, leaning toward partner. Clients are more willing to pay attention to and practice these nonverbal skills when they realize their potential impact. Their importance may be emphasized by viewing a three- or four-minute videotape of a television show or home video movie with the sound turned off. The actor's nonverbal communication, which was previously unnoticed, becomes surprisingly vivid. After a discussion about the nonverbal messages, couples are more willing to practice and be sensitive to nonverbal skills.

Couples should be encouraged to practice their verbal and nonverbal communication skills. A few homework exercises facilitate communication and also enhance the relationship. A technique for increasing positive interactions between couples was described by Stuart (1980). Caring Days (see Fig. 10-2) is a method of teaching clients to communicate discrete behaviors that their spouses can perform that are pleasing to them. The couple is then taught to watch for and record when the spouse performs the behavior. While the exercise increases the number of positive interactions in the relationship, the method requires couples to practice communicating their needs and giving supportive feedback.

Finally, Gambrill (1997) identified common errors people make when communicating. For instance, advice giving is a communication error, because people do not generally want to be given advice. Inadequate responses, such as responding with a cliché or parroting what the partner says, are not believed to be helpful. Similar errors to avoid include interruptions, tentativeness, pretending understanding, interpretations of the other's comments, and patronizing statements.

In summary, both verbal and nonverbal skills can be taught by practitioner modeling, client rehearsal, feedback from practitioner and spouse,

FIGURE 10-2 Caring Days List

John					Caring Behaviors	Marie			
7/2	7/3	7/4	7/5	7/7	Ask me how my day went.	7/1	7/2	7/3	7/6
7/3	7/6	7/7			Call me at work just to say hi.	7/7	7/8		
7/4	7/6				Sit next to me when we watch TV.	7/7	7/8	7/9	
7/2	7/4	7/6	7/7	7/9	Compliment me when I look nice.	7/3	7/4		
7/4	7/5	7/9			Talk to me at breakfast and read the paper later.	7/3	7/4	7/5	7/7

SOURCE: Adapted from R. Stuart (1980).

videotaping client's strengths and weaknesses, and homework assignments. Enhancing communication skills facilitates many areas of growth for troubled as well as healthy couples. Furthermore, these skills enable couples to learn from additional experiences. For example, Gambrill and Richey (1985) used role reversal with couples to increase their sensitivity to the opposite gender spouse. Wives can take on the protector role by helping the husband on with his coat and opening the door for him; the husband can wait for the door to be opened, or sit quietly in a restaurant while the spouse orders for them both. With enhanced communication skills, these partners are enabled to exchange feelings and perceptions in a constructive, growth-producing manner. These skills also help couples negotiate other areas of their lives.

Negotiation and contracting skills training.   When couples learn how to communicate well, they need a few additional skills to negotiate and contract areas of differences or conflict. Problem-solving techniques (Sheafor et al., 1997) may be used to look at all possible solutions. The steps include 1) writing or stating a clear description of the problem, 2) identifying each partner's stake in the problem, 3) brainstorming to come up with all possible solutions without making any judgments about any of the suggested solutions, 4) throwing out all solutions that are absolutely unacceptable to each member, 5) evaluating and ranking the remaining solutions, 6) trying out the solution, and 7) making modifications if necessary.

Some clients are reluctant to review problem solving because they presume that they already know and usually use this easy, logical strategy. They should be reminded that the ease of use and the logical steps are deceptive, because people usually skip steps or fail to use the approach all together. For example, people normally solve problems by looking for the first solution that is sufficiently logical and familiar. Unfortunately, what is logical and familiar may simply be a repeat of previously ineffective solutions or a mismatch between a perfectly good solution and the wrong problem. The problem-solving approach facilitates a clear definition of the problem and a review of alternative solutions. Clients may also be helped by a reminder that one ingredient in successful problem solving is a longer list of alternative solutions.

Contracts (Stuart, 1980) have also been used by couples to negotiate areas of conflict (see Fig. 10-3). Quid pro quo contracts make spouses' behavior contingent on their partners' performance. For example, a husband will take out the trash if (and only if) the wife cooks dinner. Quid pro quo is most helpful when emotionally distant partners need to focus on positive, contingent behavior.

The good faith, or parallel, contract makes individual performance of behaviors independent of the other spouse. For example, the wife gets to go shopping for four hours on Saturday if she completes the laundry by Friday night. The husband gets to play tennis when the kitchen is cleaned. While this approach may feel rather mechanistic to many people, couples quickly recognize contracting as an effective way to get their needs met and ensure some

FIGURE 10-3   Contract

Target behaviors: (a) *preparing food for the baby*
                    (b) *feedings*

HUSBAND:

Husband agrees to prepare food for
   evening and bedtime meals for
   baby.

Husband agrees to get up for
   nighttime feeding on even-
   numbered days

WIFE:

Wife agrees to prepare food for
   morning and lunchtime feedings.

Wife agrees to get up for nighttime
   feedings on odd-numbered days.

Rewards for compliance with terms of the contract:
   Husband gets to take one night off per week to go out with his friends.
   Wife will stay with the baby or arrange for a babysitter.

   Wife gets to have time off to go shopping on Saturdays. Husband will stay
   with the baby or arrange a babysitter.

Contingencies for noncompliance:
   Husband forfeits night out and must give wife $20 for her shopping trip.

   Wife forfeits shopping trip and must give husband one additional night out
   with friends.

SOURCE: Adapted from R. Stuart (1980).

---

equalization of power in couple relationships. The process reemphasizes the constructive necessity of stating needs and having some of them met.

While clinicians help couples negotiate contracts for various roles and responsibilities in the family, couples should be encouraged not to perceive household roles in gender-specific terms. Frequently, husbands and wives are surprised when they construct a simple chart describing the time and energy required of each person in their work outside of or inside the home. Husbands and wives may be willing to take on extra roles when they realize inequities. This is particularly facilitated when various chores are tied to clear-cut payoffs and benefits. For example, each partner may receive free time on the weekend in exchange for an equal amount of child supervision. Similarly, some wives are rather surprised when their self-described "macho" husbands are willing to accept child-care roles following a discussion about their husbands' child-hood experiences (or lack of experience) with their own fathers. In essence, the therapeutic setting helps couples contract ways to manage their harried lives and their traditional-nontraditional roles.

In contracting at home, partners who work outside the home frequently benefit from negotiating and contracting the rules for interaction with the opposite sex in business and social situations. Spouses may be concerned about their partners becoming emotionally or physically involved with another person. Rice (1999) offered guidelines that may serve as a possible contract:

1. Keep business relationships on a professional level.
2. Make a point of introducing your friends to your spouse.
3. Let your spouse know of occasions when you have seen or met (including e-mail) with the other person, whether at a business lunch or on a social occasion.
4. Never try to hide anything from your spouse, and do not have anything to hide.
5. Avoid one-on-one dates for social purposes.
6. Prefer groups of mixed company rather than dyadic encounters.
7. Recognize that many affairs develop without people intending things to happen, simply because people place themselves in compromising situations.
8. Make certain that other people whom you meet know you are monogamous (i.e., no hanky panky attitude).
9. As a couple, develop your social life with other couples, both of whom the two of you know and enjoy being with.
10. If you are having marital difficulties, get help from a professional. Many extramarital affairs develop because of a series of unresolved problems in the marriage, making the partners vulnerable to outside encounters and relationships.

Since successful marriages involve sexual exclusiveness and commitment to one person only, these steps may prove useful. To ignore them and allow friendships to go beyond the just-friends stage is to court problems (Rice, 1999, pp. 323–324).

Time-management techniques. For Greenhaus & Beutell (1985), time-based conflict may arise from conflicting roles that are impossible to fulfill without some compromise or outside assistance. For example, problems emerge as a result of workaholism, the responsibilities that come from caring for small children, spouses adhering to traditional gender roles, or a partner whose work requires significant traveling and inflexible job hours.

Time management is a therapeutic injunction to help couples prioritize their commitments and make time for important people, places, and events. The therapist can help couples structure their time by encouraging them to establish and prioritize individual, couple, and family goals (Davidson, 1978; Ferner, 1980, 1995). Clinicians will want to help clients keep in mind obstacles to effective time management such as procrastination and worry, perfectionism, fear of failure, avoidance versus confrontation, and overwhelming tasks (Curtis & Detert, 1981).

Couples should be encouraged to organize family life with a planned approach. For example, couples should be encouraged to consider that each partner has home and family responsibilities. Similarly, if there are children, they too should pitch in and perform their share of home tasks that are appropriate for their ages. Couples can list all of the individual and joint projects and rate each task. Top priority tasks receive an A, second-level tasks a B, and so forth (Lakein, 1973). Partners then negotiate and schedule A-tasks first. For example, home chores and responsibilities may be divided up on the basis of expertise. The cooking is performed by the best cook, while checkbook/financial responsibilities are given to the one who spends the most money. Cleaning tasks may be divided according to certain payoffs. For example, cleaning bathrooms may be sufficiently unpleasant (to both partners) to afford the person who volunteers for that role no other household cleaning duties (or special fringe benefits such as a modest clothes shopping budget).

On another level, some couples may need to decide which home and family responsibilities are shared by the couple and which are performed separately (Smith & Reid, 1986). One couple may choose to share meal preparation responsibilities, but each partner chooses to have his or her own checkbook or possibly keep money separate. Independently handling chores or responsibilities is an appropriate solution, especially if spouses have different standards of performance. Finally, when both partners have busy schedules outside the home, hiring outside help may be efficient in terms of cost, increased personal or family time, enhanced mental health, or simply the good feeling derived from being cared for.

Mackenzie and Waldo (1981) made the following recommendations for time management: 1) Log your time to find out where it goes; 2) admit your time wasters (i.e., not setting deadlines, procrastination, etc.); 3) set goals; 4) organize your home and office; 5) learn to delegate; 6) learn to avoid interruptions; 7) be assertive; 8) set deadlines for completion of important projects or activities; 9) practice stress-reduction techniques; 10) take time to have fun. Clinicians may provide couples with this list of steps and guide them through a planning session. The process of practicing will be as beneficial as the outcome.

Stress-management techniques.   As time management is an essential ingredient in couples' therapy, stress management is crucial for families as well as couples. Greenhaus & Beutell (1985) identified strain-based conflicts that occur when stress in one role (work) spills over into another area (family). Solutions can be structural, that is, couples can lessen the conflict by agreeing on new expectations. For example, a partner may give up one of the roles (e.g., hire a nanny to help care for the children). Also, solutions may be personal, reducing one's performance standards by prioritizing, compartmentalizing, or reducing the standards. For example, rank the tasks to be done and perform only the urgent ones.

Therapists can help individuals, couples, and family members make lists of the stress points in their lives and analyze them in terms of importance, strength, impact, and duration. This analysis often helps clients realize that the stressors previously considered temporary or transitory are actually part of a long line or chain of ongoing struggles. Couples may need to determine if the stressors are due to lack of organization or overwhelming responsibilities, and if so, they should be encouraged to develop specific strategies for solving particular problems. For example, they may hire outside help, set aside a specific time to solve a developing problem, or perhaps decide to intentionally ignore a long-lasting situation since no one in the past has had sufficient interest to fix it.

Most empirically based programs (Freidman & Dermit, 1988) for stress management contain four components: self-monitoring, daily relaxation exercises, cognitive restructuring, and environmental alteration (such as time management). Other techniques to help reduce stress include meditation, self-hypnosis, or biofeedback. Clinicians may benefit from reading Friedman and Dermit's (1988) list of recommended stress-management texts. For example, they recommend Gendlin (1978); Girdano and Everly (1986), Meichenbaum (1983), and Schafer (1996). A similar list of texts is suggested for clients (Mantell, 1988).

Clinicians should be ready to challenge irrational beliefs or unrealistic attitudes that contribute to stress. Cognitive restructuring (Granvold, 1988) is a technique that helps practitioners challenge and dispute cognitive distortions. For example, the following distortions are common in couples with distressed marriages: 1) Absolutistic/dichotomous thinking, such as seeing situations in a rigid good/bad manner; 2) overgeneralization—applying information from one situation to an unrelated situation; 3) selective abstraction—looking only at the negative information and ignoring the positive; 4) arbitrary inference—mind reading and predicting negative outcomes; 5) magnification and minimization—perceiving situations in the extreme rather than in a more realistic fashion; 6) personalization—inappropriate self-blaming; 7) negative attribution—attributing negative motivations to another's or one's own behavior; and 8) faulty interpretation—missing the intent of another's message.

Clients are usually quite willing to examine a copy of the above list and recall examples of the distortions in their own lives. When exchanged in a warm and fun atmosphere, the label of "distortions" can more readily be accepted and incorporated. The clinician should model for the client constructive ways for each partner to highlight or point out when their partner uses one of the distortions and to openly correct him or her. For example, the therapist may want to say, "All clients benefit from learning about these distortions." Then, with humor and with a sense of the double bind, the clinician may say, "Oops! Did you hear that distortion? I'm sure not 'all clients' are capable of learning from their own distortions or overgeneralizations."

Treatment Limitations

The leading technique is communication skills training. Rice (1999) reported the following types of barriers that inhibit a couple's learning to communicate: physical/environmental, situational, cultural, gender, and psychological. Physical/environmental barriers are related to space. When couples are unable to have contact because of periods of separation, their level of verbal intimacy decreases. Situational barriers, such as pregnancy, changes in job/home setting, or work schedules, may make communication more difficult. Cultural barriers include differences in style, values, religion, and so forth. Since these barriers as invisible and perhaps perceptually unavailable, spouses from different ethnic backgrounds may speak to each other from the standpoint of differing paradigms and may completely fail to communicate. For example, gender barriers relate to socialized masculine-feminine differences. Women who are socialized to be nonconfrontational and accommodating may have difficulty communicating with husbands who are more aggressive. Psychological barriers may inhibit communication if spouses do not trust each other or keep silent because of fear of rejection or failure.

Another significant treatment limitation is the clients' motivation to change. Stuart (1980) reported that couples who come for marital therapy are often taking one last chance to save the marriage. Therefore, either one or both spouses may have already made the decision to leave the marriage. Treatment should, therefore, focus on giving the couple as much hope and positive signs of change as quickly as possible to keep them in therapy. Techniques such as Stuart's Caring Days are designed to help spouses recognize and reinforce the positive behaviors of their partner.

Another limitation is generalization and maintenance of the treatment. Just because couples learn to interact on a more positive basis in your office, does not mean that they will continue a satisfactory relationship once they leave. Generalization of positive changes learned in the office must be transferred to the couple's external world by setting up homework assignments. This can help the couple to practice newly learned skills in the natural environment. Additionally, they can report to the therapist how the practice sessions went and get therapist feedback on improving skills.

Maintenance of change, that is, continuing the positive changes learned in therapy over time, can be encouraged by therapist follow-up after the conclusion of therapy. If needed, the couple can then come in to bolster their skills. Also, a recommended termination strategy is to end the treatment with a summary from the therapist to the couple reviewing changes made and skills learned while in therapy. At the final visit, the therapist may also present the couple with different situations that might occur and help the couple to think through how their newly learned skills might be applied.

GENERALIZING THE INTERVENTION TO RELATED PROBLEMS

Each element of the intervention package has been used in diverse settings. Values clarification is used with adults and adolescents; communication training is a common component of many different strategies such as group marital counseling, counseling with the chronic mentally ill, and business education. The remaining three have similar, yet less extensive exposure.

Research and practice wisdom support the generalization of this comprehensive treatment package to problem areas where interpersonal interaction is important for the maintenance of dyads or groups and for the goal of growth and development for participants. Specific populations include adolescents and their parents, teams of professionals in medical or mental health settings, and business or management groups whose function and goals require close interpersonal support and cooperation. Many of the latter groups resemble a "marriage" of personnel to each other and the task at hand.

Self-Esteem

The personal concept of the self is an important factor in therapy and this invention package. Self-esteem is a much-talked-about idea, even though people define it differently. A helpful definition of self-concept focuses on the cognitive image people have of themselves. For example, some people see themselves as succeeding at various tasks and others expect the worst of themselves. This image is largely learned from the complex array of people, life experiences, personal thoughts, and so forth, of each person. Parents are very influential when they frequently tell their children that they are smart, dull, female, male, fat, skinny, and so on. The telling of these messages is frequently verbal, yet more influential images are projected nonverbally. For example, numerous adults can recount the facial expression of their parents that signaled disapproval. Similarly, children and adults acquire the mannerisms, attitudes, and behaviors of important role models, e.g., parents, friends, teachers, movie stars, and/or strangers who are impressive for a variety of reasons. These images, attitudes, and so forth constitute the self-image or self-esteem, and yet self-esteem is so much a part of peoples' lives that they are largely unaware of it until that image or concept is questioned.

In intimate relationships the self-esteem or self-concept of each partner affects the nature of the relationship. Rarely if ever are two partners so similar or complementary that their self-concepts mesh without occasional distress or outright hostility. Whereas all partners challenge each other and sometimes question their partner's behavior, distressed couples focus on their differences and emphasize the negative aspects of their self-image, such as beliefs of unworthiness or helplessness. Unfortunately, in some destructive relationships partners may emphasize the imperfections or insecurities of their mates in order to gain an advantage. Therefore, improving the self-image or self-esteem is vitally important to healthy relationships.

The skills training addressed in this intervention package affirms the reality that insight into a person's low self-esteem is not as effective as building self-image through improved social competence. People's self-concepts improve when they gain the ability to interact more effectively with others. They see themselves as more in control of their environment when they can experience themselves getting their own needs met and meeting the needs of others.

As people's images of themselves improve, they can actively reconcile role and value conflicts with their partners. The cognitive dissonance between behaving in a new, effective manner and the old negative self-images often results in the alteration of the negative self-attitudes. Additionally, overcoming value conflicts allows partners to set new goals and interact in healthier patterns. Similarly, other people in their environment come to expect different interactions with the person and therefore treat the other person in a more positive and affirming manner.

When communication, the primary vehicle for the resolution of value conflicts, is improved, clients frequently experience an enhanced image of themselves because they are able to effectively use communication as a tool to get what they want or need. For example, partners may feel that they are being taken advantage of because they are not getting what they need. Techniques of leveling may enable partners to clearly express their needs, and, consequently, their partners know how to respond. They are frequently surprised to learn that their partners never knew of the previously unmet needs.

Similarly, negotiation and contracting skills are effective strategies for resolving long-standing disagreements or problems. Mastering these tools improves the sense of self-efficacy that comes from gaining the ability to negotiate solutions to problems. A byproduct of the contracting skill is the increased self-evaluation that they are worth the time and effort of making a contract with in order to enable them to fulfill their needs. Additionally, their partners may increasingly see them as more valuable and may treat them differently.

Finally, reducing stress and managing time greatly improve clients' ability to gain control over difficult and demanding lifestyles. Persons armed with the skills for this intervention package are persons who are much more capable of meeting their own needs, interacting effectively with their partners and family, and gaining a more satisfying self-image.

SUMMARY

The social learning–cognitive behavioral approach teaches couples to take charge of their relationships and produce changes that best fit their own needs, and it increases the rewards and lowers the costs of being with their partners. The current intervention package focuses on the following five areas: values clarification, communication training, negotiation and contracting skills training, time-management techniques, and stress management. In general, the first three interventions are recommended as a sequence because they logically develop out of each other. The last two intervention areas may be added as couples make sufficient progress in the other areas.

Values and goal clarification interventions are frequently helpful with couples who describe frustrations and conflicts over divergent opinions and perspectives. When couples complain about nonspecific frustrations and dissatisfaction, clinicians should look for underlying differences in expectations or perspectives, i.e., housekeeping standards, differences in child-rearing styles, friendships at work, gender roles, and appropriate expressions of intimacy.

Communication training focuses on partners' inability to express ideas or opinions and listen effectively to their partners. Couples who communicate about everything at once benefit from editing procedures; those who avoid intimate or disagreeable issues need methods of disclosure or leveling. Also, couples whose interactions get out of control should be taught to use time-out or stop-action procedures. Couples who frequently give mixed messages need to learn how to recognize and modify incongruent verbal and nonverbal messages.

The communication skills training helps couples develop their negotiating and contracting skills. These help couples who have recurrent problems. Techniques presented are problem-solving techniques for couples and quid pro quo and good faith contracts.

The time-management interventions give couples tools to preserve the valuable human resources of time and energy. Couples need these skills when they report being continually overwhelmed, tired, or resentful of family or work demands. The intervention requires couples to prioritize and potentially reorder their time allotments and responsibilities. They are encouraged to give up activities that require inordinate amounts of time and hire outside help to alleviate pressures on the couple and family.

Finally, the last section of intervention focuses on stress-management techniques. Clinicians are encouraged to assess the amount of stress their clients endure in terms of importance, strength, impact, and duration. The assessment can further differentiate between temporary or transitory stressors and long-term stressors. The intervention package requires practitioners to select from such methods as self-monitoring, daily relaxation exercises, cognitive restructuring, and environmental alteration (such as time management).

Couples involved in this intervention package can be expected to generalize their learning to other settings. The skills perspective enables them to apply these tools in related areas such as in work settings, in other friendships or in relationships with relatives, and in parent-child interactions. Changes in clients' self-esteem are expected to follow from the new or renewed sense of self-efficacy.

CHAPTER 11

Social Competence Promotion for Troubled Youth

Craig Winston LeCroy

In this chapter, LeCroy examines the problems that are common with troubled youth and clearly and concisely defines various risk-taking behaviors. Such problems frequently result from peer pressure, and in response to this, LeCroy shows how to help promote social competence in adolescents. The intervention is a well-defined approach that develops social skills, problem-solving abilities, and cognitive skills. LeCroy demonstrates a foundation of change by matching the particular need for interpersonal competency with the specific environment (e.g., family or school). This chapter shows how to use an intervention in a well-defined and straightforward step-by-step protocol.

INTRODUCTION

Nancy was referred by the school social worker to an outpatient clinic that specializes in depressed children. She has been feeling lonely and is frequently seen at school by herself and appears to have few friends. Her parents report that she cries often and does not seem happy with her life. Tom was suspended from school because he and his friends were caught drinking alcohol on the school grounds. Tom has plenty of friends, but they are frequently in trouble with school officials and the law. Tom's parents are concerned about his alcohol use; he has been caught coming home intoxicated on numerous occasions. John dropped out of school at 15 and has had a difficult time finding employment. He does not present himself in a very convincing manner to employers although he has had numerous job experiences. He lives with his mother and stepfather but does not feel welcome there and would like to become independent.

All of these young people lack certain social or life skills. With the necessary skills, all these young people could lead more satisfying interpersonal lives. Nancy could be helped to learn friendship skills to address her feelings of loneliness. She could also be taught coping skills to address her negative and depressing thoughts. Tom could be helped by learning about the consequences of drug use and learning the skills needed to resist peer pressure. John needs to learn how to anticipate employers' concerns, skills for presenting his qualifications confidently and assertively, and appropriate ways to follow up with prospective employers.

These methods of helping young people constitute an approach referred to as social skills training. This approach asserts that the explanation for this problem behavior in young people comes from the fact that they have not acquired the skills needed to cope with various situational demands. The emphasis is on social skills, the skills that are maximally effective in resolving the demands of problem situations while minimizing the likelihood of future problems. Human development is perceived as a process of confronting a series of tasks and situational demands rather than movement through stages. Promoting social competence in young people is an effective strategy for helping them confront stressful or problematic situations (Haggerty, Sherrod, Garmezy, & Rutter, 1996). Young people need to acquire numerous social skills because during adolescence they develop new patterns of interpersonal relationships, confront new social experiences, and learn new behavioral responses (Jessor, 1982). Without sufficient social skills, these experiences can become avenues to pregnancy, delinquency, drug abuse, and social isolation.

The extent to which adolescents successfully confront the complex demands and tasks of adolescence will have an impact on the course of their lives. Problem behaviors that begin in early adolescence are more likely to continue in later life. For example, drug use in early adolescence is a strong predictor of drug use in late adolescence and adulthood (Yamaguchi & Kandel, 1984). Young adolescents are vulnerable to serious social problems in our society: drug abuse, school dropout, unemployment, delinquency, early pregnancy, and poor mental health.

Research on the social problems of youth indicates that problems begin to develop between the ages of 13 and 16. Indeed, research on adolescent development suggests that there are important differences between early, middle, and late adolescence (Santrock, 1996). The young adolescent years mark the beginning attempts to establish friendships, high degrees of anxiety regarding peer relationships, increased conformity with one's peers, and beginning attempts to acquire social competence (LeCroy, 1983). It is also during early adolescence that young people begin to experience their vulnerability to some of society's external forces. Adolescents begin to confront many social problems, and without the requisite social and coping skills they become vulnerable to many situations that threaten their future potential.

THE NEED TO REDUCE THE RISK-TAKING BEHAVIORS OF ADOLESCENTS

The risk-taking behavior of young people is a serious national problem. Successfully confronting the pressures of sex, alcohol, and drugs is a normal part of the process of growing up in American society (Dryfoos, 1990). Jackson and Hornbeck (1989, p. 833) state emphatically, "in our society, peer pressure to engage in early sexual activity and the availability of alcohol, drugs, and cigarettes virtually guarantee that every American young adolescent will be confronted with decisions about whether to engage in behaviors that could have life-long, if not lethal, consequences." Estimates are that upwards of 25 percent of youth are extremely vulnerable and another 25 percent are considered moderately vulnerable to engaging in high-risk behavior (Dryfoos, 1990). In addition, epidemiological data indicate that up to 22 percent of children and adolescents have mental health problems serious enough to warrant treatment (Costello, 1990; Tuma, 1989).

Drugs, Alcohol, and Cigarettes

The combined effects of drugs, alcohol, and cigarette use is taking an unprecedented toll on young people. Over 12 percent of high school students report smoking six or more cigarettes a day, and over 23 percent report using alcohol two days per month or more (Resnick, Bearman, & Blum, 1997). Marijuana use has dramatically increased over the last ten years. From 1991 to 1994, marijuana use by eighth graders doubled to 13 percent, increased by two-thirds for tenth graders to 25 percent, and almost doubled for twelfth graders to 31 percent (Johnston, Bachman, & O'Malley, 1995). Although recent studies document a decline in the use of marijuana, one-quarter of all young people report having smoked marijuana at least once in their lives (Resnick et al., 1997). Studies also find large numbers of students using other drugs such as crack and cocaine. The initial use of these drugs is taking place earlier, for example, 55 percent of high school seniors report alcohol use prior to the tenth grade. Although drug use has leveled off in the last several years, reports indicate that approximately 50 percent of those who had used drugs by their senior year, initiated use prior to the tenth grade (Johnston, Bachman, & O'Malley, 1995).

Sexual Activity

Large numbers of adolescents are sexually active. By the time they graduate from high school almost half of all adolescents will have had sexual intercourse. An increasing number of them are young people under the age of 16. Girls 14 years of age and younger continue to increase their rate of sexual activity. These younger girls are engaging in high-risk behaviors because they are slow to use contraception. Almost half of these girls (42 percent) delayed using contraceptive methods for more than a year (Hofferth, Kahn, & Baldwin, 1987). In addition to the risk of unwanted pregnancy, young people face high rates of contracting sexually transmitted diseases. One-fourth of all adolescents will have contracted a sexually transmitted disease before graduating from high school (US Department of Health, Education, and Welfare, 1979).

Delinquency

Delinquency is also a concern because delinquent behavior begins and peaks in adolescence. By the age of 15, delinquent activity has reached its peak (Farrington, 1995). In one study (Institute for Juvenile Research, 1972), one-half of the 14- to 18-year-olds surveyed had shoplifted. Farrington (1995) reports that 96 percent of inner-city youth admitted committing at least one of ten common offenses. Census data show that an estimated 625,000 young people were admitted to juvenile detention and correctional facilities (Bureau of Justice Statistics, 1986). With regard to criminal offenders, one of every twenty persons arrested for a violent crime and one in seven property crimes is committed by a person less than 15 years old (Wetzel, 1987). In fact, "youths are the segment of the population most likely to be victimized by a criminal, most likely to commit a crime, most likely to be arrested, and, after their early 20s, most likely to be imprisoned for committing a crime" (Wetzel, 1987, p. 31).

School Dropout Rates and Unemployment

The overall dropout rate has decreased over time, but it is still over 10 percent (National Center for Education Statistics, 1993). Minority youth make up a disproportionate share of the total number of high school dropouts, and disparities in high school completion rates between white and minority youth did not improve between 1990 and 1996. There is reason to believe that the school dropout rate will increase because the educational system is unresponsive to the needs of non–college bound youth. Whether they graduate from school or not, many young people have early negative experiences in their attempt to find employment. The unemployment rate for adolescents (ages 16 to 19) is 15.8 percent (William T. Grant Foundation, 1988). The unemployment rate for minority youth is nearly double that of their white peers.

There has been an intensification and increase in the health and behavior problems young people must face. Americans have witnessed critical changes in families, schools, and neighborhoods during the past several decades. Major social and economic changes include increased rates of poverty, the deterioration of neighborhoods, weaker social supports available to youth and families, a deficit in positive role models, growing educational disadvantage, and increased exposure to negative media messages. In this context, we must develop realistic cost-effective strategies to impact the psychological and social needs of young people.

While multiple strategies are necessary, the promotion of social competence offers an approach that can be used for both problem prevention and problem remediation. Clearly, there is a multitude of life tasks that many young people are not prepared to address. Young people are repeatedly presented with the skills necessary to offset the influences and pressures to use drugs (Botvin, 1996). Much research has gone into programs developed to help young adolescents prevent unwanted pregnancies. Barth (1996) discovered that coping with sexual behavior and successfully using contraceptive aids involves a set of acquired social skills. Freedman, Rosenthal, Donahoe, Schlundt, and McFall (1978) validated a conceptualization of delinquent behavior that is based on situationally specific skill deficits. Disadvantaged youth can be taught a skill-building process that helps them overcome common skill deficits in seeking and and maintaining employment (Staab & Lodish, 1985). The social problems of youth, described above, document the problems young people face and the consequences for our society. It appears that the present methods of socialization are inadequate given the increasing number of youth who are involved in such problems. The promotion of social competence is of critical importance to the successful socialization of youth.

PROMOTING SOCIAL COMPETENCE

The promotion of social competence as a framework for intervention represents a distinct move away from defect or medical models and places a greater emphasis on the environmental influences on individuals. It also emphasizes the positive aspects of functioning. Bloom (1977, p. 250) notes that "of all the concepts that have been introduced to link individual problems to characteristics of the social system, the most compelling have been the concepts of competence and competence building."

The Consortium on the School-Based Promotion of Competence (1996, p. 275) suggests that social competence be viewed in terms of "life skills for adaption to diverse ecologies and settings." Wine (1981) notes that the defining characteristic of the competence approach is a concern with the individual's effectiveness with his or her interactions with the environment. Therefore, social competence deals explicitly with an individual's impact on the environment, as well as the impact of the environment on the individual. In this manner, social competence is a transitional model of human behavior.

This approach to social competence recognizes the importance of overt behaviors, cognitive capacities, problem-solving abilities and coping skills, and the ability to produce appropriate matches between behaviors and situational requirements. Although behavior is influenced by the environment, a person creates his or her own environment. Through their transactions with the environment, people help shape the social milieu and other circumstances that arise in their daily transactions. Internal personal factors (beliefs) form a reciprocal relationship with behavior to create expectations influencing behavior. In turn, environmental influences interact with behavior to affect a person's expectations of personal effectiveness or self-efficacy (Bandura, 1977a).

Such multidirectional influence is best described by an example. A youth learns skills in resisting peer pressure to smoke cigarettes through modeling and role playing with others in a smoking prevention group. Whether these skills hold up under natural conditions depends on interactions between the person, the environment, and his or her performance. Personal sources of influence provide the initial stimulus ("If I smoke a cigarette my friends won't think badly of me" or "I don't want to smoke because I know it's bad for my health"). The youth then selects a course of action ("No, thanks, I'm not smoking anymore because it's bad for one's health"). His or her peers may support this refusal by telling others the youth is no longer smoking, thereby influencing the environment by reducing the pressure to smoke. The youth's expectations are also influenced since confidence has been gained in his abilities to make and implement responsible decisions.

The social competence approach has increasingly stressed that the concept of self-efficacy provides a framework for studying stress and coping. Competence in coping with the environment is more than knowing what to do. It requires cognitive, social, and behavioral skills in dealing with situations that are ambiguous, unpredictable, and stressful. Bandura's model of self-efficacy assumes that people use four sources of information for judging their capabilities to confront environmental demands. Most important is the performance mode, which relies on information gained from previous experience in handling similar situations. In this way, experience with situations where individuals cope successfully builds efficacy. Research has found that lower perceived self-efficacy in stressful situations leads to a decrease in exertion of effort. People begin to give up easily and learn to anticipate failure. Information about efficacy expectations is gained through vicarious channels. When individuals observe success or failure of others, their perceived efficacy is influenced. The intervention task is to understand these multiple sources of influence and make appropriate matches between the individual's competencies and the demands of the environment. Figure 11-1 shows the relationship between various competencies and environmental tasks or stresses for adolescents. Interpersonal competence resolves around three areas: cognitive development, problem-solving abilities, and social skills. At adolescence, the environment presents situations that demand competencies to deal with issues such as peer relationships, school, and family relationships. A competency such as generating alternatives and thinking consequentially might be needed to address a situational demand such as deciding whether or not to have sexual intercourse when no contraception is available.

Social incompetence is the result of a mismatch between a young person's ability to perform a given certain task and the demands imposed on the person. Problems develop when this imbalance occurs between a person's abilities and the demands present in the person's person-environment system.

METHODS OF PROMOTING SOCIAL COMPETENCE

Strategies for promoting social competence consist largely of the techniques of social skills training and problem-solving training. Social skills training provides an environment for young people to experiment with new

FIGURE 11-1 Social Competence Model

Interpersonal Competence		Environment (at adolescence)
Cognitive Development		Peer Relationships
Reasoning abilities		Anxiety over friendships
Interpersonal awareness	MATCH	Pressure to conform
	COMPETENCIES	Sexual socialization
Problem-Solving		
Abilities	WITH DEMANDS	
Generating alternatives	OF THE	School
Thinking consequentially	ENVIRONMENT	Entry into new peer groups
Means/end thinking		Authority structure
		Exposure to drugs, sex, etc.
Social Skills	← →	
Prosocial behavior		Family
Resisting peer pressure	TRANSACTING	Independence from the family
Negotiating abilities		Family versus peer relations
		Family conflict

behaviors. It is usually done in a group format that provides support and a reinforcing context for learning new responses. Additionally, the group allows for extensive use of modeling and feedback, which are critical components of successful skills training. Rotheram-Borus & Tsemberis (1989, p. 299) identify seven common features of social competency training programs:

1. A set of specific skills is taught.
2. Members participate in structured activities, usually in a group setting.
3. Peers and/or adults provide social support.
4. The social skills to be acquired are practiced in the group setting.
5. An active style of coping with problem situations is encouraged.
6. A language or vocabulary for understanding one's affective, behavioral, and cognitive responses to problems is provided.
7. Programs aim to make the skills that are acquired relevant and useful to children and adolescents at various stages of development.

The following is an overview of the steps involved in social skills training.

Developing Program Goals and Selecting Skills

In order to develop a successful social skills training program, it is important to identify the goals of the program, for example, perhaps the outcome will be to manage one's anger in provocative situations. Once the goals of the program are decided on, it is important to select the specific skills that are to be taught.

Depending on the type of problem situation you are addressing, a number of different skills are appropriate. Table 11-1 presents examples of programs and the types of skills that are targeted. For example, in working with problems of aggressiveness, some common skills include recognizing that interactions are likely to lead to problems and learning to request behavior changes of others (see Table 11-1).

In identifying social skills, it is important to break them down into their component parts so that they can be more easily taught. For example, LeCroy (1994) points out that a conversation involves six parts: looking the other person in the eye, greeting the person by name and asking an open-ended question about the person, making a statement to follow up on the person's response, asking another open-ended question, making a statement about the conversation, and ending the conversation.

Constructing social situations that demand certain social skills is also an important part of social skills training. It is preferable if the social situations and skill can be determined empirically. For example, Freedman et al. (1978) constructed problematic situations that delinquents were likely to encounter, elicited responses to these situations, and then had the responses rated for competence. This allows for a clear indication of what types of situations are problematic for delinquents and what constitutes an appropriate response to those situations. However, most practitioners develop their own problematic situations for use in social skills training. For example, the following situation could be used in a substance abuse prevention program:

> You ride to a party with someone you've been dating for about six months. The party is at someone's house whose parents are gone for the weekend. There is a lot of beer and dope, and your date has had too much to drink. Your date says, "Hey, where's my keys—let's get going."

After goals have been defined and skills have been selected, the focus is on the process of teaching social skills (for additional information on assessment and selection of skills, see LeCroy, 1994).

The Process of Teaching Social Skills

The following is an overview of the process of teaching social skills. There are seven basic steps that leaders should follow. Table 11-2 presents these steps and outlines the process for teaching social skills. In each step, there is a request for group member involvement. This is because it is critical that group leaders involve the participants actively in the skill training. This keeps the group interesting and fun for the group members.

TABLE 11-1   Problem Behaviors and Related Social Skills Training

Type of Program and Resources	*Social Skills Focus*
Aggressive Behavior Elder, Edelstein, & Narick (1979) Feindler & Guttman (1994) Goldstein & Glick (1987) Bierman & Greenberg (1996)	Skills to Work On 1. Recognizing interactions likely to lead to problems. 2. Learning responses to negative communication. 3. Learning to request a behavior change.
Withdrawn and Isolated Behavior Gottman (1983) Greenwood, Todd, Haps, & Walken (1982) Hops, Walker, & Greenwood (1979) Paine, Hops, Walker, Greenwood, Fleischman, & Guild (1982)	Skills to Work On 1. Greeting others. 2. Joining in ongoing activities. 3. Starting a conversation. 4. Sharing things and ideas.
Substance Abuse Prevention Pentz (1985) Hohman & Buchik (1994) Botvin (1996)	Skills to Work On 1. Identifying problem situations. 2. Learning effective refusal skills. 3. Making friends with nonusing peers. 4. General problem-solving techniques.
Teen Pregnancy Prevention Schinke, Blythe, & Gilchrist (1981) Barth (1996)	Skills to Work On 1. Identifying risky situations. 2. Refusing unreasonable demands. 3. Learning new interpersonal responses. 4. Problem-solving techniques.
Peer Mediation for Interpersonal Conflict Schrumpf, Crawford, & Usadel (1991)	Skills to Work On 1. Communication skills. 2. Focusing on common interests. 3. Creating options. 4. Writing an agreement.

TABLE 11-2 A Summary of the Steps in Teaching Social Skills Training

1. Present the social skill being taught.
   A. Solicit an explanation of the skill.
   B. Get group members to provide rationales for the skill.

2. Discuss the social skill.
   A. List the skill steps.
   B. Get group members to give examples of using the skill.

3. Present a problem situation and model the skill.
   A. Evaluate the performance.
   B. Get group members to discuss the model.

4. Set the stage for role playing the skill.
   A. Select the group members for role playing.
   B. Get group members to observe the role play.

5. Group members rehearse the skill.
   A. Provide coaching if necessary.
   B. Get group members to provide feedback on verbal and nonverbal elements.

6. Practice using complex skill situations.
   A. Teach accessory skills, e.g., problem solving.
   B. Get group members to discuss situations and provide feedback.

7. Train for generalization and maintenance.
   A. Encourage practice of skills outside the group.
   B. Get group members to bring in their problem situations.

SOURCE: LeCroy (1994).

Present the social skill being taught. In this first step the group leader presents the skill being taught. The leader begins by soliciting an explanation of the skill, for example, "Can anyone tell me what it means to resist peer pressure?" After group members respond, the leader emphasizes the rationale for using the skill. For example, in teaching young people the skill of resisting peer pressure, the leader might say, "You would use this skill when you're in a situation where you don't want to do something that your friends want you to do and you should be able to say no in such a way that your friends can accept your refusal." The leader then asks for additional reasons for learning the skill.

Discuss the social skill. The leader presents the specific skill steps that constitute the social skill. For example, the skill steps for resisting peer pressure are good nonverbal communication (includes eye contact, posture, and voice volume), saying "no" early in the interaction, suggesting an alternative activity, and leaving the situation if there is continued pressure. Group members are then asked for examples of when they have used the skill or examples of when could have used the skill but did not.

Present a problem situation and model the skill.   The leader presents a problem situation that demands the use of the skill being taught. For example, the following is a problem situation for resisting peer pressure (LeCroy, 1994, p. 145):

> You agreed with your parents that you would be home at 9:30 p.m. It is now 9:00 p.m. You are at a friend's house, and he says, "Hey, let's go to the mall, I know Matt and Blake will be there."

The group leader chooses members to role-play this situation and then models the skills. Group members are asked to evaluate the model's performance. Did the model follow all of the skill steps? Was the performance successful? The group leader may choose another group member to model the skills if the leader believes that this group member already has the requisite skills. Another alternative being increasingly used is to present to the group with videotaped models. This has the advantage of following the recommendation by researchers that the performers in the model be similar to the trainee in age, sex, and social characteristics.

Set the stage for role playing or rehearsal of the skill.   At this point the group leader needs to construct the social circumstances for the role play. Group members are selected for the role play and given their respective parts to play. It is important that the leader review with the group members in the role play exactly what their role is to be. Group members not in the role play are asked to observe the process. It is sometimes helpful if they are given specific instructions for their observations. For example, one member may observe the use of nonverbal skills, another member may be instructed to observe when "no" is said in the interaction.

Group members rehearse the skill.   Rehearsal or guided practice of the skill is an important part of effective social skills training. Group leaders and group members provide instructions or coaching before and during the role play and provide praise and feedback for improvement. Following a role-play enactment, the leader will usually give instructions for improvement, model the suggested improvements, or coach the person to incorporate the feedback in the subsequent role play. Often the member doing the role play will practice the skills in the situation several times in order to refine his or her skills and incorporate feedback offered by the group. The role plays continue until the trainee's behavior becomes more and more similar to that of the model. It is important that overlearning take place, so the group leader encourages many examples of effective skill demonstration followed by praise.

Group members should be taught how to give effective feedback prior to the rehearsals. Throughout the teaching process, the group leader can model desired responses. For example, after a role play the leader can respond first and then model, giving feedback that starts with a positive statement.

Practice using complex skill situations. The group continues with more difficult and complex skill situations. More complex situations can be developed by extending the interactions and roles in the problem situations. Most social skills groups also incorporate the teaching of problem-solving abilities. Problem solving should take a general approach to helping young people analyze and resolve interpersonal problems. Young people are taught to gather information about a problematic situation, generate a large number of potential solutions, evaluate the consequences of various solutions, and outline plans for the implementation of a particular solution. Group leaders can give young people problem situations and have members generate alternatives and consequences, select a feasible solution, and make plans for implementing it. The problem-solving training is important because it prepares young people to make whatever adjustment strategies are needed in a given situation. It is a general skill with large-scale application. For a more complete discussion on the use of problem-solving approaches, see Elias and Clabby (1992).

Train for generalization and maintenance. The success of the social skills program depends on the extent to which young people can learn transfer the skills to their day-to-day lives. Practitioners must always be planning for ways in which to maximize the generalization of skills learned and their continued use after training. There are a number of principles that help facilitate the generalization and maintenance of skills.

The first is the use of overlearning. The more overlearning that takes place the greater likelihood of later transfer. Therefore, it is important that group leaders insist on mastery of the skills. Another important principle of generalization is to vary the stimuli where skills are learned. To accomplish this, practitioners can use a variety of models, problem situations, role-play actors, and trainers. The different styles and behaviors of the people used produce a broader base to apply the skills learned. Perhaps most important is the requirement that the young people use the skills in their own real-life settings. Group leaders should assign and monitor homework to encourage transfer of learning. This may include the use of written contracts to perform certain tasks outside the group. Group members should be asked to bring to the group examples of problem situations where the social skills can be applied. Lastly, practitioners should attempt to develop external support for the skills learned. One approach is to set up a buddy system in which group members work together to perform the skills learned outside the group (Rose & Edelson, 1987).

Treatment Limitations

Although numerous applications and research support have been presented in support of a model for the promotion of social competence among youth, it is not without problems regarding its development as a treatment modality. In particular, three issues need further clarification: the conceptualization of social competence and social skills, the content of the treatment programs, and the applicability of the training.

There are many issues in grappling with the best way to conceptualize social competence. McFall (1982) believes that "the most important component in the evolving conception of social competence is the concept of a task." Competence should be evaluated in reference to a particular task. In order to assess how adequately a person has performed a task, "one must understand these important features of that task: its purpose, its constraints, its setting, the rules governing task performance, the criteria for distinguishing between successful and unsuccessful performance, and how the task relates to other aspects of the person's life system" (McFall, 1982, p. 16). For example, with regard to setting, where does peer pressure occur? We also do not know much about the rules governing situations where young people are pressured into sex or drug use. Our attempts to address social skills should take into consideration the implicit organization and rules that govern such interactions.

Conceptual questions also arise concerning the reasons why some young people may fail to acquire social skills. It may be that these young people never developed the necessary skills, or they may possess the skills but may have substituted alternative behaviors that are dysfunctional. These conceptual questions require much more work and investigation.

Another issue is what behavioral units should be analyzed in attempting to understand problematic situations. Social skills training content has focused on narrow units (e.g., eye contact), as well as on broadly based units (decision-making skills). What impact is there on effectiveness and generalization when narrow or broad units are taught in social skills programs? A similar issue is the emphasis on overt skills versus cognitively based skills. Is an integration of both overt and cognitive skills the most desirable treatment package?

Although social skills programs have been applied successfully to numerous social programs, there is a need for more research on the effectiveness of social skills training. For example, can social skills training programs produce additional treatment outcomes when used in conjunction with other treatment methods? What is the relative effectiveness of social skills training and family therapy for different adolescent problems? Future work is needed to address these issues.

In conclusion, the promotion of social competence in adolescents is a promising treatment model for helping young people. It has direct relevance to the tasks and demands that young people must face in our society. It focuses on positive aspects of functioning and emphasizes the development of needed skills for young people. Social skills training has good empirical support, and its application is clear and direct. Furthermore, the techniques of social skills training are applicable to various populations and problem configurations. Young people need skills to adapt and cope with an increasingly complex society. To prepare our young people for the future, we must teach them the necessary skills to confront, with self-confidence, the difficult social circumstances that await them.

CHAPTER 12

An Eclectic Approach for Persons with Substance-Related Disorders

Joel Fischer

In this chapter, Fischer shows how to use an eclectic approach with persons who have problems resulting from drug or alcohol abuse. As an eclectic approach, the intervention draws from several different theories and emphasizes the effectiveness of social learning theory. Fischer shows how to reach a well-defined understanding of the specific problem, one that is amenable to monitoring client change, and how to establish realistic goals. These components of structure are of particular concern with a controversial issue such as abuse of drugs and alcohol. The treatment plan Fischer illustrates tends to have well-organized and well-explicated components and is a comprehensive approach to problems of drugs and alcohol. There is clear and unquestioning emphasis on the need for active participation of the client and contracting to help facilitate change. Fischer presents a variety of well-explicated techniques.

INTRODUCTION

There is little question that substance abuse is one of the hot topics from the 1980s up until today. Both the lay and the professional literature are rife with references to the problems and dangers associated with substance use and abuse—and rightly so. The direct and indirect costs of substance abuse—in terms of dollars and lives—are enormous.

However, the real issues involved sometimes are lost in the virtual national hysteria that has arisen since the days of the Reagan administration. The hysteria regarding drug usage in the United States has been well documented by Abbie Hoffman (1987) in his book *Steal This Urine Test*. Hysteria also can be seen, perhaps, in the statement of a graduate social work student who announced in class that an alcoholism expert in a lecture had asserted that 80 percent of human service professionals either have problems with alcohol themselves or come from families where at least one member does. Finally, the national preoccupation with substance abuse can be seen in President Bush's declaration in September of 1989 that "the gravest domestic threat facing our nation today is drugs" (*Honolulu Advertiser*, September 6, 1989, p. A-4).

Obviously, then, there is a great need for social work practitioners to get some kind of handle on the enormous range of problems associated with substance abuse and perhaps to carve out some area of special understanding (or expertise) as a way of addressing some of these problems.

This chapter provides the basis for doing just that. Because of the complexity of and enormous literature on substance abuse problems, and the space limitations inherent in a book such as this, this chapter will not be a general treatise on the nature of substance abuse. Thus, many important and fascinating issues will not be explored, such as,

1. Theories and research about the etiology and maintenance or continuation of substance abuse.
2. The existence of the addictive personality.
3. The concept of addiction, per se (Peele, 1989).
4. Total abstinence versus limited use of some substance for those recovering from abuse.
5. The pros and cons of twelve-step programs (Herman, 1988).
6. The disease model controversy (Fingarette, 1988).
7. Substance abuse prevention (Nathan & Gorman, 1998) and education (Milgram, 1987) programs.
8. Public policy issues (Fraser & Kohlert, 1988).

Many of the references cited in this chapter, however, do address these issues, especially such recent books as Donovan and Marlatt (1988); Miller and Heather (1986); Lewis, Dana, and Blevins (1988); Bratter and Forrest (1985); McCrady and Sher (1985); Galatner (1983); and Nirenberg and Maisto (1987).

Instead of addressing the issues listed above, the focus of this chapter (in keeping with the purposes of this book) is on clinical implications of substance abuse. Substance-related disorders will be viewed essentially as a variety of problems in living that are manifested in biological/physiological, social, and psychological realms of human functioning. The use of the term "problems in living" is not intended to deny the powerful and significant effects of substance abuse. Rather, it is an attempt to destigmatize and delabel the problem and is linked to the approach to intervention that will be described later in this chapter, especially in regard to the need for development of individualized goals and interventions.

Subsequent sections of this chapter describe some dimensions of the problems of substance abuse, both epidemiologically and clinically; present some assessment and evaluation guidelines; and focus most intensively on describing a program for clinical intervention with the problems of, and problems associated with, substance abuse.

PROBLEM IDENTIFICATION

Several substances typically are considered to have the potential to be abused, including alcohol, licit and illicit drugs, food, caffeine, and the nicotine in smoking and smokeless products. There are a number of commonalities among all these substances: all can be used by some people without any problems, whereas other people experience serious problems with their use; all involve short-term pleasurable activities with potential for long-term negative consequences; all involve biosociopsychological phenomena; and all, when abuse is most extreme, seem to involve some aspect of compulsiveness on the part of the abuser in his or her attachment or involvement with the substance (see Miller, 1987).

This chapter focuses mainly on just two of the substances—alcohol and drugs. This is largely because of space limitations, but it is also because the assessment and intervention strategies for alcohol and drug abuse are relatively similar, and because social work practitioners apparently see more instances of alcohol and drug abuse—as identified problems, at any rate—than the other forms of substance abuse. However, it should be pointed out that the intervention techniques to be discussed in this chapter can also be applied to abuse of other substances and that simply because they are not covered here, the problems associated with abuse of these substances are not viewed as less serious than those associated with alcohol and drug abuse.

Definition of Substance Abuse

Perhaps the most widely used definition of disorders associated with use of substances such as those described above is the one contained in the *Diagnostic and Statistical Manual* (DSM-IV) of the American Psychiatric Association (APA, 1994; see also Maxman, 1986). This definition distinguishes between two major conditions associated with dysfunctional use of substances: substance dependence and (the more commonly used term) substance abuse. The DSM-IV also identifies certain substance-induced disorders, including substance intoxication, substance withdrawal, substance-induced mental disorders included elsewhere in the DSM-IV, and a variety of disorders related to each of the specific substances (e.g., alcohol, amphetamines, etc.). This chapter focuses mainly on the overarching categories of substance dependence and substance abuse.

Substance dependence refers essentially to a cluster of cognitive, behavioral, and physiological symptoms that indicate that a person has impaired control in the use of one or more substances and continues use of the substance despite adverse consequences (APA, 1994). The primary symptoms of dependence, according to the DSM-IV, include, but are not limited to, physiological tolerance and withdrawal. Tolerance refers to either the diminishing effects over time of a fixed amount of a substance or the need to increase amounts of a substance in order to maintain the same effect. Withdrawal refers to the symptoms that occur when use of the substance is reduced or stopped. The symptoms of tolerance and withdrawal vary according to the specific substance and the frequency, amount, and chronicity of its use.

Substance dependence can show up in a variety of ways. The DSM-IV lists seven symptoms, three of which must be present for at least a month or have occurred repeatedly over a longer period for substance dependence to be present.

Substance abuse is referred to in the DSM-IV as a residual category in that maladaptive patterns of substance use are present that do not meet the criteria for dependence. These criteria, one of which must be present for one month or occur repeatedly for a longer period, are 1) failure to fulfill major role obligations; 2) use of the substance in hazardous situations (e.g., driving while intoxicated); 3) legal problems; and 4) persistent social or interpersonal problems.

There are at least two problems with the DSM-IV view of substance abuse. One is that it focuses mainly on the abuse, per se, and not on the myriad problems that could be associated with it. Thus, it implies that substance abuse is a more or less homogeneous problem, and, correspondingly, that treatment can be a more or less homogeneous activity (focused only on the abuse). The second problem is that the seven diagnostic criteria for substance dependence (of which at least three must be present) and the four for abuse all are indicative of very severe problems of substance use. By no stretch of the imagination can the presence of any of those criteria be construed as mild (e.g., the main criterion for evaluating both dependence and abuse is "a maladaptive pattern of substance use, leading to clinically significant impairment or distress . . ." (APA, 1994, pp. 181, 182).

It is especially important to recognize that substance abuse and the problems associated with it vary tremendously in severity from person to person. It would be overly simplistic to say that a person does or does not abuse some substance. A far more useful perspective—for both assessment and intervention—would be to view the use of substances on a continuum from nonproblematic to extremely problematic. In other words, deciding who has or does not have a problem with substance use depends on a variety of factors related not only to use (or misuse) of the substance, but also to the ways in which that misuse affects total functioning. Just such a continuum regarding problems with substance use has been proposed by Lewis et al. (1988), who conceptualize disorders associated with substance abuse as ranging along the following continuum:

1. Nonuse
2. Moderate, nonproblematic use
3. Heavy, nonproblematic use
4. Heavy use; moderate problems
5. Heavy use; serious problems
6. Dependence; life and health problems

This continuum allows for greater individualization in goals and techniques of intervention and avoids overgeneralized or stereotypical thinking about the supposed homogeneity of substance abusers.

The complexities of all of the above, then, necessitate some working definition of substance abuse that can help guide practitioners' activities. Such a working definition might be as follows: when use of alcohol or drugs (or, for that matter, any substance) affects an individual's biological/medical, social, behavioral, or psychological functioning, that problem can be viewed as one of substance abuse. This definition allows for the wide variety of problems typically associated with substance abuse to be viewed on the continuum described above. Thus, at one end of the continuum, few if any problems are associated with substance use, while at the other end of the continuum, serious problems exist in one or more areas of the individual's life. These problems could include dependence and/or abuse (as defined by the DSM-IV) and could also include the pattern that often brings people to the attention of professional helpers (voluntarily or involuntarily) and the overwhelming involvement or attachment to the substance—the compulsiveness and inability to control its use that was mentioned earlier as a common characteristic of serious abuse of all substances.

In line with the DSM-IV, this chapter focuses on the following classes of substances, individually or in combination: alcohol; amphetamines (e.g., speed and certain appetite suppressants); caffeine; cannabis (e.g., marijuana, hashish); cocaine; hallucinogens (e.g., LSD); inhalants (e.g., glue sniffing); opioids (e.g., heroin); phencyclidine (PCP); and sedatives, hypnotics, and aniolytics. Throughout this chapter, the term "substance abuse" will be used in the general sense of problems associated with the use of any of the above substances, rather than the more narrow use described in the DSM-IV. Perhaps an even more appropriate general term might be "substance misuse," although this typically is taken to mean a less severe set of problems than substance abuse.

Prevalence of Substance Abuse

The United States is a society of alcohol and drug users: some 90 million adults use alcohol on a regular basis (Miller, 1987). By the time they reach their mid-twenties, up to 80 percent of Americans have tried an illicit drug, and at any given time some 37 percent of high school seniors have had five or more drinks in one sitting within the preceding two weeks (Johnston, O'Malley, & Bachman, 1986). In other words, alcohol and drugs seem to be as American as apple pie and ice cream.

It is difficult to know precisely how many of the users of these substances actually have problems of abuse or dependence or misuse. Some estimates are available, however, from a community survey of three metropolitan areas that was conducted in the early 1980s (Robins et al., 1984; see also Helzer, 1987). This survey examined lifetime prevalence of fifteen DSM-III psychiatric disorders, with lifetime prevalence being the proportion of people in a representative sample who had ever experienced the disorder up to the time of assessment. Of all the disorders, by far the most prevalent was substance abuse, with 15 to 18.1 percent of the population being diagnosed. Of these, alcohol abuse ranged from 11.5 to 15.7 percent of the population, and drug abuse from 5.5 to 5.8 percent. These percentages translate into hefty numbers of the American population; with 1987 census figures showing roughly 185 million adult Americans, these data suggest that some 3 million or more adult Americans, at some time in their lives, may have been affected by alcohol and/or drug abuse. Given that the 1987 census figures show roughly 89 million households, this means that up to 37 percent of American households may be affected.

The prevalence of alcohol and drug abuse appears to be substantially higher for whites than other racial and ethnic groups, despite the common perception that substance abuse is mainly a "minority problem" (Smith, 1993). There are few differences related to education regarding prevalence of substance abuse (again with one exception in one city that showed higher rates of alcohol abuse among non–college graduates). There are clearer differences according to gender: most data show higher rates of substance abuse for men than women, with this difference being greatest for alcohol abuse (a ratio of up to 5 to 1).

Although these data are startling, their true meaning becomes clear when examining the implications of these problems for everyday life. The direct and indirect costs—both in health terms and financially—of alcohol and drug abuse are immense. One of the leading experts on the topic, J. Danforth Quayle (1983), estimated, perhaps conservatively, that the price paid for health care, days away from work, and lost productivity amounts to approximately $70 billion per year. The medical risks are even more frightening, with a huge variety of illnesses associated with alcohol and drug abuse (Wartenberg & Liepman, 1987; Segal & Sisson, 1985). More importantly, estimates are that drug and alcohol abuse are related to the deaths of up to 130,000 people per year, including the many innocent victims of people who drive while under the influence of some substance (Hoffman, 1987; Wartenberg & Liepman, 1987).

Add to all this the incalculable toll of substance abuse on individual functioning, family life, and employment, and it can be clearly seen that substance abuse is indeed one of the major problems of the era. Indeed, when the categories of substance abuse are expanded to include nicotine and food, with some 50 million smokers and 40 million overweight Americans (Miller, 1987), the enormity of the problem becomes even more apparent, with countless billions of dollars added to the nation's costs and hundreds of thousands of deaths added every year to the number of deaths associated with alcohol and drugs alone (Wartenberg & Liepman, 1987; *Honolulu Advertiser,* April 4, 1989, p. D2).

Clinical Manifestations of Substance Abuse

Despite the many myths about the "typical alcoholic" or "typical drug addict," it would be inappropriate to try to characterize the clinical manifestations of substance use as though they apply to all people with substance abuse problems. The dangers here are stereotyping and overgeneralizing; it is perhaps better to err by individualizing than by assuming that all people are alike. This is not to say that there are not some commonalities among the manifestations of substance abuse. Rather, it is to say that the range of possibilities of clinical manifestations of substance abuse is so great that the real need for assessment and intervention is to be able to precisely pinpoint areas for change that are specific for each individual. This is one more rationale for use of the continuum of abuse—ranging from nonuse to misuse to serious abuse—described earlier.

Problems related to substance abuse can show up in all realms of human functioning. As mentioned earlier, the DSM-IV describes seven possible diagnostic criteria (or patterns of behavior) related to dependence (e.g., a great deal of time spent in trying to get, use, or recover from the substance; persistent desire or one or more unsuccessful attempts to cut down or control substance use), and four criteria or patterns related to abuse. Not all of these need to be present either for the formal diagnosis to be made or for serious problems as a result of substance use to be present.

Similarly, the DSM-IV lists several categories of disorders caused by the direct effect of various substances on the nervous system that could be present in any given case of substance misuse. These include intoxication, withdrawal, delirium, withdrawal delirium, delusional disorder, mood disorder, and other syndromes. Thus, the clinical manifestations of abuse could include one or more of these disorders as well.

In addition, any individual who misuses or abuses some substance could be suffering from any one of a number of medical problems associated with the abuse (Wartenberg & Liepman, 1987). These problems run the gamut from malnutrition to cancer to respiratory and cardiovascular problems to a variety of infections, such as hepatitis or even AIDS.

Finally, Lewis et al. (1988) list numerous problems that typically, but not uniformly, are associated with substance abuse. These include employment problems; problems with friends or neighbors; problems with spouse, children, parents, or other relatives; problems with arrests and the criminal justice system; financial problems; problems of belligerence, depression, anxiety, and so on. These numerous problems all are ways in which the clinical manifestations of substance abuse can be seen.

Practitioners who work exclusively with individuals who abuse only one substance may see more commonalities among presented problems than those who work with abuse of a range of different substances. However, when substance abuse as a whole is examined, it is obvious that it can manifest itself in so many ways, and in so many realms of human functioning, that it requires the practitioner to be especially sensitive and to be able to carefully assess each individual for the unique ways in which the problems may be manifested. The next section presents some guidelines and tools that emphasize the importance of such individualized assessment.

ASSESSMENT AND EVALUATION

This chapter emphasizes the idea that problems associated with substance use should be viewed as problems in living, leading to the necessity of individualizing goals and interventions. It is, therefore, probably not an overstatement to say that the assessment of the client is the most important phase of the clinical process. This is because the assessment identifies the specific problems of each client, sets specific goals for each case, selects specific interventions tailored to the problems and goals, and develops a plan to monitor and evaluate the success of the intervention. Even though initial goals and interventions are selected, however, the assessment does not stop there; substance abuse involves such a complicated set of problems that goals and interventions may have to be reformulated constantly on the basis of new or better evidence, changes in the problems, or the appearance of new problems. Indeed, the very complexity of the assessment process requires mastery of a great deal of material, much of which can be obtained from comprehensive guides to the assessment process (e.g., Donovan & Marlatt, 1988; Lewis et al., 1988; Baker & Cannon, 1988; Miller, 1981; McCrady & Sher, 1985; Sobell, Sobell, & Nirenberg, 1988; Nirenberg & Maisto, 1987; Bratter & Forrest, 1985).

Assessment in this chapter is used for the purposes described above rather than for diagnosis. Diagnosis serves important purposes, including agency or insurance requirements. However, for reasons described earlier regarding problems with the DSM-IV categories, the diagnosis, per se, is downplayed here in order to focus on the broader perspective of clinical assessment of not only the substance abuse itself, but also of the context and problems associated with that abuse.

Basic Principles

A number of basic principles underlie the assessment methodologies discussed here.

1. Substance abuse is a biopsychosocial problem that is very complicated and requires a multivariate assessment process to properly understand it. Thus, a variety of assessment methods must be utilized.
2. The problems of, and associated with, substance use occur on a continuum, from nonproblematic to severely problematic. Thus, the purpose of assessment is not to make a simplistic determination of whether or not an individual abuses some substance, but to examine the problem in all its manifestations.
3. There are a variety of interventions available to deal with the diverse problems associated with substance abuse. It is crucial for the practitioner to be aware of these interventions so that the best interventions available can be selected for each component of the problem.

4. The focus of assessment for substance abuse is largely on the present, especially on factors that might be maintaining the abuse. This is because factors that might be associated with the original development of abuse may not be the ones maintaining it; in fact, they may no longer be present at all.

5. The practitioner must be aware of the importance of socioeconomic, ethnic, and cultural variables in conducting an assessment. The basic principle is, the greater the difference between the practitioner and client (in values, attitudes, socioeconomic status, etc.), the greater the sensitivity required of the practitioner to properly understand the client's situation (see Lum, 1986; Schare & Milburn, 1996) for frameworks for conducting assessment that are attuned to sociocultural issues).

6. Assessment for substance abuse is very complex. Misconceptions associated with abuse, poor professional education in this area, difficulty of gaining cooperation from some clients, variability of problems associated with abuse, need to understand prior treatments with relapsed clients, and the covert nature of some problems of abuse all have been cited as reasons why assessment for substance abuse is especially difficult (Sobell et al., 1988). Thus, the practitioner must take even more care than with other problem areas to ensure that he or she has done as thorough and sensitive a job as possible.

7. Despite the need to know as much as possible about the problem so that one can make a rational decision about the best available intervention, reality suggests that this must be balanced with the amount of time available to the practitioner, i.e., the cost efficiency of the assessment process (Donovan & Marlatt, 1988). In order to avoid practitioners becoming overwhelmed with assessing each case, Donovan & Marlatt (1988) describe the use of clinical hypothesis testing (generating hypotheses based on data collected) and segmented assessment strategies (funneling from very broad to increasingly specific foci in the assessment).

8. The practitioner who works with substance abuse needs an extensive body of knowledge to aid in understanding the variety of factors associated with the abuse. This includes not only knowledge that all practitioners might have about dealing with social and psychological problems (employment difficulties, depression, cognitive distortions, anxiety, and so on), but also knowledge about the specific substance of concern, including biophysiological factors, behavioral factors, cognitive-expectational factors, and social factors (Donovan & Marlatt, 1988).

Areas for Collection of Information

There are a number of areas about which practitioners should collect information to help in goal formulation and treatment planning. These have been hinted at above but will be described in a little more detail here. Although the most common focus of assessment for substance abuse is the pattern of the abuse itself, the other elements described here are viewed as no less important in developing a comprehensive understanding of the client and the client's problems.

Medical information. Because of the numerous possible medical complications that could be associated with substance abuse, it is crucial for every client to have a thorough medical evaluation. In addition, it is important for practitioners to solicit information from clients about any physical problems as early in their contacts as possible in the event that referral to a physician is necessary.

Presence of related social/psychological disorders. In addition to the several substance abuse–related disorders described in the DSM-IV mentioned earlier, there are a number of problems about which practitioners must be aware. These include the behaviors, thoughts, and feelings associated with disorders involving depression, anxiety, sleep, eating, sex, and impulse control. Problems in any of these areas pose serious complications in the lives of clients who abuse some substance and will need attention if a comprehensive treatment program is to be developed.

Life stresses. In addition to the above, there are any number of events that could complicate substance abuse patterns and, indeed, could even be associated with maintaining the abuse. These life stresses must be carefully assessed. They include problems with family, income, housing, and peer relationships.

Prior treatment history. The practitioner must be informed about the client's attempts to receive treatment for any of the problems described above, or for the substance abuse itself. The practitioner then should determine the reasons for the success or failure of those programs and try to build on the successes and not duplicate the failures.

Client motivation and expectations. The client may have a number of preconceived notions of what treatment may be like. These expectations can have a serious impact on the success or failure of treatment, and it is crucial for the practitioner to elicit these expectations from the client and to create positive expectations of success as part of treatment. Similarly, it is important to know and understand the client's motivation for seeking treatment. Obviously, the client's commitment to the process could be influenced by any number of factors, ranging from genuine desire for change to the desire to avoid some legal problems or dissolution of a marriage. This information allows the practitioner to make judgments about the extent to which he or she will need to emphasize enhancing the client's motivation as a major or minor part of the intervention.

Availability of social supports.   In making decisions about the type of treatment that will be recommended, the practitioner will have to understand the client's social support system, if indeed he or she has one (McCrady & Sher, 1985). The presence or extent of social support could have a bearing on the type of treatment (i.e., in- or outpatient), types of tasks and homework assigned the client, type of maintenance program, and so on.

Functional analysis of the pattern of substance abuse.   Ultimately, of course, the practitioner will have to do a careful assessment of the pattern of substance use and factors that may be associated with it, including antecedents that may be eliciting substance abuse and consequences that could be maintaining it. Sobell et al. (1988) have provided a comprehensive list of areas to be examined in such an assessment, including the following:

1. Specific quantities and frequency of use of the substance.
2. Usual and unusual substance-use circumstances and patterns.
3. Predominant mood states and situations antecedent and consequent to substance use.
4. History of withdrawal symptoms.
5. Identification of possible difficulties the client might encounter in refraining from substance use.
6. Extent and severity of previous substance use.
7. Multiple substance use.
8. Reports of frequent thoughts or urges to use substances.
9. Review of positive consequences of substance abuse.
10. Risks associated with nonabstinence treatment goal.

Other areas.   In addition to the areas described above, Shaffer and Kauffman (1985) offer a number of hypotheses to be tested in assessing substance abuse. These hypotheses—actually partial formulations—include biological hypotheses (e.g., can the substance use be understood as an attempt to reduce dysphoria?), sociological hypotheses (e.g., does the substance use occur in limited or varied environmental contexts?), and behavior hypotheses (e.g., can the problems be understood as contingent upon the reinforcing properties of the substance?).

Methods of Data Collection

In order to collect information on the wide range of activities, behaviors, patterns, thoughts, and feelings described above, a number of different methods of data collection must be employed. These methods include interviews with clients and others, self-report measures, direct observation (influencing analogue measures), biochemical measures, and records.

Interviews. The interview is, of course, the major medium for the collection of the information described in the previous section. This is as much the case in the area of substance abuse as it is in any other clinical area. Thus, standard social work intervention strategies are used to elicit and analyze this information. However, there are some specifics that differentiate interviews in this area from those in other areas (see, e.g., Shaffer & Kauffman, 1985). A summary of interviewing conditions that provide the most useful information in the area of substance abuse has been provided by Sobell et al. (1988, pp. 29–30) and includes the following: 1) when the client is alcohol and drug free; 2) when rapport is developed both by the practitioner's style and by stressing confidentiality and the importance of the information; 3) when the terminology used is clearly understood by both parties; 4) when the focus of the interview is information gathering rather than social labeling; 5) when the client's self-reports are checked out against other sources; and 6) when data are gathered, to the extent possible, in a clinical research setting.

The interview typically contains both structured and unstructured portions. A very useful guide for the initial interview was developed by Lewis et al. (1988), along with a psychosocial and substance-use history form and a behavioral assessment and functional analysis interview form. A widely used structured interview format for assessment of alcohol abuse is the Comprehensive Drinking Profile (Marlatt, 1976), and a structured interview format for drug abuse, called the G-DATS, has been described by Boudin et al. (1977). Another structured interview format for both drug and alcohol abuse is the Addiction Severity Index (McClellan et al., 1980

Self-report measures. Especially important areas for the collection of data on substance abuse are self-report measures and self-monitoring. These measures range from simple oral reports the client might make during the interview to the use of standardized questionnaires. For the purposes of this chapter, these two types of self-report measures will be divided into two categories: standardized scales and self-monitoring.

Standardized scales. One of the fastest growing areas of assessment for substance abuse is that of standardized scales. Many of these measures have reported fairly good reliability and validity data. Standardized measures cover not only problems of abuse, but also problems that could be related to abuse, such as depression, anxiety, and cognitive distortions (see Corcoran & Fischer, 2000a, 2000b, for a collection of over 400 short-form measures for clinical practice; and see Hersen & Bellack, 1988, for a dictionary of well over 400 assessment procedures). Some of the most useful standardized self-report scales developed for assessing substance abuse are the Substance Abuse Problem Checklist (Carroll, 1984), the Michigan Alcohol Screening Test (Selzer, 1971), the Drug Abuse Screening Test (Skinner, 1982), the Hilton Drinking Behavior Questionnaire (Hilton & Lokane, 1978), and the Callner-Ross Assertion Questionnaire (Ammerman & Van Hasselt, 1988).

Self-monitoring. The second major type of self-report measure is called self-monitoring. Self-monitoring refers essentially to the client routinely recording, via diaries or logs, problems and behaviors related to abuse. This includes recording not only actual use patterns, but also problems associated with use and the urges and consequences related to use. Essentially, the process of self-monitoring involves training the client to record a variety of factors related to abuse, including some or all of the following: time, date, and amount of the substance; antecedents and consequences, including thoughts, feelings, and behaviors of self and others; and activities associated with substance use. These data are collected before, during, and after treatment and can be used as a basis not only for assessment, but also for evaluation. Of course, the practitioner's response to the client's efforts at self-monitoring can play a major role in how useful and accurate these data are (Sobell et al., 1988).

Reliability and validity of self-report data. A major concern about self-report data in the area of substance abuse is their reliability and validity. The prevailing myth is that such data are almost always suspect. In fact, a substantial amount of research shows that self-reports in the area of substance abuse can be both reliable and valid (Sobell et al., 1988; Ridley & Kordinak, 1988), including good agreement between self-reports and reports by collaterals (Sobell et al., 1988). The main cautions about these conclusions are that they apply mainly when the client is interviewed under the following conditions: he or she is substance free, he or she is in a clinical/research setting, and he or she is assured of confidentiality.

Direct observation. Although rather difficult to implement in clinical settings, direct observation has been used in some instances to provide information on use of some substances (Foy, Cline, & Laasi, 1987). One type of direct observation involves the use of analogue measures, in which tasks are developed that are considered analogous to the natural environment in which a person must work to obtain a substance (typically alcohol). Another type of direct observation is where the client is placed in a simulated bar or living room environment and provided with the substance (again, typically alcohol), and then observed as to the patterns and amounts ingested.

Biochemical measures. A wide range of biochemical measures typically are used in comprehensive substance abuse programs. Although many of these are not available to the individual clinician (especially without research/medical supervision), they nevertheless add an important dimension to understanding the patterns of clients' substance use. These measures have been reviewed by Sobell et al. (1988); Foy et al. (1987); and Wells, Hawkins, and Catalano (1988a, 1988b) and include blood-alcohol level analysis, liver function tests, Antabuse monitoring, urinalysis, breath alcohol tests, alcohol dipstick (for ethanol concentrations), and the sweat patch. Some of these tests are used for assessing recent use (e.g., breath and urine tests), and others for extended use (e.g., liver function tests).

Records.   A final source of data is official records (Sobell et al., 1988). These records could include police, hospital, and school reports. Of course, these data may be incomplete or even biased (e.g., member of a minority group may be picked up by police for apparent illegal behaviors far more frequently than members of the majority group or upper-income people displaying the same behaviors). Nevertheless, official records can form part of the basis for a comprehensive assessment, especially when used in context as only one source of data about the problem as a whole.

Integrative Formulation

The last part of the assessment process is to develop an "integrative formulation" (Siporin, 1975). The integrative formulation consists of a summary of the information collected by the practitioner, plus the practitioner's analysis of that information. The integrative formulation pulls together disparate pieces of information collected during the assessment, allowing the practitioner to reflect on that information and decide what it all means. If the practitioner is required to make a formal diagnosis, say, based on the DSM-IV, this is where he or she would do it, adding to that diagnosis, ideally, the concept of the continuum described earlier in this chapter. The integrative formulation would then be used as the basis for goal setting and for the development of treatment plans.

Goal setting.   Goal setting is a particularly sensitive area for substance abuse treatment because it raises a number of difficult issues, foremost among them the issue of abstinence versus controlled use (especially of alcohol). Although the literature is too extensive to be covered thoroughly here (see recent reviews by Lewis et al., 1988; Maisto & Carey, 1987; Foreyt, 1987; Brownell, 1984), there does appear to be sufficient evidence to suggest that controlled use may be an appropriate goal for a small percentage of clients under very select circumstances.

Be that as it may, the setting of goals in the area of substance abuse should

1.   Reflect the broad ranges of problems identified in the assessment (not just the substance abuse, per se).
2.   Be clear and precise.
3.   Allow evaluations.
4.   Include long- and short-term goals.

5. Add to specificity by identifying *who* is to change, what will be changed, *to what extent*, and under what *conditions* (Gottman & Leiblum, 1974; Brown & Brown, 1977). This will allow the practitioner to be as specific as possible in identifying specific areas of change.

Treatment plan.   The final part of the assessment process is developing a treatment plan that will address each of the problem areas and goals that have been identified. (One model of a treatment plan for substance abuse—including some very useful forms—is presented by Lewis et al., 1988.) The idea here is to select those intervention techniques that have the best evidence of effectiveness and apply them in a systematic way to each of the problems identified in the assessment. Although this may not always be possible, it is this effort to link previous research on effectiveness with a given client's individualized problems that is a hallmark of the eclectic approach.

Obviously, a number of factors in addition to previous research play a part in developing a treatment plan for substance abuse. These include issues such as, Will the treatment be in- or outpatient? How motivated is the client? To what extent are environmental factors involved? How extensive are the abuse and the problems associated with it? How familiar is the practitioner with the techniques recommended by the research, and does he or she have the commitment to learn them?

The final step in the assessment process is putting everything into a written contract with the client. Not only will the contract itself be a positive force in structuring the treatment, but it also will clarify goals, time limits, mutual tasks and responsibilities, monitoring and evaluation activities, and precisely how and by whom the treatment will be implemented.

Interventions for substance abuse can be evaluated with every client using a type of evaluation approach called single-system designs (Bloom, Fischer, & Orme, 1999). These designs rely on the use of repeated measures on target problems/behaviors, stretching from a baseline/assessment (nonintervention) phase through the intervention and maintenance phases. Any of the measures discussed in the section on methods of data collection, above, can be used to track changes in the target, whether these measures are collected by the client, practitioner, or relevant other. These designs allow for monitoring of change on a daily basis so that the intervention program can be changed if the results are less than optimal. All single-system designs allow for a clear determination of whether the practitioner's interventions might have produced those changes. A comprehensive yet practical approach to these designs is in the book by Bloom et al. which discusses how to conceptualize and identify problems and goals, as well as how to measure client problems. The book also discusses the designs themselves and methods for analyzing the data collected with single-system designs, including easy-to-construct charts for visual analysis of changes over time.

ECLECTIC INTERVENTION

This section focuses on specific intervention techniques that could be incorporated in a comprehensive treatment program for substance abuse. There is, in fact, no single specific treatment (or theory) of choice; rather, a number of different interventions can be applied, depending on the individual client, problem, and situation.

Research and Practice Support

Unfortunately, in the area of substance abuse there is no single intervention program with unequivocal support, nor is there a single source of literature that one can turn to that clearly illustrates empirical support for one or more intervention programs. Indeed, the interventions described in this section are derived from several sources, including recent research.

1. Review of evaluation research on substance abuse (Matuscha, 1985; Merbaum & Rosenbaum, 1984; Nathan & Gorman, 1998; APA, 1995; Thyer & Wodarski, 1998, chs. 9–11; Hester & Miller, 1989; Miller & Hester, 1986; Maisto & Carey, 1987; Stitzer, Bigelow, & McCaul, 1983; Ingram & Salzberg, 1988; Cox, 1987; Miller, 1985; Colletti & Brownell, 1982; McCrady & Sher, 1985). The upshot of all this research is that there are several techniques that have been effective with some substance abuse clients under some circumstances, but no techniques that are effective with all clients under all circumstances. Further, although it appears that (with alcohol abuse at least) some treatment is better than no treatment, the type of treatment is not always crucial. However, there are many commonalities regarding treatment techniques in some of the most successful programs. The recommendations in this chapter will focus mainly on techniques that have been used successfully in several programs.

2. Less rigorous research, case studies, and practice experience. The literature on substance abuse is replete with hundreds of references to innovative programs, new techniques, small-group studies, and case studies, many of which can be found in the references cited throughout this chapter. Although this literature is too immense to be reviewed comprehensively here, some of those reports are incorporated in the recommendations later in this chapter (see, e.g., *Social Casework*, 1989).

3. Adaptations of effective techniques. There are a number of techniques with substantial evidence of effectiveness in areas other than substance abuse (see Fischer, 1976; Nathan & Gorman, 1998; Pikoff, 1996; Roth & Foragy, 1996; and Chambless et al., 1998, for reviews of some of these techniques). Because the perspective of this chapter is that problems associated with substance abuse can be as serious as the abuse itself, and a number of these related problems have been treated successfully inde-

pendent of treatment for substance abuse (e.g., problems of anxiety, depression), a number of these treatment techniques are incorporated in the recommendations here.

Basic Principles of Intervention

There are a number of basic principles of intervention that underlie the treatment recommendations here.

1. Treat the whole person. It is crucial to remember, first of all, that substance abuse is usually not an independent problem—many other problems typically are associated with it; and second, that substance abuse rarely occurs in a vacuum. People exist in environments, and the successful treatment of substance abuse requires attention to the environmental context.

2. There is no single best treatment. The treatment always must be tailored to the individual client and problem. This matching of treatment to client is perhaps the key ingredient of an effective program.

3. Be prepared for failure. Work in the area of substance abuse is usually difficult and frequently unrewarding for the practitioner. On the one hand, it is easy to begin blaming clients and/or feeling burned out, especially when clients are uncooperative or even disruptive. On the other hand, the intrinsic rewards of success are so great that they may make all the effort worthwhile. Typically, practitioners working in the area of substance abuse are unusually committed and have abandoned the rescue fantasy of being able to help everyone with everything. Indeed, sometimes they can reframe the difficulties as challenges, thus leading to a more positive, self-reinforcing outlook.

4. Attend to diversity in clients. In addition to the variations in client problems in this area, there is a tremendous diversity in other characteristics: race, gender, ethnicity, socioeconomic status, sexual orientation, and the like. Many of these variations can become barriers to successful interventions, especially if the practitioner views the client as an alcoholic or a drug addict and does not take into account his or her other human characteristics. This individualizing includes being aware of the client's world views; being sensitive to his or her culture, values, and norms; working to understand different patterns of communication; and using all this knowledge and awareness to create more individualized and sensitive intervention programs.

5. Use a variety of roles. One of the great strengths of social work is the wide variety of roles that can be employed on the client's behalf. If the practitioner views intervention as taking place solely in the clinical role, he or she could be undercutting the effectiveness of the program. Problems associated with substance abuse often involve the need for intervention with significant others and in the environment in such practitioner roles

as consultant, advocate, and broker. Case management is an important option for clients with multiple needs (Brindis et al., 1995).

6. Attend to client motivation. Although poor client motivation frequently is used as an explanation (and sometimes as an excuse) for treatment failures, motivating the client to continue in treatment can be viewed as just one more challenge to the expertise of the practitioner. Indeed a number of successful strategies for enhancing client commitment in the area of substance abuse have been reviewed by Miller (1985), who describes several techniques that have been successfully used to enhance client motivation. These include giving advice, providing feedback, setting specific goals, role playing and modeling, maintaining continuity of contact, manipulating external contingencies, providing choice, and decreasing the attractiveness of the problem behavior. (A number of other procedures for enhancing client commitment are described by Meichenbaum & Turk, 1987; and Shelton & Levy, 1981.)

7. Focus on a positive relationship. Any intervention program should be grounded in the core interpersonal skills of effective practice. Empathy, warmth, respect, and genuineness—ingredients of a positive relationship— are the heart of all practice, but are especially important when working in the area of substance abuse. First, practitioners will find that the clients are more willing to work and cooperate with practitioners who communicate high levels of these skills (Meichenbaum & Turk, 1987). This is particularly critical in the area of substance abuse. Second, there is clear evidence that the effectiveness of many intervention techniques will be increased when the practitioner implements them with high levels of interpersonal skills (Fischer, 1978). Thus, interpersonal skills—the relationship—and techniques bolster each other in enhancing overall practice effectiveness.

8. Use clinical guidelines. Clinical guidelines involve recommendations for clinical intervention based on the results of research and the consensus of experienced practitioners. Just such a set of guidelines has been developed by the APA (1995). These guidelines discuss choices regarding treatment settings as well as both pharmacological and psychosocial interventions. The strength of the evidence for each recommendation is provided. Guidelines such as these can indicate what the state of the art is at any given time and can be used to optimize the effectiveness of our interventions.

Intervention Techniques

The interventions described here, none of which rely on electrical or chemical interventions and thus can be used by social workers, have been synthesized from a variety of sources, as described earlier. Although, of course, these are not the only successful treatments, it is likely that combinations of these techniques, systematically applied to individualized components of clients' problems, constitute some of the more effective strategies available as of the early 1990s. Indeed, some of these treatments, when combined, have been called "ideal services" (Nathan & Gorman, 1998). Obviously, because this is a multidimensional treatment program, not all of the techniques will be applied with all clients. Thus, the key, once again, is judicious matching of individual intervention components with client problems.

The individual components of this program are divided into twelve separate categories: detoxification and motivation enhancement, self-regulation and self-control, contingency contracting, stress-control training, aversive treatment, cognitive coping strategies, coping and social skills training, education about the substance, lifestyle intervention, marital and family counseling, community enforcement, and group support and self-help groups.

Detoxification and motivation enhancement.   One of the axioms of treatment is that clients cannot be using or abusing substances if treatment is to be successful. Thus, a first step in treatment is to help the client withdraw from the substance he or she is using. This is usually a short-term process, but the period may also be an intense one, as the client may be experiencing some discomfort. There are several options for detoxification, depending on the extent of use, level of dependence on the substance, degree of social support, and resources available (McCrady & Sher, 1985; Lewis et al., 1988). The detoxification process could occur on an outpatient basis without involvement of a detoxification center; or in either a nonmedical (social) or a medical detoxification center, with both types of centers involving either partial or full hospitalization. Detoxification is the first step in a comprehensive treatment effort; however, a substantial part of the assessment, goal setting, and treatment planning could take place during this first step, and the detoxification effort can be coordinated with subsequent treatment to produce a more comprehensive and integrated approach for the client.

To the extent that the client becomes able to participate, this early stage begins the process of assessing and enhancing the client's motivation for treatment, using some of the techniques described in the previous section. In addition, if the client appears to be uncooperative, perhaps denying that he or she has a problem, specific intervention strategies to overcome this denial should be considered. Frequently, these strategies involve planned confrontations by family members, friends, or perhaps other group members in a detoxification program. These confrontations should be carefully planned and supervised, and could involve such techniques as family members making a list of specific incidents in which they were hurt by the client's substance abuse and then rehearsing how to present these to the client. Other, more recent, variations of planned family confrontations include programmed confrontation and programmed request by the client's spouse, as described by Thomas and Yoshioka (1989).

Self-regulation and self-control. There is little question that after termination of the formal substance abuse program, the client will have to take control of his or her own program. The self-regulation, self-control component not only is intended to prepare the client to do just that, but also provides in-treatment benefits.

The very terms self-control and self-regulation imply that it is actually the client who generates and designs a unique self-improvement program, although this is not typically the case (Merbaum & Rosenbaum, 1984). In fact, the self-control package really is just one component of an overall comprehensive program in which the client learns certain techniques that he or she will continue to apply once the formal part of the program is completed.

A number of techniques for self-control components have been suggested by Nathan & Gorman (1998), Merbaum and Rosenbaum (1984), and Kanfer (1986). Some of these techniques are

1. Self-monitoring. Clients are taught to keep track of any substance-related thoughts, behaviors, or feelings, as well as amounts and circumstances of any substance use. The goal here is to increase awareness of patterns and urges so that the client can eventually engage in some change activity. It also may be that the recording itself will have a (positive) reactive effect.

2. Self-evaluation. Although related to self-monitoring, the focus here is on setting goals and encouraging self-evaluation of adherence to these goals.

3. Self-reinforcement. A crucial component of any intervention program, self-reinforcement involves teaching clients to reinforce themselves— covertly (through thoughts) and overtly (through desired activities) for successful adherence to goals, successful completion of tasks, or even partial successes.

4. Self-control manual. Clients are given training manuals that help them develop comprehensive self-control programs.

Contingency contracting. The use of contracts is increasingly a part of everyday practice in many social work organizations. Contracts have numerous advantages, including ensuring explicitness, adding to structure, enhancing the client's commitment, clarifying goals, and clarifying client and practitioner responsibilities. Contingency contracts, per se, go a step further by actually spelling out relationships between desired behaviors and reinforcement for those behaviors (see Epstein & Wing, 1984). They provide for reinforcement of desired activities, such as self-monitoring or adhering to a program of abstinence, and sometimes punishment for undesired activities or behaviors, such as nonadherence.

Contingency contracts for health and substance abuse problems were recently reviewed by Epstein and Wing (1984). They describe numerous characteristics of these contracts, including the variety of potential patterns of reinforcement, their use with several substance abuse problems, inclusion of third parties in these contracts, and the use of behaviors that are incompatible with substance use. Contingency contracts can be used in a variety of ways to deal with problems of abuse, per se (e.g., adherence), as well as those only indirectly related to abuse (e.g., relationship problems). As such, they are a flexible and important part of the practitioner's armamentarium.

Stress-control training. A key factor in helping clients overcome problems of substance abuse is training them to deal with anxiety and stress. It is not uncommon for practitioners to hear clients who have abused alcohol or drugs for many years state that they never experienced any anxiety in all that time; the alcohol and drugs prevented the anxiety from occurring or killed it quickly when it did occur. Indeed, a major theory of the etiology of substance abuse is that it serves a tension-reducing function.

The goal here, however, is to help clients deal with tension and stress once they have stopped using alcohol and drugs. Many Americans think nothing of using a glass or two of wine or a tranquilizer to help them navigate through a stormy emotional period. However, people with problems of substance abuse, once they complete treatment, usually have to control stress and anxiety without resorting to drugs and alcohol.

In these circumstances, clients can be taught to use a variety of relaxation and stress-control techniques. Many of these have been spelled out by Cormier and Cormier (1985). They include meditation and muscle relaxation, systematic desensitization, stress inoculation training, and emotive imagery. All of these techniques focus on providing the client with a variety of ways of dealing with stress and anxiety reactions, with stress inoculation training providing the broadest range of potential responses. In addition, all of these techniques can be taught by the practitioner during the treatment program and can then be used as self-control techniques by the client once the formal treatment program is completed.

Aversive treatment. Aversive treatments have a long and substantial history in the treatment of substance abuse. Some degree of success in at least limiting consumption has been found for both chemical (the drug Antabuse) and electrical aversion therapies. A technique called covert sensitization (Cautela, 1967) produces an effect similar to other aversive therapies, but does so without the use of chemical or electrical aversion.

Covert sensitization pairs aversive images with images involving substance use. Clients are instructed to imagine a scene in which they are about to use alcohol or drugs, and to incorporate realistic, unpleasant information about the antecedents, location, and so on, in the scene. In this way, clients are taught to imagine another scene—one of disgusting or repugnant responses, such as vomiting all over oneself—that, through repeated practice, becomes paired with the first scene. Clients also are instructed to imagine feeling total relief upon leaving the first scene and refraining from substance use.

Covert sensitization appears to be a moderately successful way of helping clients reduce urges to consume and levels of consumption. The research, however, is neither rigorous nor extensive enough to suggest that this should be more than one technique in a more comprehensive program.

Cognitive coping strategies.   The way people think about their problems is often strongly related to what they do about them. Thus, clients' self-statements, expectations, and beliefs may be critical factors in maintaining patterns of substance abuse. A number of cognitive techniques are available to help clients develop ways of coping with both life problems and urges to use some substance.

Cognitive restructuring.   Cognitive restructuring is a complex technique (some might say an entire approach to therapy) that focuses on identifying and altering clients' dysfunctional beliefs and negative self-statements or thoughts (Cormier & Cormier, 1985). Often a number of such dysfunctional beliefs and self-statements are uncovered in the assessment process (e.g., "I can never stop using"; "I need [substance X] to keep functioning"), and cognitive restructuring can be directed to altering those beliefs. This not only is beneficial in and of itself, but also can ease the way in other areas of the program by reducing resistance.

Guided imagery.   The focus of guided imagery techniques, such as covert modeling (Cormier & Cormier, 1985), is on helping the client rehearse adaptive rather than maladaptive (using the substance) responses to problem situations. Guided imagery can also be used to rehearse any task or activity that the practitioner suggests as a homework assignment.

Thought stopping.   The key components in a pattern of substance abuse often are the thought processes, which include obsessive thinking about the need and desire for a substance. This obsessive thinking typically takes place in the interval between the last use of the substance and the possible next use and is one of the features of compulsiveness in substance abuse that was discussed earlier. Thought stopping is a fairly simple technique to implement and works to control unproductive, obsessive, or self-defeating thoughts by suppressing or eliminating them and teaching the client to switch to productive or reinforcing thoughts (Cormier & Cormier, 1985).

Coping and social skills training.   One of the keystones of effective treatment of substance abuse is a broad-based coping and social skills training program. Such programs foster a greater sense of self-efficacy (Bandura, 1977) or perceived control in clients by teaching them to cope more effectively with everyday problems in living (Marlatt, 1979). There are any number of social skills that might be the focus of such a program, and the determination of which skills are missing from the client's repertoire is based on information obtained from the assessment.

A number of skills have been the target in substance abuse programs: assertiveness, communication skills, job-hunting and interview skills, refusing the invitation to use a substance, and so on.

Most social skills programs incorporate similar techniques: modeling, coaching, rehearsal, reinforcement, and feedback. These techniques are applied in various ways and to varying degrees in developing an overall social skills training program that best meets the needs and aptitudes of individual clients. Social skills training is particularly amenable to implementation in groups, because groups provide greater potential for rehearsal opportunities. As such, social skills training has been a major focus of intervention in both residential and outpatient treatment centers (Monti, Abrams, Kadden, & Cooney, 1989; Ingram & Salzberg, 1988).

Education. One component of a comprehensive substance abuse program typically is education about the substance itself and especially about the negative health and social effects of use of the substance. This education usually takes place through films, readings, lectures, and group discussions. Educational programs operate on two assumptions: 1) that the substance user may not know about the negative effects of substance use; and 2) that even if the client does know about such effects, it is a good idea to reinforce or update that knowledge.

Actually, evidence of the effectiveness of education as a sole or even just one component of a treatment program is rather skimpy. One way of bolstering its effectiveness is through the use of emotional role play, a technique with some evidence of effectiveness with smokers (Janis & Mann, 1977). In emotional role play, the client role plays some emotionally devastating scene (e.g., telling relatives that he or she has cancer of the liver brought on by too much drinking and will die in two months) as a way of breaking down defenses about use of a harmful substance. Such an experience can produce a change in the client's feelings of personal vulnerability, thereby opening the door for more serious consideration of the educational content.

Lifestyle intervention. This is a catch-all phrase for using a number of interventions that focus on other problems in the client's life, whether or not they are related directly to the substance abuse (Marlatt, 1979). The idea here is that bringing these other elements of the client's life into balance (or within tolerable levels for the client) cannot help but have an overall impact on the client's level of well-being and self-efficacy. Lifestyle intervention can consist of a number of components, including the following:

1. Supplementary counseling. This would include using any or all of the techniques discussed here plus others to deal with problems in the client's life. Such problems could include depression, anxiety, problems at work,

money problems (perhaps calling for a referral for income supplementa-
tion programs), and so on. This also could include supportive counseling
to help the client as he or she proceeds through the treatment program.
2. Exercise and hobby programs. Once the client is cleared by a physician for
participation, an exercise program can be a particularly useful antidote to
substance use. Similarly, a hobby can occupy time that a client might otherwise spend thinking about or engaging in substance use.
3. Substitution. The client can be taught to substitute desired alternative
activities (e.g., jogging) for substance use.

Marital and family counseling.   For those clients who are married or
living with a family, consideration of that context is a major priority in a comprehensive program. As Lewis et al. (1988) state, "No substance abuser—in
fact, no client—can be treated effectively unless his or her social interactions
are taken into account" (p. 157). Attention to the client's social support system can be a major factor in attaining optimal effectiveness.

A focus on the marriage and family has numerous benefits: it can reduce
pressures on the client so that he or she can be more successful in the program; it provides support to family members, who also may be suffering
through the treatment program; it enhances follow-up and maintenance by
teaching the spouse and family how best to deal with the client once he or she
is discharged; and it enhances overall family functioning.

Because marital and family therapies and attention to environmental
supports are trademarks of social work, there is little need to expand on this
topic here except to note that there are several intervention programs available that focus on marital and family therapy in the area of substance abuse,
per se (e.g., Lewis et al., 1988; Schlesinger, 1988; O'Farrell, 1987; McCrady &
Sher, 1985). Recent research shows family therapy is particularly useful for
adolescent substance abuse (Waldron, 1997).

Community reinforcement.   Because all clients operate in an environmental context, community reinforcement has shown particular promise
as a way of enhancing the client's social support system. Although there is
more than one variation of the program, community reinforcement is
designed to restructure family, social, and vocational reinforcers in a manner
that reinforces nonuse of the substance while discouraging further use (Miller
& Hester, 1986). The components of community reinforcement programs
range from buddy systems to family training to attendance at social clubs
where the problematic substance is not available. But in all such programs,
the focus is on reinforcing nonuse and helping clients avoid or deal successfully with situations that could result in use of the substance.

Self-help groups.   One of the more controversial but most widely used
interventions is the self-help group support operation, such as Alcoholics or

Narcotics Anonymous. These organizations often are called twelve-step groups because they typically follow the twelve-step program outlined by the founders of Alcoholics Anonymous.

The controversy about these groups runs the gamut from scattered accusations of lack of evidence of effectiveness, to criticism from professionals who do not like to be out of control of treatment, to complaints from group members who do not approve of the philosophy and methods, and so on. But there are few professionals in the field of substance abuse who do not know numerous clients who say, "A.A. (or N.A.) saved my life."

Thus, it seems reasonable to consider such programs as important adjuncts to professional treatment programs. In the first place, they provide group support, not only during treatment but also on a permanent basis, long after the formal treatment program has been terminated. Second, they operate on a twenty-four-hour basis, with the client being able to phone a sponsor at any time of the day or night. And third, the absence of evidence does not automatically mean that such programs are not effective. The task of research (which is particularly complicated with such groups) may be to attempt to discover the characteristics of clients and twelve-step programs that are most optimally matched and to make referrals on that basis.

MAINTENANCE AND GENERALIZATION

Of what use is an intervention program that is successful during the formal treatment, but is unsuccessful once that treatment is terminated? That key question is addressed by maintenance programs in the area of substance abuse. Indeed, relapse—an uncontrolled return to drug or alcohol use—is perhaps the most important issue that the substance abuse practitioner must confront.

One report stated that almost 90 percent of clients treated for substance abuse relapsed within one year after termination of formal treatment (Polich, Armor, & Braiker, 1981). Although rates of relapse vary by substance, program, and other characteristics, it is almost a cliché to say that substance abuse remains one of the problems that is most refractory to successful treatment. Thus, it becomes the task of the practitioner to work into the client's treatment program a comprehensive antirelapse program that is geared toward maintaining treatment gains and generalizing them into the client's everyday life.

A Relapse Model

Much of the work on relapse has been pioneered by Marlatt (1979; Marlatt & Gordon, 1985; see also Lewis et al., 1988). Among his contributions are the identification of determinants of relapse and the development of a model of relapse that leads to specific intervention strategies.

Relapse episodes were classified by Marlatt and Gordon (1985) into two categories. The first is intrapersonal/environmental determinants, which is subdivided into categories of coping with negative emotional states (e.g., frustration or anger), coping with negative physical/physiological states, enhancement of positive emotional states, testing personal control, and giving in to temptations or urges.

The second major category is interpersonal determinants. This is subdivided into coping with interpersonal conflict, social pressure, and enhancing a positive emotional state (in an interpersonal situation).

In a study of these factors as determinants of relapse for alcohol, smoking, and heroin, Marlatt and Gordon (1985) found that 76 percent of all relapse episodes fall into just three categories: coping with negative emotional states (37 percent), social pressure (24 percent), and coping with interpersonal conflict (24 percent). The remaining 24 percent of all relapses fell in increments of from 3 to 7 percent into the other five categories.

These and other data led Marlatt to develop a model of the relapse process (Marlatt & Gordon, 1985). The model is based on the notions of self-efficacy and personal control in that it assumes that a client who is refraining from using a substance experiences a sense of personal control that leads to a sense of self-efficacy. This perception continues until the person meets a high-risk situation, one that poses a threat to the client's sense of control and increases the risk of potential relapse. This high-risk situation is affected by covert antecedents, beginning with a possible lifestyle imbalance leading to the desire for indulgences or immediate gratification. This can lead either to urges or cravings mediated by expectancies for immediate effects of the substance, or to rationalization, denial, and apparently irrelevant decisions (choices that enhance the probability of a relapse).

Once the high-risk situation exists, if the client is prepared with a coping response, the result will be increased self-efficacy and lower probability of relapse. However, if no coping response is available, the result will be decreased self-efficacy plus positive outcome expectancies for the effects of the substance. This will lead to initial use of the substance followed by an abstinence violation effect (AVE) that would include dissonance, conflict, guilt, and perceived loss of control. All of this then results in the increased probability of a relapse.

The whole model, then, from start to finish, follows the following steps:

1. Lifestyle imbalance
2. Desire for indulgence or immediate gratification
3. Urges or cravings
4. Rationalization, denial, and apparently irrelevant decisions
5. High-risk situation
6. No coping response
7. Decreased self-efficacy

8. Initial use of substance
9. AVE
10. Increased probability of relapse

Use of this model in understanding determinants of relapse can be aided by the use of four new instruments that were developed to help predict clients' relapse potential. The first is the Relapse Precipitants Inventory (Litman, 1986), a twenty-five–item measure that appears to distinguish between relapses and nonrelapses. The second is the Coping Behaviors Inventory (Litman, 1986), a thirty-six–item inventory that evaluates a person's ability to develop coping strategies. The third is the Inventory of Similar Situations (Annis, 1986), a 100-item questionnaire designed to assess situations in which a client drank heavily over the past year. The last is the Situational Confidence Questionnaire (Annis, 1986), a 100-item instrument designed to assess self-efficacy in relation to a client's perceived ability to cope effectively with alcohol.

One of the major contributions of this generic relapse model is that it suggests a number of points for intervention that lead to several of the maintenance strategies discussed below.

Maintenance and Generalization Strategies

The literature increasingly reflects a good deal of concern about ensuring maintenance and generalization of interventions in all problem areas (Goldstein & Kanfer, 1979; Karoly & Steffen, 1980). This literature has produced a number of general principles regarding maintenance of therapeutic gains, including the following:

1. Make sure that the behavior or activity is being performed at the desired level prior to termination.
2. Try to approximate as much as possible the conditions of real life in your intervention program.
3. Use more than one intervention agent (e.g., have the client rehearse with other practitioners, clients, etc.).
4. Try to find events in everyday life that will help maintain the desired activity and build these into the program.
5. Decrease the program gradually (do not end it all at once).
6. Train the client to continue the activities in real life by having him or her practice them in advance of termination.
7. Use real-life homework assignments throughout the intervention process.
8. Gradually decrease the similarity between the artificial and real situations.
9. Train others in the client's environment to maintain the desired behavior or activities (e.g., train in the use of contingency management). This is an especially important strategy for ensuring generalization.

In addition to these general principles, a number of maintenance strategies, have been developed specifically in the area of substance abuse. A recent review of the outcome research for aftercare in the treatment of alcohol abuse shows that such programs contribute significantly to overall positive outcome (Ito & Donovan, 1986). Although several different aftercare or maintenance strategies were evaluated, the findings were consistent and substantial enough to suggest that such maintenance strategies be made a major part of every intervention program with substance abuse.

Several of these maintenance strategies have been described succinctly by Lewis et al. (1988, ch. 6; see also Daley, 1986). Many of them consist of continuing parts of the intervention program described in the previous section, so they need only be mentioned here. In addition, many also fit the specific stages of Marlatt's relapse model and will be briefly described.

Strategies related to relapse model.   These strategies can, of course be used at any time, but there is a particularly neat fit between the stages of the model and selection of an intervention. The idea here is to prepare the client in advance for dealing with any of the situations indicated in the model.

1. Lifestyle imbalance requires development of a balanced daily lifestyle, including jogging, hobbies, meditation, and so on.
2. Desire for indulgence requires substituting positive indulgences, such as recreational activities.
3. Urges and cravings can be countered by preparing the client with coping imagery and stimulus control techniques.
4. Rationalization, denial, and apparently irrelevant decisions can be countered by labeling these phenomena as warning signals and by teaching the client to use a decision matrix in which he or she lists immediate positive and negative consequences for using or not using the substance.
5. High-risk situations can be dealt with by having the client use self-monitoring and self-evaluation skills that teach him or her to recognize those situations and by teaching a variety of avoidance strategies.
6. The absence of a coping response is dealt with by the use of skill training plus a technique called relapse rehearsal. Relapse rehearsal teaches clients to imagine a relapse situation in which they successfully use a coping technique to avoid using the substance.
7. To counter decreased self-efficacy and positive outcome expectancies for using the substance, the client can be taught to use relaxation training, stress management, and efficacy-enhancing imagery. In addition, the client can be educated about immediate versus delayed use of the substance.
8. To avoid initial unplanned use of the substance, clients can be taught the techniques of programmed relapse. This is a fairly tricky technique to use and is not recommended for most cases because it involves program-

ming the first relapse (e.g., the first drink of alcohol) under the supervision of the practitioner. Other techniques include a contract to limit the extent of use plus a reminder card for what the client should do if he or she has a slip.

9. For AVE, with its risk of relapse, clients can be taught through cognitive restructuring that a slip is actually a mistake to be learned from and does not have to lead to a complete relapse.

General maintenance strategies.   In addition to the strategies above that fit the Marlatt model, a number of other strategies and techniques could be considered, including the following:

1. Use of booster sessions and follow-ups. These should be scheduled in incrementally increasing intervals following termination (e.g., at two weeks, one month, three months, six months, one year).

2. Use of problem-solving training to help clients deal with life problems in a functional way without having to turn to substance use.

3. Use of exercise programs to maintain the benefits of physical health.

4. Continued membership in a self-help group with periodic follow-ups from the social worker (phone calls will do) to encourage the client's attendance.

CONCLUSION

As this chapter has illustrated, the problem of substance abuse and its modification is very complex. The essence of successful treatment is two-pronged: 1) critical use of the available literature to be informed about what works (with the awareness that new developments are appearing daily); and 2) careful individualizing of clients and problems so that specific treatment programs can be developed. It is hoped that the assessment and intervention guidelines presented here will be of use to students and practitioners who have made a commitment to working in this area. In the long run, it is this commitment that will lead to the greatest satisfaction and increasingly more effective treatment.

CHAPTER 13

Working with People with HIV Disease

Harvey L. Gochros

Gochros discusses the changing nature of HIV disease and suggests approaches to working with infected individuals and others who are impacted by the disease. Although many people with AIDS are still dying, we may be witnessing the final phases of the AIDS epidemic as we have known it. Gochros defines the problems that HIV-infected people continue to face in the various stages of the infection and then focuses on life planning for each specific phase. He also focuses on the impact of the disease on the family, lovers, and friends of those who are infected. As Gochros illustrates, the person adjusting to the progression of AIDS faces different issues at different stages. The interventions range from stress management and will preparation to issues relating to death, dying, suicide, sex, and dealing with loved ones. Clearly, these issues reflect the importance and usefulness of matching the client's current concerns with particular interventions. Using a task-oriented perspective, Gochros shows the importance of active participation by both social worker and client.

INTRODUCTION

HIV disease underwent dramatic changes as the twentieth century drew to a close (Stine, 1998). Although there are still people dying of AIDS, "the Plague"as we knew it in the past is largely over, at least for mid-Americans and western Europeans. Death rates have dropped dramatically: the death toll in 1999 was 62 percent lower than in 1998, and infected individuals are living longer and healthier lives (Centers for Disease Control [CDC], 2000).

The source of many of these changes has been the success of medical research in combating the virus and forestalling, if not preventing, its lethal consequences. While giving hope to those infected with the disease, these changes also produce further complications and pose new challenges for those who are HIV infected and those who care for them.

Toward the end of the nineteenth century, William Osler, a renowned pioneer in medical education, stated that to know syphilis was to know medicine in all its aspects. It might be similarly stated today that to know AIDS is to know social work. Social work practice with people with AIDS calls forth virtually every aspect of the profession, including our underlying values of supporting populations that are socially oppressed, our professional ethics, the need to work cooperatively with other disciplines (especially medicine and law), and our range of intervention skills with individuals, families, groups, organizations policy makers, and communities.

AIDS is an epidemic that has profoundly affected almost every aspect of our lives and has a devastating impact on everyone involved with the infected person. It is still a new, evolving disease, virtually unknown until the mid-1980s, and it has killed an estimated 430,000 men, women, and children in the United States (CDC, 2000, Table 22) and countless millions around the world, especially in Southeast Asia and sub-Saharan Africa.

The number of those who are infected but surviving is difficult to assess. HIV reporting (as opposed to reporting on AIDS itself) is currently required in only thirty states. These states report 92,000 cases that have not yet resulted in full-blown AIDS (CDC, 1997, p. 32). Many tens of thousands of other cases doubtlessly exist in these as well as in the nonreporting states.

All states, however, report cases of full-blown diagnosed AIDS cases. Most recently, 733,000 people were reported to be diagnosed with AIDS in the United States. From the beginning of the epidemic through December 1999, more than 430,000 Americans died from AIDS (CDC, 2000, Table 22). AIDS statistics are complicated by the extremely long incubation period between infection by the HIV virus (which causes the disease) and the actual appearance of the life-threatening consequences of the disease. It is the opportunistic diseases contracted because of an impaired immune system that cause death. Detectable physical damage or even symptoms of AIDS may not occur for many years, if at all in some cases, following infection by the virus. This extended latency period has contributed to underestimating its long-range impact on the thousands of people who already are infected but are not yet aware of their condition.

To better understand treatment approaches for people affected by HIV, some of the troublesome circumstances of the disease must be taken into account:

1. Despite exaggerated fears among many people, AIDS is not easily transmitted. Infection occurs only when bodily fluids from an infected person that contain high concentrations of HIV enter the bloodstream of another person. Yet unfounded fears of casual transmission persist. AIDS elicits irrational fears of contagion even among many people in the helping professions, including physician, nurses, dentists, and other health-care personnel who are called upon to care for those who are infected. Homophobia can still be found even among the physicians who may be called upon to treat AIDS (Schatz & O'Hanlan, 1994.) The genesis of these fears may be found in an association of the causes of infection (notably male-to-male sexual contact and drug use) with social disapproval and therefore those involved directly or indirectly in these activities are seen as deserving of rejection. These reactions are thus a product of guilt by association.

2. AIDS continues to attack primarily populations that are already socially unpopular and stigmatized—homosexual men, drug abusers, the poor, and people of color—and is usually contracted through voluntary pleasurable acts (sexual activity and intravenous drug use) that may be illegal and/or considered immoral.

3. AIDS most often attacks young people, who are ill prepared, as are those around them, to deal with their mortality.

4. Despite recent advances in the medical treatment of the opportunistic illnesses that attack the impaired immune system of HIV-infected individuals, along with progress in defeating the virus itself, there are still no cures or vaccines available or in sight. At best, given current therapies, AIDS might be reduced to a chronic and only potentially fatal disease.

5. AIDS has forced those helping professionals dealing with the social and emotional sequelae of the disease to discuss and deal with not only such social taboos as sex and death, but also with controversial and anxiety-producing subcategories of these taboos: homosexuality and suicide.

6. Because the major behaviors leading to infection (sex and psychotropic drug use) are among the most highly reinforced of human behaviors, both produce powerfully pleasurable experiences and both have deeply entrenched symbolic meanings. These factors contribute to the difficulty in modifying behaviors that contribute to HIV infection.

7. The AIDS epidemic has uncovered the extent of previously hidden homosexual and bisexual behavior and has forced society and the helping professions to reexamine their ethical and moral stances on these behaviors. The epidemic has also led to a decrease in the fear and repugnance of these behaviors on television and in the motion pictures. Despite this progress, however, there is still abundant homophobia in the nation.

In addition to these unique features, there have been additional problems for social workers and others concerned with preventing the disease and serving those already infected. The very character and basic assumptions about the disease are changing rapidly.

Just a few years ago, AIDS was considered an incurable, terminal disease with a life expectancy subsequent to diagnosis of just months or, at best, a few years. Relatively recent medical and pharmacological advances have significantly changed the prognosis for many Americans with HIV. As noted above, the death rate from the disease has dropped dramatically, and the life expectancy of infected individuals has greatly increased.

Despite this optimism, it is still likely that many people with HIV infections will eventually advance to having full-blown AIDS. HIV-infected individuals are still dying. Despite the many near-miracle drugs that have become available, there are many who are not able to benefit from them. Others are resistant to the new medications or are unable to follow the rigid regime of pill taking required if the drugs are to prove effective. It is not unusual for people with AIDS to have to take sixteen to twenty pills a day, including a protease inhibitor "cocktail" to ward off opportunistic diseases as well as to combat the virus itself. Some must be taken with meals, some without, all on a rigid time schedule. (New drugs have been promised, however, that can be taken in fewer numbers.) Still other infected individuals—especially the millions in developing countries as well as some in the United States—cannot afford these expensive medications.

With the emerging improved drug options to match the needs and characteristics of individual patients, it is possible that in the not too distant future AIDS will no longer be necessarily fatal, but instead will become a life-threatening but treatable condition, similar to diabetes or heart disease. Meanwhile, there remains considerable uncertainty about the disease's progress for any particular individual.

The emotional reactions of people who have lived with AIDS over extended periods are complex. One long-term survivor of AIDS described his experience with AIDS as being similar to Alice in Wonderland's reaction to falling into the rabbit hole:

> . . . either the well was very deep, or she fell very slowly, for she had plenty of time as she went down to look about her, and to wonder what was to happen next. First she tried to look down and make out what she was coming to, but it was too dark to see anything. (Carroll, 1960, p. 26)

Like Alice, most people with HIV infection are not quite sure what is coming next.

Emerging Needs of AIDS Survivors

Not only are many people with AIDS living longer, but they also are experiencing relatively good health in the absence of, or in the lengthening periods between, opportunistic disease. This trend toward longer, healthier lives is having a major impact on the kinds of services that social workers have to provide. Already the emphasis of social work treatment of clients with AIDS is shifting from "death planning" to "life planning" with a heavy emphasis on helping the newly recovering or symptom-free populations reenter the world of work and relationships. This reentry process may call on the skills of vocational rehabilitation counselors to help clients return to satisfying productive employment appropriate to their skills, past experience, and energy levels.

Many healthier, more energetic clients are also experiencing a return of their libido, despite the libido decrease associated with some drugs, along with possible depression. Obviously, most will make adjustments to minimize the risks of infecting potential sexual partners. Many men encounter discomfort as they contemplate sexual activities that involve orgasm: ejaculation used to be an enjoyable climax to a sex act—now orgasm might involve the ejaculation of the seed of infection and death.

In contemplating the renewal of sexual activities people infected with HIV also confront options for how to reveal their HIV condition to potential sexual partners. Many clients, however, are less interested in seeking out sexual opportunities than they are in becoming interested again in romantic bonded relationships.

Changing Client Population

Another shift in AIDS is the changes in the proportions of the populations newly infected with the disease. AIDS was originally considered a gay plague, with most of those afflicted being young white gay males. Largely because of effective AIDS education within major gay communities, along with saturation of the host population, members of that population who were going to become infected had been infected by the 1990s. Thus, the rate of new HIV infections among gay and bisexual men has generally decreased. Despite the optimism that these data invite, however, male-to-male sex still accounts for the largest proportion of AIDS cases, and there is concern that condom use may be decreasing among younger gay men. This raises the question whether we will see a resurgence of AIDS in the coming generation of gay white men. Regardless of these trends, many thousands of gay men who are already HIV infected will continue to need attention for years to come.

Preventative and treatment services are gradually retooling to better serve other populations: urban black and Hispanic gays, bisexuals, IV drugs users, their sexual partners, and heterosexual women and their children (Gant, 1996; Gillman, 1996; Stine, 1998.) Preventive programs such as drug education for adolescents, needle-exchange programs for IV drug users, and outreach to homosexually active members ethnic minorities require further development and evaluation.

Ethnic Populations at Risk

The major targets of new HIV infections in the United States are such underclass ethnic minorities as blacks and Hispanics, particularly those who are IV drug abusers, as well as those whom they have infected through birth, shared needles, or sex. Although the public still generally perceives AIDS as a disease primarily of white homosexuals, people of color have been disproportionately affected by it (Raine, 1989). Black Americans make up 12 percent of the US population, yet 35 percent of AIDS cases reported through December 1999 were in the black population (CDC, 2000, Table 21).

When Hispanics with AIDS are added, the percentage of people with AIDS from these two ethnic minorities rises to approximately 50 percent (CDC, 2000, Table 21). Furthermore, 76 percent of women with HIV disease are black or Hispanic, as are 71 percent of heterosexuals with the disease. Finally, 85 percent of infants under 5 years of age with AIDS belong to ethnic minorities.

These high percentages reflect the poverty and associated high incidence of IV drug use among these populations.

Being a member of an ethnic minority and being gay are not, of course, mutually exclusive. Of the 436 cases of AIDS among black men reported in San Francisco through February 1989, 294, or 67 percent, were gay men. Another 59, or 14 percent, were both gay and IV drug users (Raine, 1989). Although social workers must certainly address the complex world of IV needle sharing among blacks and Hispanics, they must not lose sight of those heavily closeted, hard-to-reach ethnic minority gays and bisexuals whose cultures generally reject men perceived to be less than "macho."

Another population requiring greater attention is the increasing number of children and adolescents of color with AIDS. As with their adult counterparts, these individuals and their families must deal with isolation, stigma, and rejection, along with the basic struggle for life and survival (Stine, 1998). In addition to offering individual and group support and counseling to these children and their families, social workers must consider legal and ethical issues associated with placing these children in institutions and foster care, develop culturally sensitive ways to address the specific concerns of minority ethnic families, and improve service delivery systems to the rising number of underclass families affected by the HIV epidemic. The HIV crisis forces us to try to understand the impact of poverty, ethnocentrism, racism, and homophobia on clients and on social work treatment and prevention efforts.

Perhaps the largest population needing attention in the HIV epidemic are people whose HIV infections have not yet manifested themselves in troublesome or potentially fatal opportunistic diseases. There is no reliable count available of Americans who are infected with HIV but are unaware of their condition.

As noted earlier, in the past, HIV infection was considered to be a death warrant, with an inevitable march to a variety of potentially fatal opportunistic diseases. With recent significant medical advances in the treatment of the opportunistic disease—particularly AIDS drug cocktails, including protease inhibitors—there has been a major shift in the outlook for those with HIV infections. In 1998, the FDA approved a drug, Sustiva, that is taken once a day, in contrast to previous "wonder drugs" that were taken several times a day. The rigidity of these schedules created compliance problems for many individuals (*Advocate Internet*, September 18, 1998). The new drug is another step forward in providing effective and manageable drug treatment of AIDS. Unfortunately, these "miracle drugs" are available only to those who can afford them or are in a location where such drugs are provided at no or minimal cost through insurance or clinical trials. These costs can take a heavy toll on the income of HIV-infected people, who may no longer be able to work and who may lack or have insufficient insurance coverage. Petamidine treatments for one of the most common life-threatening opportunistic diseases, for example, can cost about $1,800 a year, and drug cocktails designed to fight HIV (now frequently prescribed for people in the early stages of infection) can cost thousands of dollars a year.

Stages of the Disease

The very definitions of the "stages" of the disease are undergoing change, reflecting the rapid evolution of the AIDS epidemic. In the late 1980s, AIDS was thought to be a disease that divided AIDS sufferers into three distinct categories according to the stage of the disease:

1. Asymptomatic, HIV-antibody positive—people who had been tested and found to have antibodies created by the immune system to ward off an invasion by HIV, but who had not yet manifested any physical symptoms of the disease.
2. ARC (AIDS-related complex)—people who had some physical manifestations of the infection, such as swollen glands, oral thrush, night sweats, weight loss, and so on, none of which were necessarily life threatening. (It should be noted, however, that some people died in the ARC stage.)
3. Full-blown AIDS—people who were HIV antibody positive and who had been diagnosed with a potentially life-threatening opportunistic disease, such as pneumocrystis carinii pneumonia or Kaposi's sarcoma, or other manifestations, such as AIDS-related dementia, that "take the opportunity" of a weakened immune system caused by the HIV infection to attack the body.

The CDC designated certain diseases that attack people with a compromised immune system as diagnostic of full-blown AIDS. In 1993, the CDC added a T cell count of less than 200 as another diagnostic criterion for AIDS.

Many people who work with AIDS, however, have done away with what they consider artificial and unhelpful labels for these three stages. Rather, from the detection of HIV infection onward, the condition could more logically be referred to simply as HIV disease.

The elimination of staging labels, however, is not meant to imply that many people with HIV infections go through some identifiable, although increasingly indistinct, phases as the disease progresses. Indeed, these phases determine which social work tasks and intervention might be anticipated as the social workers assist their clients in dealing with the various concerns, issues, and problems that the disease ordinarily creates.

GENERAL CLINICAL MANIFESTATIONS OF AIDS

Physical Manifestations

The physical manifestations of AIDS vary from individual to individual and over time, as the disease progresses, depending on a number of variables, including whether various drug regimes succeed or fail. The multitude of life-threatening as well as relatively minor but troublesome physical opportunistic diseases can include rare forms of pneumonia and cancer, blindness, diarrhea, fatigue, peripheral neuropathy, dementia, and dermatological problems. In recent years, considerable progress has been made in treating many of these opportunistic infections.

Psychological Manifestations

It is not surprising that a high incidence of anxiety, depression, alcoholism, and other major psychiatric disorders are found in people infected with HIV. Learning that one has a still potentially fatal disease that may have painful and protracted physical, social, financial, sexual, and mental sequelae, as well as attendant social biases and stigma ("AIDS is the punishment of God!" some religious practitioners have said), can have severe psychological consequences.

Neurological infections of the brain and spinal cord may also cause severe psychological problems. Indeed, dementia is a frequently encountered diagnostic indicator of an advanced stage of AIDS and is often one of the most feared consequences of the disease. Suicidal ruminations are common, and actual suicides are not rare at crisis points in the progression of the disease.

INTERVENTIONS IN THE POTENTIAL PHASES OF HIV PROGRESSION

HIV can cause problems in almost every sphere of the lives of infected individuals: physical, social, emotional, sexual, economic, vocational, and spiritual. Indeed some people with AIDS feel bombarded by such a range of problems that they seem to spend whatever remains of their lives going from one crisis to another!

The dramatic changes that occurred in the treatment of HIV in the late 1990s, including both the treatments for the opportunistic infections associated with HIV as well as the availability of a growing number of medications that attack the virus itself, are having a profound effect on the prognoses for infected individuals. There is cautious optimism for the long-term benefits of these new medications. However, it may still be too premature to predict the long-term effects—physical as well as psychological—of these medical advances.

Although each person with AIDS encounters a unique cluster of physical and social situations, reactions, and support systems, some common concerns and problems can be identified. The following suggests some of the crisis points still typically encountered by many infected individuals and some interventions that might be helpful.

1. Interventions for At-Risk Persons Having an Uncertain HIV Status

Because of extensive public education efforts, it is unlikely that anyone who engages in high-risk sexual behaviors (e.g., receptive anal or vaginal intercourse without a condom with a potentially infected partner) is unaware of the possibility of HIV infection. Yet much confusion remains as to just what is safer sex. The social worker can be helpful by passing on current, accurate information that will enable clients to better understand the routes and risks of HIV infection and be better prepared to reduce risks. It cannot be stated with certainty what particular sexual activities are absolutely safe or the degree of risk of others. Sexually active people must understand the relative levels of safety of activities in the wide range of sexual options that exist between handshakes and intercourse.

The situation of HIV needle sharers is more complex and poses far more difficult problems both in prevention and in treatment. Many addicts consider the long-range risks of HIV infection to be secondary in importance to getting a fix. Also, there is nothing among IV drug users that is comparable to the gay communities' own cooperative efforts to change risky behaviors through education (Stine, 1998).

IV drug use is often a byproduct of poverty and racism, both of which remain related and unsolved problems. Needle-exchange programs—proven to be effective in reducing infection in several cities as well as in the state of Hawaii—are opposed by many governmental bodies, including the US Congress, because of the moral concerns of certain segments of politically powerful groups.

Despite their concerns, there is overwhelming evidence that needle-exchange programs reduce the incidence of infection and do not encourage drug usage. Social workers should lobby their legislatures to make these lifesavers available in localities where they are not yet sanctioned.

Persons at risk for HIV infection who have not yet sought antibody testing often experience anxiety regarding their drug use and sexual behavior. Given the stigma, shame, and serious consequences of HIV infection, many sexually active gay men and IV needle sharers are confronted with two major decisions: whether to seek testing to determine their antibody status or whether to modify or abstain from their high-risk behaviors.

Interventions.   The decision of whether to take an antibody test is simpler and more weighted toward the positive than it was just a few years ago. Initially, it was feared that the test might give false negative and positive results and that one might subject oneself to discriminatory practices such as loss of job, insurance, or housing should a positive HIV result become publicly known; and finally, it was argued, why subject oneself to the pain of knowing one is HIV positive if there is nothing one can do about it anyway?

Now, however, existing tests are known to be reliable, anonymous testing is available in many locations, and antidiscrimination laws are now in effect in many, but, unfortunately, not all localities and are buttressed by federal legislation on the rights of the disabled. Also, there are now medications that, if taken soon after infection, may delay (but perhaps not stop) the progression of AIDS.

Thus, after a discussion of the pros and cons of testing with a client at risk, and an assessment of the individual's support systems and anticipated behavior in the event of an HIV-positive result, the social worker might well support testing if anonymous or at least confidential testing is available. Indeed, the arguments for testing continue to grow stronger.

Another category of client who might be supported in seeking testing is made up of overanxious individuals, sometimes referred to as the "worried well," who are at low risk for HIV infection but have a high degree of guilt and anxiety, and who, despite reassurance about their low-risk status, can only be put at ease by being tested. Krieger (1988) has suggested a five-step counseling approach to assist clients experiencing dysfunctional "AIDS anxiety."

1. Prepare the client by providing accurate, up-to-date information about the disease, its transmission, and its prevention.

2. Assess realistically the client's risk of prior exposure to the virus. Has the individual really been at risk?

3. Instruct the client in procedures to minimize or eliminate risks of future infection.

4. Help the client find peer support to avoid patterns of both extremes of denial and despair in response to HIV risks.

5. Address issues directly and indirectly related to the clients' AIDS anxiety, such as guilt about sexual or drug behavior, attraction to atypical dangerous sexual activities, concealment of risky behaviors from sexual partners, and latent or manifest homophobia.

When working with clients who consistently or even occasionally engage in high-risk behavior, the practitioner should explore clients' motivations for these behaviors and try to provide them with an understanding of relative sexual risks and the value of eroticizing safer sex. To do so, the social worker should also explore and overcome his or her own sexual biases and learn to directly and casually discuss explicit aspects of clients' sexual motivations, decisions, and behaviors (Gochros, Gochros, & Fischer, 1986; Gochros, 1992). Education and treatment programs to modify risky sexual behaviors raise complex pragmatic and value issues. Preventive strategies that rely on simple "just say no" approaches are usually no more successful with sex than with drugs. Discussions with sexually active individuals at risk for infection should focus on modifying but not eliminating all sexual activity. The use of both sex and drugs is too powerfully reinforced and carries too much symbolic meaning to easily will away. Decades of efforts to curb adolescent sexual expression have shown the failure of simple moral persuasion. Further, in the case of sex, there are reasons to believe that attempts at abstinence may prove hazardous. Fortunately, there are a number of relatively safe alternatives to abstinence (Gochros, 1988).

The social worker's approach to drug-related behavior that puts clients at risk for HIV infection is more complex. It is difficult to modify the drug addict's needle-sharing behavior when he or she is high on drugs. There is some evidence—albeit controversial—that supplying bleach kits to clean used needles and/or providing clean needles through carefully monitored needle exchange programs might reduce IV-transmitted HIV infection. Ultimately, however, reducing infection among IV drug users requires drug rehabilitation, harm reduction programs, behavior change therapies, and social policy changes that go beyond the scope of this chapter.

2. Interventions with Persons Who Are HIV-Antibody Positive but Are Asymptomatic

As more and more people take antibody tests, many will discover that they are indeed infected with HIV, even though they display no symptoms of the disease. These people are confronted with an agonizing paradox: their body contains the seeds of its own potential destruction, and there is no known way to get rid of the invaders, and yet they feel fine!

Further, there is no way to predict when, how, and even whether destructive manifestations of the illness in the form of opportunistic infections will occur. Typically, people who are diagnosed as asymptomatic, HIV positive will alternate between feeling fine, especially if they deny the diagnosis, and feeling anxious, depressed, guilty, and irritable.

Some individuals, however, report a feeling of relief upon learning their antibody-positive status. Some had been expecting the illness to hit for some time and were relieved when it finally does. Others report relief that they could now remove themselves from what they perceive as the arduous and often unrewarding world of "anonymous sex and one-night stands."

Contradictory reports on "cures" and a constant procession of new drugs for AIDS can also add to the confusion of newly infected individuals: "Just how much *should* I worry?" Still others feel almost grateful that they now have no excuse for not coming out as gay to their family and friends. The person who has just learned his or her antibody-positive status may begin to integrate a new identity, however, it may be an identity that will set him or her apart from others in his or her own mind and perhaps in the minds of others.

For many gay people, acknowledging that they have AIDS is a "second coming out" that is comparable to the "first" coming out as gay. Indeed the way people carry out and respond to their first coming out may be a good predictor of how they will handle dealing with informing others that they have AIDS.

Upon learning that they are infected, many people will experience reactions associated with crisis: denial, withdrawal, random impulsive behaviors, and fears of "going crazy." Some will seek out alternate explanations for their test results or begin doctor shopping. Others will consider suicide.

Interventions.   The major tasks during this period for people with HIV are seeking a doctor they trust and with whom they feel comfortable, learning what they can about their physical status, cognitively incorporating this new information, carefully appraising its significance, and developing a balanced perspective on the infection that includes both an awareness of the risks and of the hope associated with emerging medical advances. The most difficult task they confront is living with the uncertainty of when, how, and even whether the disease will progress.

Guilt is a factor that may become an issue among some AIDS clients. Most of those who developed full-blown AIDS in the first half of the 1980s and earlier contracted the infection at a time when they, their physicians, public health officials, and the popular media did not know that their behavior could lead to a life-threatening disease. It can be anticipated, however, that people who became infected with HIV after the mid-1980s, and into the new century, when the media had made AIDS and its routes of transmission well known, may well experience a higher degree of guilt, shame, and emotional trauma: "I should have known better."

These clients pose a challenge for social workers because of the feelings of guilt engendered by their belief that their "unacceptable" behavior brought about their HIV infection. The social worker often must deal with the crisis that an HIV-positive diagnosis generates. Standard crisis intervention strategies may well be called for (Golan, 1979).

The social worker must also try to keep up to date on the rapid medical advances and other information that may impact their clients. It may not be appropriate, of course, for the social worker to advocate for certain drugs, explain their use in detail, or even offer advice except in general terms. But it is important for social workers to have general AIDS-related medical knowledge in order to better understand, in an objective manner, their clients' medical situation and choices. It will also help to base interventions on a sound assessment of the significance to the client of his or her diagnosis and of the extent and accuracy of the client's understanding of his or her medical status, especially, as is often the case, if the client's physician does not take the time or effort to explain important medical matters to patients.

In this phase, as in subsequent phases, the social worker must be aware of the possibility of suicidal ruminations. These thoughts may simply be an effort by clients to take control of their lives in a period in which everything seems out of control. Although they are common, suicidal thoughts should not be discounted. The social worker should deal with them calmly and objectively. In later phases of AIDS, suicide may be either a rational or irrational choice of an HIV-infected individual. However, as the prognosis for people with AIDS continues to improve, suicide may become a less rational and less frequent choice.

Contact with a physician should be initiated by the client as soon as possible after diagnosis, as there is growing evidence that early medical treatment, including the use of new medications, may well delay the progression of AIDS. The social worker should be aware of the physicians in the community who are experienced at and capable of treating people with HIV infections and not assume that all physicians are AIDS phobics, who unfortunately are not unknown in the medical profession (Schatz & O'Hanlan, 1994). AIDS is a complicated syndrome that requires skill, empathy, sensitivity, and time on the part of physicians.

3. Interventions with Persons Who Have Begun to Experience Symptoms of HIV Infection

The first physical symptoms of HIV infection, such as weight loss, lymphadenopathy, diarrhea, and night sweats, cut through clients' denial of being infected and can be experienced as a major trauma. The disease becomes real. Some individuals react with a frantic search for a cure, including medical, holistic, and nontraditional therapies.

People in this phase are less able than they were to deny the significance of the disease for their lives. They must make important decisions about medical treatment, reevaluate their long-term planning, and consider in great depth and detail the impact of the disease on their work and career, interpersonal relationships, and sexuality. Some will need to reevaluate now or later where to live and perhaps consider a return to their family and home community. At this point, many will want to decide whom to tell about their disease and when and how to tell them.

Interventions.   This phase, like all of the significant phases of AIDS, requires active listening and emotional support from the social worker, who must be knowledgeable about both the disease and the client's current situation. The social worker should explore the client's perception of his or her future, correct any misinformation, and, if necessary, interpret the client's medical situation and treatment.

Of prime importance, as they may begin to lose control over their lives and even their bodies, is the need to empower clients in as many areas of their lives as possible. Clients should be encouraged to take an active role in health and medical planning. The clients' right to know what is going on in their treatment and to share treatment decisions with their physician should be supported—including their right to make use of alternative approaches to western medicine.

Anxiety management and social skills training might be offered to deal with the interpersonal challenges that may be ahead (Guay, 1989). Clients also may be responsive to explorations of philosophical and spiritual matters, either with the social worker or through referral to individuals or support groups within the community.

4. Interventions with Persons Who Have Developed Their First Opportunistic Disease

The actual diagnosis of AIDS is made only at the onset of an opportunistic disease that is recognized by the CDC as clearly indicative of AIDS or a T cell count under 200. However, the client and others may have erroneously labeled their condition as AIDS much earlier. Clients may manifest a wide range of reactions to their illness, often rapidly going through and repeating the classic phases of grief, including shock, denial, anger, bargaining, depression, and acceptance (Kubler-Ross, 1987). The social worker should anticipate that the onset of a life-threatening opportunistic disease likely results in a crisis situation not only for the client, but possibly also for family, friends, and lovers.

Depression and panic are common reactions, along with recurring obtrusive thoughts about illness and death, including suicidal ruminations. People who are experiencing a first opportunistic illness, and the people who are important to them, must be given realistic hope.

Interventions.   In working with clients in this phase, the social worker must carry out the tasks that are associated with a client confronting a major crisis (Golan, 1979). The client should avoid such impulsive decisions as moving, divorcing, and quitting work. Social workers may have to help clients sort out insurance and public welfare procedures and seek competent medical care and funding for expensive medications.

Discussions of future financial planning, including making a will, and perhaps a living will that articulate clients' wishes for their care and medical management during their potential last days, may be initiated but should not be forced—these activities may be premature at this point. Social workers may also act as brokers and advocates, if necessary, with the diverse agencies that will be involved in the client's care.

On the one hand, to impress upon a client with AIDS that an opportunistic disease is no longer usually fatal, the social worker may want to ask a case manager or volunteer who has survived his or her first opportunistic disease to visit the client in the hospital and demonstrate that most people with AIDS are now surviving their opportunistic diseases and go on to live fulfilling and enjoyable long lives. On the other hand, to further help in dealing with the psychological trauma of facing what could be a life-threatening illness, the social worker can also teach clients how to use the techniques of thought stopping, relaxation training, and visualization to manage potentially overwhelming feelings.

5. Interventions with Persons Who Have Had Repeated Opportunistic Disease

Because of significant progress in medical care and pharmacology, people with AIDS are increasingly likely to survive most opportunistic diseases. Often, however, the progress of AIDS is characterized by chronic fatigue and other painful and annoying, if not disabling, symptoms such as peripheral neuropathy. Occasionally the social worker may note that a client is slowly and subtly "winding down" or "wasting away." These clients (a minority of today's HIV-infected individuals) must deal with two conflicting pressures. On one hand, they may need to prepare psychologically, philosophically, practically, and spiritually for the possibility of death. On the other hand, they must reevaluate and readjust their life planning to take into account that they may live a full life for many more years.

Whereas the goal for many people with AIDS used to be to "live day by day," expanded life expectancies may now necessitate long-range life planning. Those who have regained their strength and optimism may need help in thinking through the problems of reentry into the world of work and relationships. Others may need to review their hopes and ambitions and accept that they may never accomplish some of their life goals that they had set for themselves prior to their infection. This can be a painful process.

There is a danger, however, that formerly active and accomplished clients may withdraw prematurely, when they could still maintain an active and rewarding lifestyle. Finding "alternatives" to former life satisfactions and new avenues in love and work calls upon the creativity of clients and social workers alike.

Despite the improved prognosis for people with AIDS, many may still face numerous difficulties and losses. They may no longer be able to work, with a resulting loss of a sense of productivity and independence, not to mention loss of income. They may have lost their interest in sex as a result of the opportunistic diseases, depression, or medications. (Some clients have reported success with the erection-stimulating drug Viagra, although one client reported that Viagra gave him an erection, but, unfortunately, he did not have the energy to do anything with it!)

Even if they still have erotic urges and appropriate physiological responses, clients may still be reluctant to seek partners or engage in any sexual activity that could conceivably lead to infecting a partner. Systemic symptoms (such as diarrhea and cramps) and disfiguring dermatological problems may well impair their physical attractiveness and sense of well-being. Most difficult and important to people with AIDS, however, is their loss of identity and an uncertain sense of a future. Many now see themselves or are seen by others only as a "person with AIDS."

It should be noted, however, that many clients at this point in their disease progression do quite well and see this as a high-quality period of their life.

They have survived life-threatening disorders and now experience a new perspective on life. Some report enjoying their lives as they never had before. They treasure each day and celebrate every joyful aspect of living. Some report a rapprochement with family and friends and a spiritual reawakening. Often, however, this "high" sets the client up for discouragement and depression if new physical evidence of the HIV infection emerges.

Two tests.   At all stages of the disease progression, two medical tests often take on considerable significance to HIV-infected people. People with AIDS generally take a great interest in their T cell counts and their viral load. The T cell test reflects the losses or gains in the body's immune system, and the viral load reports the quantity of HIV in the person's vascular system. Many see a dropping T cell count and a rising viral load as portents for their future. While the reliability of these two tests in precisely predicting disease progression can be questioned, there is no doubt that the tests have great psychological meaning in terms of clients' fears and hopes.

Intervention.   The social worker's role with clients who have experienced a succession of serious opportunistic disease may be varied and complex. Some clients may choose to defend themselves against anxiety or depression through denial and choose to avoid what they may consider morbid preoccupation with the disease. For many, this is an effective and positive self-treatment that the social worker should not challenge.

Many, however, choose to talk about the seriousness of their situation if they can find someone willing to listen. For such clients, the social worker can facilitate grief work to deal with the diverse losses clients are or are anticipating experiencing (Kubler-Ross, 1987). At the same time, social workers can help clients maintain as active and fulfilling a life as possible within the constraints of their illness.

Support groups for people with AIDS are important resources. They reassure clients that they are not alone and provide information, models for behavior at various stages of the illness, and a potential friendship network.

Most people infected with HIV need to continue to feel useful. Generally, they should be encouraged to continue to work as long as they enjoy their work, have a supportive work environment, and are physically able to do so. Even if clients must leave their work and seek other sources of support, there are ways for them to maintain a sense of usefulness. Many are able to learn enough about their illness and its treatment to take an active role in their medical care decisions. Many have been active in coalitions that advocate for the rights and needs of people with AIDS. Others act as volunteer AIDS educators or do other work with AIDS caregiving organizations. Social workers can help their clients determine their needs for productivity and discover creative outlets for expressing them.

Sexual concerns. Social workers should create an atmosphere in which clients can freely discuss their sexual needs and concerns. Although, as noted earlier, some clients, as a result of medication or chronic depression, will experience reduced or no sexual energy, many will still have a sexual release that can help to reduce this stress. If a person with advanced AIDS has a sero-negative sexual partner, however, it is possible that conflict might develop over sexual choices. There may well be asymmetrical sexual interest: Clients may need information and challenges to or confirmation of their beliefs about safer sex when they are considering continued sexual activity.

Social workers may also help clients think through the dilemmas posed by revealing their HIV status to potential sexual partners. The complex issues of how, when, and whether potential partners should be informed require careful consideration by both clients and social workers. Clients also may benefit from information about erotic enhancement of safer sex activities.

Throughout these discussions of sexual behavior, social workers should keep in mind that sexual expression carries with it considerable symbolic meaning for people with AIDS, as it does for everyone. Many people with AIDS have learned to use their sexuality not only to achieve pleasure and intimacy, but also to enhance their self-esteem, solidify interpersonal relationships, confirm their desirability, or overcome their loneliness.

AIDS creates a number of obstacles to sexual fulfillment, however. The majority of infected individuals are concerned that they not pass on their disease to sexual partners. Some perceive themselves as hopelessly contaminated. Those who do not have regular sexual partners may be torn between the desire for new partners and the need to tell them of their infection, recognizing that informing potential partners may lead to rejection.

Some social workers may, of course, find sexual activity for people with HIV infections inappropriate and disturbing. For many people, however, including persons with AIDS, sex is an important aspect of life and, indeed, may well be a celebration of living. Social workers should be supportive of clients' explorations of safe and responsible avenues of sexual expression.

In interactions with clients, social workers may choose to support clients' positive denial of the possible fatal nature of the disease. Clients and those who are close to them will need occasional breaks from focusing on the problems and the psychological stress generated by the disease. Some refer to these as "AIDS-free days," in which they think and act as if they were free of the disease. Clients can be taught various behavioral techniques to help them handle the chronic, recurring tension described above. These techniques may include assertiveness training, relaxation training, cognitive restructuring, and social skills training (Guay, 1989).

The need for case management may well increase as housing, financial, and insurance problems emerge or intensify. Medical and drug bills may become overwhelming. Clients may need help in expressing themselves more assertively to physicians in order to get their questions answered and their needs understood and met. Social workers must support their clients' efforts to receive adequate health care services.

In an era in which potential cures for the disease seem "just around the corner," it is difficult to deal with the possibility of death. Some clients may no longer be able to deny that their illness is progressing and that they might die from it. The "honeymoon" that may have followed overcoming earlier major opportunistic diseases may come to a sudden halt. Their psychological seesaw of hope and despair can be stressful. People experiencing a reoccurrence of earlier opportunistic disease may once again have to work through their grief. There may be specific plans that clients want to make for their dying and death. Some may want to disengage slowly from life, gradually withdrawing from family, friends, and their daily activities.

When clients have not been able to profit from the emerging medical advances for physical or psychological reasons, and are in advanced phases of AIDS, their social worker will need to assist the client and his or her loved ones in carrying out grief work. To the extent that the social worker feels comfortable and competent, he or she may also help the client explore spiritual and philosophical perspectives of their situations. Whether they are long-term survivors or people who are resistant to the new life-saving drugs, clients often ask "why me?" It is a difficult question to answer. As in earlier stages, many people with AIDS, and those in their social environment, experience waves of anger that may be aimed in almost any direction. It is difficult to express one's anger toward a virus, and thus clients may direct their rage at family, friends, social service agencies, doctors, the president, or even God.

Once again, discussions of suicide initiated by clients should not be avoided. Indeed, it may be advisable to ask depressed clients in this phase of the illness whether they have considered suicide. The question will not cause the act. For some clients, preparation for suicide becomes the ultimate opportunity to exercise control over their lives, even if they never carry out their plans.

Suicide may be a difficult topic for some social workers to deal with, however, because of their own value system, religion, or fear of shared responsibility for such a serious act. A nonjudgmental, supportive listener, however, may be invaluable to clients who have found no one with whom they can calmly discuss their thoughts and wishes.

The social worker may be called upon to carry out new case management tasks, including exploring terminal care facilities. Work with the family may also come into greater focus (Lynch, 1996). The client may wish to try to "make things right" with family, friends, and present or past spouses or lovers. This may involve working through a family's unresolved feelings about the client's homosexuality or drug use. There is no reason to believe, however, that a terminal disease will bring the family together and resolve conflicts, rejection, and emotional distance that has existed for decades. Deathbed resolutions of long-term conflicts occur more often in movies and on television than in real life. AIDS affects not only those who are HIV infected but also their lovers, spouses, and families, especially if they act as the caregivers (Lynch, 1996).

Couple conflicts.   If people with AIDS encounter a series of serious opportunistic diseases, difficulties in relationships with spouses or lovers may come to a head (Shelby, 1992). Couple counseling may be necessary to deal with the strains on the caregiving partner, especially in a relationship where one partner is HIV positive and the other is not. An important ingredient in this counseling is an assessment of the relationship, using a review of the characteristics of the relationship before and after one or both partners became infected. This might help to shift perceived responsibility for problems in the relationship from either the infected partner or the uninfected partner alone to both partners. Couple conflicts often simply repeat relationship problems that preexisted the HIV infection.

Both partners may need the social worker's support to understand each other's needs and fears as they communicate feelings directly and sensitively. The couple might choose to renegotiate their relationship, including allowing, perhaps, sexual expression outside the relationship if the infected partner is no longer interested in sex. If both partners are infected, the healthier partner might also profit from the social worker's permission to express his or her feelings about being in a relationship with a person in an advanced stage of the disease. An often expressed concern is, "If I get sick and my partner has died, who will take care of me?"

Temporary or permanent separation may also have to be negotiated, with the social worker urging a slow and careful examination of the factors that led to the need for separation. Sometimes the partner with AIDS chooses the separation because he or she feels that whatever gulf has separated the couple in the past has been widened by the progress of the disease. If the couple stays together, the social worker might teach the couple new relationship strategies, including ways to argue fairly and effectively and how to deal with tensions and conflicts (Caldarola & Helquist, 1989).

6. Interventions with Persons in the Terminal Phase of Illness

For the reasons noted above, there has been a dramatic drop in the likelihood that HIV-infected individuals will die from the disease, and many if not most will live out a "normal" life span. Some, however, will unfortunately be unable to profit from recent medical advances because they are resistant to the drugs, the side effects are prohibitive, or compliance is too difficult. For this minority, physical deterioration may be rapid or progress erratically. Often as the client's defenses weaken, he or she may experience dementia, blindness, and a host of other major and minor physical complications. Clients also may experience considerable pain, loss of control over body functions, confusion, and psychological withdrawal.

Although improved medical treatment may save most Americans with

AIDS from an early death, in some cases it has also prolonged their dying. The fact that many people with AIDS were young and in good health and possessed strong bodies prior to their infection tended to prolong the dying process. People with AIDS often experience repeated close calls with death and surprise their doctors, families, and themselves with unexpected rebounds from the deathbed.

Unfortunately, the bleak side of these rebounds and the associated psychological seesaw is the often unexpressed exhaustion experienced by family and friends, especially if they serve as caregivers. Even burned out professional helpers may experience this reaction. Some may secretly and guiltily wish that the client "would get it over with." This can be disturbing not only to the family, but to the medical staff and the patient as well. It is not unusual that people in the terminal stages of AIDS, whose doctors had informed them that they were in their final days and given them "permission to let go," suddenly rebound and are back on their feet in days.

Intervention.   For those who will still die from the disease, the major task in this phase is to help clients make the transition from life to a physically and psychologically comfortable death and to help the client and those who are close to him or her achieve peace of mind. Just as interventions in the earlier phases of the disease focused on enhancing the quality of life of people living with the disease, towards the end of life, the interventions focus on enhancing the quality of dying.

Dying with dignity has become increasingly difficult in the technological age, and social workers may need to help their clients achieve this. Social workers often are confronted with a medical staff that is committed to keeping patients alive as long as possible, yet is unwilling or unable to adequately ease their pain. The social worker should attempt to overcome physicians' reluctance to prescribe adequate pain medications. Fear of causing addiction and other rationales for withholding adequate pain medications from dying patients are unconscionable.

Social workers may need to act as their clients' advocates in carrying out their clients' wishes as to where and how they want to die. Most people with AIDS would prefer dying quickly and painlessly at home to dying gradually and alone in the hospital, hooked up to life-extending tubes and machines. If the patient chooses, the social worker may express his or her wishes about when and whether to continue or stop life-saving procedures. The existence of a living will or right of attorney is helpful in doing so.

It is more important than ever in this phase for the social worker to be a good listener. Physical touching and holding may be all that is wanted and needed toward the end. The social worker also may help the client assess whether he or she has finished his or her "work" and then give the patient permission to let go and peacefully die. Sometimes the best we can do is listen to our clients and hold their hands. The social worker's final efforts may be with family, spouses, lovers, and friends, dealing with unresolved guilt, anger, and other unfinished grief work.

SOCIAL WORK STRESSES IN AIDS WORK

In the words of one social worker, "We are overworked and overloaded and we don't seem to be making much of a difference. . . . And nobody had told us about death. . . . Nobody has told us how to grieve or what to expect" (Pollatsek, 1994, p. 38).

Social workers are often ill prepared for the complicated legal, emotional, and medical aspects of AIDS work. As in many other areas of social work practice, social workers in AIDS work are underpaid, overworked, and under-appreciated (Gochros, 1996). Even if they value serving persons with AIDS (PWAs), social workers in AIDS service agencies and other settings may resent the demands of case management tasks that limit their time to provide counseling for their HIV-infected clients about evolving relationships with caregivers, families, and others who are close to them, as well as making important life decisions and dealing, perhaps, with their mortality.

Social workers and case managers are often expected to serve as brokers with uncaring bureaucratic local, state, and federal welfare organizations with complex, vague, and ever-changing rules. They may also be expected to serve as confidants, advocates, and friends to the PWAs in their caseload. They frequently work with angry clients from diverse cultures and lifestyles that they hardly understand. They are expected to find medical and dental care as well as furniture and transportation for their clients and accept the blame when things go wrong. They may be called upon at any hour to deal with a plethora of unanticipated emergencies. Finally, despite months or years of caring for their clients—and often enduring their depressions and anger—they are constantly reminded, at least they were in the past, that many of the clients they serve will die. Burnout is common (Gochros, 1996).

Avoiding Burnout

Although professional and volunteer caregiver burnout is understandable in the stressful situations in AIDS work, it is possible to reduce the stresses and increase the satisfactions of the work. It would, indeed, be unfortunate if the most experienced professional AIDS practitioners and other caregivers who may have the most to offer chose to withdraw from AIDS work. Some stresses that lead to burnout are endemic to AIDS and may be almost inevitable, while others can be reduced or eliminated (see, for example, Gochros, 1996; Lynch, 1996; Monette, 1988; Shelby, 1992; and Boyd-Franklin, Steiner, & Boland, 1994).

Common Stresses Associated with AIDS Caregiving

There are a number of common stresses encountered by practitioners working with AIDS patients; they often find themselves involved in the daily lives of their clients to a far greater degree than they would with other clients

(Curtis & Hodge, 1995). Inevitably, this intense involvement can lead to diverse problems for both the practitioners and their clients. Among the stresses commonly experienced by social workers are the following:

1. Observing irreversible and disturbing mental and painful physical deterioration and the threat of death.
2. Dealing with and openly discussing sex and death, including homosexuality and suicide (Gochros, 1992).
3. Encountering anger in oneself as well as in clients: AIDS is a cruel disease that teases its victims by its unpredictability. AIDS-related rage may be understandable, but it can easily overpower professional helpers who may interpret the anger as criticism or proof of their ineffectiveness (Winiarski, 1991).
4. Feeling a strong need to "fix" the PWA and experiencing frustration and guilt when they cannot end the psychological, spiritual, and physical pain or possible death of those they are caring for.

Despite these practitioner and caregiver challenges, there are ways to minimize stress. People wanting to work with AIDS sufferers should be screened for their motivations for working in this area and their ability to deal with the stresses that are likely to occur. They should then be helped to anticipate some of the stresses they are likely to encounter.

Caregivers are not helpless in the war on AIDS: "They can help the client live a better life, attain goals, come to terms, and confront dying and death. But often feelings of helplessness, spoken or not, are communicated . . . resulting in a therapist's loss of faith in himself or herself" (Winiarski, 1991, p. 128). They can be helped to think through, develop, and maintain boundaries for their involvement with their clients. To do so they must establish limits and realistic goals for their work (Gochros, 1996). It is essential that workers meet their intimacy needs through outside relationships and find and use a trained confidential listener. "To take care of others well, one needs to take care of oneself first" (Rosica, 1995, p. 4).

People working with AIDS sufferers may often need to grieve. America is a death-denying society, however. Most caregivers are ill prepared to deal with, let alone discuss, death, whether it is their own or that of others. Yet in order to keep going in AIDS work without burning out or becoming hardened, one has to allow oneself the opportunity to grieve—sometimes over and over again.

The key to long-term survival for the HIV caregiver is to learn about grief through reading, participating in in-service discussions, attending a caregivers' bereavement support group, and finding someone to listen as the caregiver expresses his or her grief. Practitioners must give themselves permission to grieve. Grieving allows caregivers to accept the reality of those losses, separate emotionally from the dead, and move on with their lives (Pollatsek, 1994). Caregivers should not be afraid of their tears.

Searching for Meaning

Despite the changing consequences of HIV infection, AIDS work still often brings up spiritual, religious, and existential issues for caregivers as well as clients as they struggle with their spirituality and the meaning of life and death. This spiritual process of evaluating our place in the universe can have benefits for caregivers beyond their caregiving role. It can help to enrich their own lives.

CONCLUSION

As can be seen from this chapter, the complex and varied tasks associated with HIV disease require a diverse and rapidly changing collection of social work roles and skills.

Case management is required to meet the basic human needs of people with AIDS, including advocacy and brokerage to help the client obtain adequate nutrition, housing, medical care, hospice, or long-term nursing care, and financial planning and assistance.

Support groups with skilled group leaders provide invaluable assistance to people in the various stages of AIDS as well as to their families, spouses, and lovers. Such groups help AIDS sufferers avoid feeling alone and provide participants with models for resolving many of the common problems they are likely to encounter.

Social workers can support and help the coalitions of people with AIDS that increasingly are acting as their own advocates to protect and assert their rights, demand a better level of service, and attack bureaucratic obstacles to their well-being. Such coalitions serve a latent function of providing another means of empowerment for people with AIDS, who often feel that they have lost some degree of control over their own lives. These coalitions can serve as major allies, as well as occasional critics, of social workers with people who have AIDS.

Both professional and volunteer caregivers for PWAs have a crucial role in coping with the AIDS epidemic. This can be gratifying work, but at the same time potentially stressful. Some of the stresses associated with caregiving for PWAs are inevitable. There are, however, ways discussed in this chapter in which many of the stresses can be eliminated or, at least, minimized.

Finally, social workers must continue their efforts to meet the needs of the growing number of people living with AIDS and resist the temptation to see the AIDS epidemic as over. AIDS remains a serious ongoing, but evolving, epidemic. Social workers can use their skills to assure that the basic human needs of people with AIDS continue to be met, not only through AIDS service agencies but also through all relevant organizations of professional helpers and through humane and supportive public policy and legislation.

CHAPTER 14

Treatment for Persons with Borderline Personality

Kevin Corcoran

Cele Keeper

In this chapter, Corcoran and Keeper review one of the most clinically complex and challenging client problems, the borderline personality. The interventions reflect the dominant theoretical approach to this personality disorder, an egodynamic approach, and the most evidenced-based intervention (a cognitive behavioral approach). The authors emphasize the importance of accurate assessment and appropriate short- and long-term goals. The long-term needs of persons with this problem require that the intervention be adjusted to the client's particular borderline symptom.

INTRODUCTION

One of the most complicated and confusing clinical problems social workers face is the client with a borderline personality disorder. Although the borderline personality has been the topic of study for nearly three decades, it only received conventional recognition from the American Psychiatric Association by inclusion in the third edition of the *Diagnosis and Statistical Manual* (DSM-III-R), as a result of political pressure (Kutchins & Kirk, 1997). The topic itself is often spiritedly debated. Is it a disorder that reflects the development of a more formal psychotic condition, such as schizophrenia? Is it sufficiently different from other personality disorders to warrant diagnostic consideration? Does it actually exist at all?

The confusion is a consequence in part of the very nature of personality disorders; most have unclear and overlapping boundaries making differentiation from other disorders difficult. The borderline personality disorder is very similar to the schizotypical, antisocial personality, an identity disorder, and has features of cyclothymia, which is a condition characterized by mood instability. In addition, persons with personality disorder often have more than one type. For example, narcissistic and histrionic personality disorders often present sufficient borderline symptoms to warrant both diagnoses. The borderline client, moreover, is confusing and controversial because of the primary theory underlying development and treatment of borderline personality disorder; namely, ego-oriented, psychodynamic theory and treatment, which are complex and are questioned by many other theorists. In sharp contrast, empirical evidence tends to support a cognitive behavioral approach. We will consider both in this chapter. The reason for considering both is because the psychodynamic view affords the best understanding of the borderline personality, while the cognitive behavioral provides the best intervention.

PROBLEM IDENTIFICATION

A person with a borderline personality is characterized by pervasive patterns of instability in several aspects of life. He or she may show instability in identity, interpersonal relationships, and mood. The pattern of instability tends to be consistent across the client's interaction with different people, in different social environments, and over time. In other words, you will see instability in the person's emotional, behavioral, cognitive, and interpersonal domains (Linehan & Kehrer, 1993). The symptoms are numerous and occur in a variety of contexts. The unstable identity tends to be the most common symptom and may be seen in the client's self-image, acceptance of values, sexual orientation, and long-term commitments, including interpersonal relationships and career goals. The client may also complain of boredom or feelings of emptiness. You might observe that the client has intense involvement and emotional investment in a person he or she just met, a new lover, for example. Yet the client may quickly disdain this person because of a seemingly inconsequential event.

You might find this client complimenting you for helping so much, and yet at the very next session he or she may be enraged at you, claiming the money and energy spent on coming to you for help are wasted. The person with a borderline personality might seem anxious and irritable with you and then both affective states may seem to pass in a few hours or a day or so. In periods of high stress, transient psychotic symptoms may appear. At times it might seem that the more you try to oblige this client, the more difficult he or she becomes. Like most social workers, you might find yourself at a loss for what to do to help this client.

The reason for this potential response to the borderline personality is the very nature of the problem as it is manifested in the treatment process. The struggle with what to do in the intervention is due, in part, to the complexity of the borderline character, as well as the interpersonal dynamics that often occur in the course of treatment. You will need to be particularly sensitive to issues of transference and countertransference, regardless of whether you are using a psychodynamic approach, a cognitive behavioral approach, or a combination of both. The treatment may seem to lack well-established, structured techniques. The components of treatment often are quite conceptual and are not always easily replicated. Further, little empirical evidence is available about specifically when to do what in the treatment process. We know what some of the components of helping effectively are (for example, a constant holding environment where the social worker consistently responds with unyielding limits and acceptance of the client), but we may not know how to actually do this or when in treatment it is optimal.

Determining how to work effectively with a person with a borderline personality can be facilitated by being flexible about the specific borderline characteristics of attention during a session and establishing concrete treatment goals, both short term and long term. For example, a meaningful short-term goal might simply be to keep the client in treatment, because persons with borderline characteristics tend to prematurely terminate treatment more than do most other clients, especially if the problem does not warrant hospitalization (Gunderson, Franks, Runningstam, Wachter, Lynch, & Wolf, 1989). A meaningful and relatively concrete long-term goal might be to enhance the client's identity, as manifested by improved self-esteem and lessened feelings of emptiness.

You can enhance your ability to work effectively with this problem by achieving a thorough understanding of the development of the borderline personality and the dynamics of clinical work, which often relies on the transference relationship. In this chapter we provide an introduction to both the theoretical development of the borderline personality and effective methods for helping this type of client. We encourage you to learn more because of the complexity of the topic and the limitations of a single chapter.

Theoretical Considerations

The two most widely accepted perspectives on the borderline client are based on the psychodynamic development of the individual and cognitive behavioral therapy of emotional, behavioral, cognitive, and interpersonal dysregulation. The psychodynamic theory is an ego-oriented one, which emphasizes the development of the ego and ego functions, such as judgment and reality testing; this contrasts with more traditional Freudian theories, where the emphasis is on the id. The theory, then, is neo-Freudian and integrates such work as Margaret Mahler's psychological development theory, Erik Erikson's psychosocial development theory, and Jean Piaget's cognitive development theory.

The essential features of the psychodynamic theory concern the developmental failure in which one's ego functions are not fully acquired. Ego functions allow for adaptive capacity, or the ability to respond adequately to the environment. For example, perception and judgment influence reality testing and are ego functions. If a person misperceives the environment or uses bad judgment in response to the environment, then the ability to adapt may be impaired. The borderline syndrome is characterized by gross fluctuations in perception, cognition, and affect in terms of self-perception and the perception of others (Kernberg, 1976).

Generally, the borderline personality has an intact ego, but it is impaired and lacks sufficient ego strength. Ego strength refers to one's adaptive capacity, the autonomy of the ego from the id, and thus the ability to tolerate frustration and anxiety in order to resist regression. Because of the absence of sufficient ego strength, the borderline personality may regress and use functions of the id and primary processes. Consequently, at times the borderline personality may be out of touch with reality and show psychotic features. At other times the person may adapt well to the environment, reflecting good ego functioning. An illustration of impaired ego functioning is a client's poor judgment and lack of established cause-and-effect relationships. For example, a young man may know the risks of intravenous drug abuse but continue to use intravenous drugs nonetheless. Alternatively, he may recognize the need for treatment, a sign of the ego's adaptive capacity, but seek treatment while under the influence of drugs.

The lack of ego strength results from insufficient mastery in one's early development. The basic position of the theory is that the borderline personality has not successfully mastered developmental issues that begin at birth and continue through adolescence (Masterson, 1976) and thus has an impaired ability to adapt to the environment. Early development is most important to the theory, and lack of ego strength results when the infant is not allowed to develop a basic sense of trust in himself or herself or others, particularly parents (Kernberg, 1975, 1976). Because the infant lacks a basic sense of trust, he or she in turn is not able to develop a sense of autonomy; "pseudo-autonomy" develops instead. This occurs at a time in cognitive development when the infant is acquiring a sense of the permanency of objects, called object constancy. The borderline has not had sufficient nurturance and opportunities to interact with a psychologically safe environment to develop the full realization of object constancy in interpersonal relationships. The sense of mistrust and pseudo-autonomy are the foundations of the borderline personality. This is further seen in the separation individuation process, in which the infant gradually emerges from a symbiotic mother-child unit to become an autonomous person (Mahler, Pine, & Bergman, 1975). If the infant is not allowed to experience adequate trust, development of the ability to tolerate frustration and anxiety is thwarted. During this phase, the child develops representational thought and symbolization (Piaget, 1953), which are used to maintain the image of one's mother while she is absent. If the infant lacks trust and object constancy, he or she will become overwhelmed and frustrated by the mother's absence. In order to preserve the positive images of his or her mother, the child will dissociate from these images and see himself or herself as a "bad" child abandoned by the mother (Kernberg, 1975, 1976). The child consequently experiences rage and separation anxiety and develops a negative self-image, all of which are characteristics of the adult borderline personality disorder. This dynamic process is the basis of the defense mechanism of "splitting" (see below) and is used throughout the borderline personality's life (Masterson,

1976). Additionally, the infant's feelings of abandonment result in the reactive fantasy, "If I grow up, I'll be alone," which helps explain the immaturity characterizing the borderline personality.

Winnicott (1969) suggests the continuation of the borderline development may be thwarted by having a parent who responds consistently, setting firm limits and sticking to them, and yet maintaining a loving, nurturing, and soothing relationship. This "constant holding environment" strengthens the child's positive image, allowing him or her to see the parent as both gratifying and frustrating. It helps the child learn impulse control, which decreases the fear of his or her own aggressive tendency (Kernberg, 1975).

These developmental issues are seen again during adolescence, when the separation individuation themes are recapitulated (Masterson, 1972). Here the child struggles with dependency on and independence from the family. If the child lacks an adequate sense of trust, acts of autonomy (or pseudo-autonomy, as real autonomy requires basic trust) are again experienced as abandonment, leading to what Masterson (1976) calls "abandonment depression."

Defense Mechanisms

To understand the borderline personality, it is important to be familiar with common defense mechanisms. Defense mechanisms are used to control anxiety and frustration. The four most common ones seen in a borderline person are splitting, acting out, projective identification, and denial (Kernberg, 1975, 1976; Masterson, 1972).

Splitting, as alluded to above, is the polarization of two images and the disowning of the positive one and acceptance of the negative one. Kernberg (1975, 1976) sees the core cause to be the borderline person's inability to integrate the loving and hating aspects of one's self-images and the images of others.

Acting out is the predominant symptom of borderline adolescents, according to Masterson (1972). It is a dysfunctional coping mechanism that is employed when anxiety cannot be tolerated and is warded off by acting out the egodystonic impulse. Acting out may be manifested in negativity, school truancy, running away, aggression, stealing, and other forms of antisocial behavior.

Projective identification is the dissociation of uncomfortable features of the personality and the projection of these features onto another person, which results in an identification with the other person because of the perceived similarity. The borderline person also tries to get the other person to conform to the projected qualities. For example, a teenage boy who hates his father will believe his father actually hates him. The youngster may continuously misbehave in order to get his father's disapproval, resulting in behavior that confirms the projected impulse. This is something you will need to be particularly sensitive to in treatment, as your client may try to facilitate negative transference by getting you angry, frustrated, and ineffective.

Denial, the fourth common defense mechanism, is when the client denies to himself or herself, and frequently to others, the existence of an emotion, thought, or action that is unacceptable to the ego; the impulse to feel, think, or behave is called egodystonic or ego-alien.

This rather complex theory contrasts with the cognitive behavioral theory. The psychodynamic theory emphasizes dysfunctionality, while the cognitive behavioral theory considers dysregulation. The borderline personality disorder symptomatology is chiefly a matter of inadequate and ineffective regulations of one's emotional system. This dysregulation is manifested as emotional instability and a lack of control over one's emotions. The poor regulation of the emotional system, in turn, has an impact on the regulation of one's behaviors (such as impulsivity and sensation seeking) and one's interpersonal regulation (such as love-hate/hot-cold friendships). As noted above, at times and under certain circumstances, a person with a borderline personality disorder may experience psychotic symptomatology. An example is a client who manifests brief reactive psychosis at the marriage of an ex-spouse, even though the client had been divorced for a number of years. This is seen as cognitive dysregulation from the cognitive behavioral perspective (Linehan, 1993a).

The distinction between dysfunctionality and dysregulation is important for at least three reasons. First of all, dysregulation is more of a state of an individual and more amenable to change than a dysfunctional trait of one's personality. Secondly, dysregulation is a result of interaction of the person and the social environment. This is a reciprocal view of the individual, who interacts with the environment, and not just love objects. As such it is similar to social work's premise of the person-situation configuration (Woods & Hollis, 1990), which is emphasized in every human behavior and social environment course at the undergraduate and graduate level.

And finally, the cognitive behavioral theory considers the emotional dysregulation as the core of the borderline personality disorder. Similar to the dynamic development view, the cognitive behavioral theory holds that emotional dysregulation results from an invalidating environment, experienced by the client both as a child and as an adult. The invalidating environment may be a harsh and punitive parent or the trauma of sexual abuse, which is reported disproportionately by persons with borderline personality disorder (Linehan & Kehrer, 1993). In essence, the client mistrusts his or her emotional states as a result of an invalidating environment. This is considered a result of never learning to accurately label and regulate one's emotions, how to tolerate emotional distress, or how to find comfort with one's emotions and consider them as appropriate or valid (Linehan, 1993a). The treatment, then, is a systematic intervention to develop and enhance skills for regulating one's emotions.

Assessment and Monitoring

The above theoretical discussions, although brief, illustrate that the borderline personality is truly complex and elusive. It is easy to overlook the personality pattern because of the variety of clinical symptoms, as well as the person's tendency to function well at times. Accurate assessment is critical because, as we will discuss in the section on treatment, it is important to establish goals and be consistent throughout the intervention process. It is helpful to diagnose and monitor the client problem with standardized assessment tools and rapid assessment instruments for specific symptoms.

The first issue, of course, is to identify or diagnose the borderline personality. The DSM-IV requires that the client be an adult (i.e., over the age of 18) and meet at least five of the following nine criteria:

1. Unstable and intense interpersonal relationships.
2. Impulsivity in two or more areas in life, such as drug or alcohol use or sexual behavior, that is self-damaging.
3. Unstable affect that lasts anywhere from a few hours to a few days.
4. Inappropriate anger or the inability to control anger.
5. Suicidal threats or self-mutilating behavior.
6. Disturbed identity in two or more areas, such as self-image, values, or career choice.
7. Chronic feelings of emptiness or boredom.
8. Efforts to avoid abandonment.
9. Stress-related, but transient paranoid ideations or severe disassociative symptoms.

These criteria have numerous possible manifestations. Because of this, you might find certain semistructured interview schedules helpful in reaching a diagnosis. One that is most widely used and has had some empirical support for its reliability and validity is the Diagnostic Interview for Borderline (DIB; Gunderson, Kolb, & Austin, 1981). The DIB is a 160-item interview that takes approximately an hour to complete. The interview has a high degree of sensitivity and specificity for differentiating clients with borderline personality from nonborderline clients (Kolb & Gunderson, 1980), as well as for differentiating borderline persons from depressed or schizophrenic patients (Gunderson & Kolb, 1978). It also has been shown to have good concurrent validity by correlating with such criteria as depression, hostility, and impulsivity (Soloff, 1981). There have been some mixed results with the concordance with other methods of diagnosing the disorder (Nelson et al., 1985), but the DIB generally identifies borderlines as well as—if not better than—other methods (Tarnopolsky & Berelowitz, 1987). Other useful methods for evaluating clients for borderline personality are checklists, including the DSM-III criteria

(Sheehy, Goldsmith, & Charles, 1980), the Ego Functions Inventory (Perry & Klerman, 1980), and two self-report measures (Conte, Pluthnick, Karasu, & Jerrett, 1980; Hunt, Hyles, Frances, Clarkin, & Brent, 1984).

In addition to a semistructured interview, you might find it helpful to monitor specific symptoms of your client. Because the borderline client often requires long-term treatment (from two to three years with a psychodynamic approach), you will find that different symptoms are the focus of your sessions at different times in the treatment. For example, abandonment depression may be the focus early in treatment, when you and your client are establishing a meaningful therapeutic alliance, and again during termination; thus you might want to monitor your client by measuring his or her depression, with the Depressed Mood Scale (Radloff, 1977) early in and toward the end of treatment.

You might also decide to monitor symptoms more specific to the borderline personality, such as impulsivity, distorted perception, or defense mechanisms. Eight instruments you might find valuable are

1. The Cognitive Slippage Scale (Miers & Raulin, 1985), a thirty-five–item measure of cognitive distortion.
2. The Intense Ambivalence Scale (Raulin, 1984), a forty-five–item measure of the existence of simultaneous and rapidly interchangeable positive and negative behavior.
3. The Magic Ideation Scale (Eckblad & Chapman, 1983), a thirty-item measure of beliefs, including invalid causation.
4. The Splitting Scale (Gerson, 1984), a fourteen-item measure of the defense mechanism that involves the radical shift in evaluation of self and others.
5. The Borderline Syndrome Index (Conte et al., 1980), a fifty-two–item self-report of symptoms of the borderline personality, which includes a cutting score to distinguish patients likely to have the disorder.
6. The Questionnaire of Experience of Dissociation (Riley, 1988), a twenty-six–item instrument designed to measure dissociation of thoughts, feelings, and behaviors.
7. The Dissociative Experience Scale (Bernstein & Putman, 1980), a twenty-eight–item assessment of the extent and frequency of experiencing dissociation.
8. The Separation-Individuation Process Scale (Christenson & Wilson, 1985), a thirty-nine–item assessment of disturbances in the childhood process of separating and individuating one's self from other love objects.

When using these or other monitor devices, it is important to keep your work in perspective. First of all, clients with borderline personality are notorious for quitting treatment before much success has occurred (Gunderson et al., 1989); consequently, you may need to monitor your initial goals frequently earlier in treatment until the borderline client is indeed committed to continuing. Secondly, once you have the client's commitment, it is important to remember that change does not occur quickly; thus, you might administer your measures every few weeks or so.

TREATMENT OF THE BORDERLINE PERSONALITY

Research Supports

The research on the borderline personality has tended to focus more on the reliability and validity of the construct than on the effectiveness of different treatment methods. This focus has been from the perspective of the value of the psychoanalytic model, as recently reviewed by Shapiro (1989), and more conventional research methods, as reviewed by Tarnopolsky and Berelowitz (1987). There have, however, been several in-depth case reports, although these procedures are beyond the focus of this section. The basic outcome of the research into the construct has been the creation of assessment tools, as discussed above.

The most noted controlled study compared supportive psychotherapy, psychoanalysis, and expressive psychotherapy (Kernberg, Burstein, Coyne, Applebaum, Horwitz, & Voth, 1972). The study was conducted on an inpatient unit, and borderline clients were reported to respond well. Other, less complicated studies have focused on pharmacotherapy. As Tarnopolsky and Berelowitz (1987) summarize, the effects of medication on the psychotic-like symptoms and affective symptoms were noted when the client was experiencing those dimensions of the condition. They suggest that future research needs to include the impact of psychotherapy.

The majority of the research has focused on the validity of the construct and thus the ability to measure the borderline personality. The above discussion of the Diagnostic Interview for Borderlines is an illustration of these efforts. It has been shown to be reliable in actual interviews (Kroll, Pyle, Zander, Martin, Lari, & Sines, 1981) and case notes (McGlashon, 1983) and for agreement between interviews and notes (Armelius, Kullgrean, & Renberg, 1985). Research also has supported the value of the DSM-III criteria for identifying the borderline construct (e.g., McGlashon, 1983) and a DSM-III–derived structured interview (Stangl, Pfhol, Zimmerman, Bowers, & Corenthal, 1985). As reviewed by Tarnopolsky and Berelowitz (1987), the lengthy interview process, usually six sessions, used by Kernberg and his associates (Kernberg, Goldstein, Carr, Hunt, Bauer, & Blumenthal, 1981) has not had adequate support for its reliability. In part this is because of the level of pathology the process attempted to measure and the length of the assessment, which may reduce reliability.

The research on the assessment and measurement of the borderline construct tends to identify rather clear characteristics. As Tarnopolsky and Berelowitz (1987) summarize, the core characteristics include "unstable interpersonal relationships, with idealization and denigration of others, intense unpredictable feelings, and impulsive, often self-destructive behavior" (p. 726). Some of the other most defining characteristics are stress-related psychotic symptoms and regression. More promising empirical evidence has emerged for the cognitive behavioral intervention.

Foundations of the Treatment

There are five general approaches to treating the borderline client: psychoanalysis, analytically oriented psychotherapy, dynamically oriented psychotherapy, supportive psychotherapy, and cognitive behavioral therapy. Goldstein (1988) defines the four psychodynamic approaches on a continuum from insight oriented and exploratory to supportive and care giving. Let us briefly consider each of the four approaches.

Psychoanalysis involves four or five weekly sessions, and is frequently conducted by having the client recline on a couch and free associate. All three of these components (frequent sessions, reclining, and free association) facilitate an intensive transference relationship. In essence, the client transfers or displays feelings and thoughts, as well as defenses against them, to the clinician. The emotions and cognitions may be real or fantasy. The crucial component of change is considered to be the resolution of the transference relationship by means of insight; consequently, the clinician relies on interpretation of the transference. This form of treatment is the least advisable for a borderline client because the regression is far too great for the client's weak ego functions.

Analytically oriented psychotherapy involves less frequent sessions than psychoanalysis, usually two a week. The clinician uses interpretation as much as possible, but does not rely on free association or a couch to develop the transference relationship. Transference is encouraged so that the client can gain insight and change. The borderline personality's tendency to regress and to distort the relationship with the clinician is seen as facilitating the transference relationship.

Dynamically oriented treatment focuses on the client's daily activities, with particular attention given to how these events correlate with the client's past. Assuming a fairly active stance, clinician and client together try to understand the current interactions from the basis of the client's sensitivities, vulnerabilities, and distortions. The clinician uses techniques similar to those of the support approach (see below) but may include partial interpretation. The role of transference is minimized in dynamically oriented treatment.

Supportive treatment is especially appropriate for persons with disturbed ego functions; its purpose is to help build a weak ego. Supportive psychotherapy uses education, suggestion, clarification, reassurance, and instructions; it rarely includes interpretation, because the client's ego is not sufficiently strong to tolerate the anxiety and frustration that facilitate insight. The clinician attempts to maintain his or her neutrality, and the sessions tend to focus on the daily activities that resulted from the client's impaired ego functions.

Supportive psychotherapy may be particularly useful in agency settings because all too often there is not sufficient time for the long-term treatment needed to help change the enduring traits of the borderline personality. Further, in agency settings you, the social worker, may be the first professional a person with a borderline personality encounters. This may be because of the crises the client experiences and the fact that borderline clients are often ordered to treatment by the legal system because of antisocial behaviors. However, as Freed (1980, p. 3) points out, "limitations of time and staff, treatment methods and the client's lack of motivation contribute to the despair of the social agencies in treating these people."

Therefore, even though the therapeutic need of the borderline client is for substantial change in the personality structure and interpersonal behaviors, in agency settings it is very likely that the initial treatment will need to be supportive. It will also be beneficial to direct your attention to concrete social services. Here you should not rule out or discount the value of goal-directed short-term treatment. Your focus should be on small, manageable immediate issues, such as arranging placement in a day treatment program or referring the client to services where long-term treatment is available. As Freed notes, providing concrete services can be "a means of reaching the client" (1980, p. 554). However, it may follow that the client does not receive the treatment services needed. Even if you make a referral in good faith, the borderline person may very well feel neglected, abandoned, or "passed on" in spite of your well-meaning intentions.

In contrast to these dynamic treatment approaches, the cognitive behavioral intervention is rather structured, including three stages plus a pretreatment role induction phase (Linehan, 1993b). The first phase is designed to stabilize the person with a borderline personality disorder and assure he or she is safe from self-harm and suicide; this phase also addresses those behaviors that are likely to disrupt treatment, such as substance abuse or sexual acting out. The final goal of the first phase of treatment is to facilitate the development of a number of coping behaviors, including emotional regulation skills and distress tolerance. During the second phase of the cognitive behavioral intervention, the focus of treatment is on decreasing symptoms of posttraumatic stress and allows for the exploration and insights about past events. The third phase is a period of synthesis with the goals of increasing the client's self-respect and capacity to achieve individually initiated goals. A number of particular and specific clinical techniques are available for each phase of treatment, and fortunately a skills training manual for implementing this cognitive behavioral intervention is also available (Linehan, 1993b).

Choosing your approach. When long-term treatment is available, you must take an approach that facilitates the development of the client's ego functions (i.e., ego building). It will be necessary for you to use your own ego to act as an auxiliary one for the borderline client (Eckrich, 1985). For example, you will need to use good judgment and constancy to facilitate such client ego functions as judgment and the sense of object constancy. In this sense, it is important for your client to identify with you and transfer the feelings and thoughts, along with the accompanying defenses, to your clinical relationship. Needless to say, this requires 1) that the agency permit long-term treatment and 2) that you have the capacity to work with very difficult persons.

Forming a therapeutic alliance. Freed (1980) elaborates on the capacities a social worker must have to work with a borderline client. She suggests that you reach out to form a therapeutic alliance and offer support and understanding that were missing from the client's early relationships. You must not be passive, and you must establish yourself as someone who will focus on reality issues and problem solving. It is necessary to establish an atmosphere of mutual respect and an expectation of achieving successful results. It is also helpful to set up ground rules and a contract with the client that state that impulsive acting out will cease and that the pressures to do so will be discussed in treatment. You must be caring and nurturing and must make this evident early in the course of treatment. If the client has a family, Freed believes strongly that you should engage them in the treatment process.

Freed further asserts that to effectively help a borderline client you must be flexible and creative. You must have a feel for when to get close to the client and when to honor the client's fear of intimacy. Setting limits and having clear and well-defined expectations are very important. A reality orientation is necessary in order to give the client the positive modeling needed to work through the splitting of good and bad object representations. Finally, the borderline client can then integrate these into a whole and gain the ability to appreciate that people can have some good and some not-so-good qualities.

Even after the borderline client has made a commitment to continue treatment, you should bear in mind that these clients have high dropout rates (Gunderson et al., 1989). It is critical to decrease the intervening-interfering of this treatment-interfering behavior (Linehan & Kehrer, 1993). Once the client has established a meaningful level of trust in you, long-term work may begin. Numerous issues will be presented once you have established the necessary trust. Rage, depression, fears of abandonment, a history of unstable personal relationships, lack of identity, feelings of emptiness, complaints of nonreality, gripes about past social workers by whom the client felt deserted, and constant job friction all will be grist for the therapeutic mill. They should be discussed, with your client ventilating and then receiving reality-based feedback.

Setting goals.   There are many long-term goals for the borderline client. Freed delineates ten:

1. Integrate good and bad splits.
2. Accept the primary ambivalence rather than fight it.
3. Bring primitive idealizations and projective identification within reality contexts and develop normal repression.
4. Develop mature dependence through the therapeutic relationship.
5. Establish efforts at mastery, impulse control, and frustration tolerance.
6. Engage the ego in realistic planning and healthy coping behavior through the problem-solving process.
7. Feel better about oneself, accept these good feelings, and achieve an improved self-image by reducing self-defeating behaviors and recognizing accomplishments.
8. Accept one's separateness and wholeness.
9. Establish the capacity to relate to others and allow others to relate to oneself with trust and warmth; permit closeness without fusion, separateness without abandonment, and individuality within the social and family context.
10. Meet concrete needs and use the therapeutic experience to build relationships and trust (Freed, 1980).

These goals are useful for clients in cognitive behavioral as well as dynamic interventions.

Effective interventions.   With such a complex client problem and elusive goals, you might ask, "What can I actually do to help the borderline client?" In the past two decades, the approach to treatment of the borderline personality has, in fact, developed from a highly supportive approach (e.g., Zetzel, 1971), where the client was thought to be unable to internalize a sufficiently stable ego identification, to use of interventions that are much more encompassing. The current mode of thinking, supported by Kernberg (1975), Masterson (1976), Buie and Adler (1982), and others, is aimed at the resolution of the pathological distortions through the use of intensive psychotherapy. Essentially, as Freed asserts, you will want to use "confrontation, insight, interpretation, supportiveness, availability, crisis intervention and transference" (Freed, 1980, p. 555).

Adler (1985) outlines a three-phase intervention. The first phase is concerned with establishing and maintaining a dyadic relationship in which the therapist can be used by the client as a holding self-object. The second phase facilitates the resolution of the transference so that the borderline client sees the clinician more realistically. Assuming the success of these two phases, in the third phase the client generalizes the knowing, esteem-building, and loving experience from the clinician to a significant other.

More specificity to the components of effective treatment is delineated by Waldinger (1987). The eight basic components discussed below tend to be accepted by most authors working with borderline clients, even though there is disagreement about the use of the four approaches outlined earlier.

1. Establish stability in the framework of the treatment. This means setting regular appointment times and expressing your expectations that the client will keep the appointments and pay the fees. Feelings about missed or changed appointments must be addressed openly and honestly and without exception. If you make exceptions, the borderline client may very well distort this and perceive you as manipulatable, weak, and not a constant holding environment. That is, you will be seen as an untrustworthy and unconstant object relationship; and such relationships were, theoretically, part of the origin of the client's problems.

2. Keep increasing your activity as a clinician. With the borderline personality you must always be active. This serves to emphasize your presence, anchor the client in reality, and minimize the distortion of the transference relationship. A couple of ways to establish yourself as active are to verbally support self-enhancing relationships and confront self-defeating behaviors.

3. Tolerate the client's hostility. You must be able to withstand verbal assaults from the borderline client without withdrawing or retaliating. This enables the client to begin to examine and master his or her pattern of relating to others. Remember, as was mentioned in the discussion of projective identification, often the borderline client will actively try to get you to confirm the projected qualities. If you get angry and tell the client off, you are simply confirming a distorted perception, for example, that "you never really did care." The ability to tolerate your client's behavior requires that you are secure in your own sense of self and not internalize or overreact to the client's behavior.

4. Make self-destructive behaviors ungratifying to the borderline client. Borderline clients are very skilled at remaining unaware of self-destructive behaviors that they use to gratify wishes and allay anxiety. For example, a client might mistreat a date such that the person never calls again; after all, the client "knows" that the other person really was not interested in him or her anyway, and the fact that the other has not called just confirms it. It is your job to point out repeatedly to the client the adverse consequence of such self-defeating behaviors. Other self-destructive behaviors that are commonly seen with borderline clients include sexual acting out, drug and alcohol abuse, and inappropriate bursts of anger, either in terms of the intensity of the anger or the circumstances stimulating the anger. In confronting the self-defeating behaviors you should focus on the outcome of the behavior rather than on the client's stated intent. This will help the borderline client learn cause-and-effect relationships and object consistency, which were not mastered in his or her early development.

5. Establish a connection between the client's action and affect in the here-and-now. Because the borderline client's actions frequently serve as a defense against the awareness of uncomfortable feelings, you must aid the client in acknowledging and understanding that his or her communication through action has a defensive function. For example, the ungracious dating behavior mentioned above defends the client against feeling fears of abandonment.

6. Block acting-out behaviors. The borderline client uses acting out as a resistance to awareness of transference and, therefore, to growth. It will be necessary for you to set limits on behaviors that threaten the safety of your client, yourself, or the treatment. For example, you should refuse to see the client if he or she arrives for treatment under the influence of drugs or alcohol.

7. Focus early clarifications and intervention on the here-and-now. That is, similar to the dynamically oriented psychotherapy discussed above, you should avoid being manipulated to examine the past for the past's sake. Early family interpretation, for example, will be counterproductive. It is important for you to focus on immediate and dangerous acting-out behaviors. You might want to use current behaviors to illustrate the influence of past development, but keep the focus of your attention on the immediacy of how the client is behaving.

8. Pay careful attention to your countertransference feelings. This component is often one of the most difficult, especially to novice practitioners. By constantly monitoring your countertransference reactions you will minimize your own acting out of feelings. In this sense, you must strive to be neutral. Neutrality is difficult with borderline clients, however, because they are masters at manipulation. You should use your countertransference feelings to further help your client change by confronting him or her and illustrating how he or she provokes others.

This last component has been a source of controversy, especially in terms of when in the sequence of the treatment process it should be used (Goldstein, 1988; Waldinger, 1987). Clinicians who work with borderline clients disagree over whether transference interpretation is actually helpful early on in the treatment or whether creating a holding environment is the style that is essential. A few words on these two positions may be useful.

Kernberg (1975) maintains that the primitive defenses of the borderline client (e.g., splitting and denial) will ensure that he or she will distort your comments. He further asserts that by clarifying such misperceptions early in the session, primitive defenses can be replaced by higher-level ones, a stronger ego will result, and the client can then make use of the comments. Masterson (1976) agrees and sees the main task as controlling the acting out by repeatedly clarifying the self-destructive nature of such behaviors. By doing so, you are making the behavior egodystonic, which means that it is alien to the wishes of the ego. Masterson further asserts that when this is accomplished, the client is able to accept your comments without gross distortions.

The ability of the borderline client to make use of your interpretation may be dependent on other variables. For example, the client's level of anxiety, how he or she relates to you, and whether there is some current stress between the client and you (such as might be the case with an upcoming vacation), all can affect the intensity of the client's transference and his or her tendency to distort interpretations. This is why, in part, Freed (1980) stresses the need for you to be flexible and creative and to use your own good judgment in working with a borderline client.

The holding environment position is dramatically stated by Buie and Adler (1982) and Adler (1985). They claim that the core of the borderline pathology lies in a failure to develop holding and soothing introjects as an infant. They, therefore, do not propose to "undo what is already there and malformed (as Kernberg and Masterson propose) but to create what never existed" (Waldinger, 1987). This position requires the client to use the clinician as a holding self-object that performs the soothing and holding functions the client cannot perform on his or her own. You might provide a soothing and holding function by such supports as hospitalization, telephone contacts between sessions, and additional appointments. While on vacation, you might send a postcard. Freed (1980) cites a case example in which the social worker made herself available for telephone interviews and occasionally called the client "just to keep in touch." This may also help to facilitate the transference relationship such that the client's affects and thoughts can be discussed in treatment. It is not the content that effectively helps the client, Buie and Adler (1985) claim, but that the clinician is stable, caring, consistent, nonpunitive, survives the client's rage, and continues to serve as a holding object that was absent in the client's early development.

As for direct empirical evidence, there is little to allow the conclusion of what is a best practice. The psychodynamic approach is useful for understanding the borderline personality disorder, but it difficult to implement. The cognitive behavioral intervention has specificity and is, therefore, easier to accurately implement. Research is proving that this intervention is quite promising and combined with the dynamic understanding should help the client change.

GENERALIZING THE INTERVENTION TO RELATED PROBLEMS

Much of what we have discussed above is applicable to work with other personality disorders. Clients who are maladaptive, who suffer from feelings of dissatisfaction, despair, and emptiness, and who make the rounds of therapists hoping to find relief from their pain, fall into the antisocial, borderline, histrionic, and narcissistic personality disorder classification. At times it is not easy to differentiate entirely among the four, and indeed clients present overlapping characteristics and features that make the diagnosis that much more difficult.

There are a few relational capacities that you should look for when generalizing the dynamically oriented treatment to any of these personality disorders. Silver (1985) favors looking at relational capacities as a means of determining therapeutic strategies. Has the client sustained an important relationship for at least a year, or could he or she do so? If not, chances are this client is too fragile for intensive psychotherapy. Can the client develop an empathetic therapeutic bridge with the therapist? If the early developmental damage experienced is too extensive, this capacity may not be there and crisis intervention and short-term treatment approaches may be the preferred interventions. Does the client have the capacity to soothe, comfort, and solace others and, in turn, be comforted and solaced by others? If this capacity is present, long-term treatment has a better chance of success. In all cases, negotiating a therapeutic contract is essential to minimize undesirable effects. Borderline clients tend to expect magic from their social workers, and "they impose on them the fantasy of original nurturer" (Silver, 1985, p. 366). It is imperative, then, that the client knows what can realistically be expected from your social work intervention.

Because repression is not a very stable form of defense for these clients, Silver goes on to assert that a great deal of unconscious material is also available from the beginning of assessment. It is wise to be cautious about making interpretations too early, however, as this can be devastating for these clients and may contribute to mild psychotic symptoms. This, in fact, is why psychoanalysis is rarely warranted with borderline or other personality disorders.

There has been a great deal of discussion regarding the differentiation of borderline from narcissistic personalities. A few words to differentiate borderline and narcissistic disorders for the purpose of treatment may be in order. The borderline is brittle, self-devaluing, erratic, and full of rage. The narcissistic personality fears humiliation, is cold, relates poorly, and covers it all with grandiosity. The borderline is hostile and may direct it toward himself or herself, but more likely directs it toward others (Freed, 1980). The borderline client is clingy, demanding, angry, and dependent. The narcissistic client may bore the social worker with self-preoccupation and be aware of the social worker only when idealizing, mirroring, or attempting to seduce him or her. You will need to keep these differences in mind when working with both the borderline and the narcissist. Empathy is essential when treating the narcissistic person. However, if you are seduced into becoming an idealized figure for the narcissistic client, he or she may distort or change perceptions and turn against you.

SUMMARY

This chapter reviewed the theoretical considerations of the borderline personality disorder, although briefly, and outlined some of the more salient features of working with clients with this clinically challenging disorder. The research in this area tends to be more idiographic than monothetic, with a reliance on case studies and clinical observations. Sample-based research is beginning to emerge, especially in the area of assessment and diagnosis. Research on the cognitive-behavioral approach is more encouraging.

Our examination of the treatment strategies for the borderline client reveals several general characteristics: creation of a constant holding environment, use of supportive techniques, the availability of the social worker's ego as an auxiliary ego for the client, the use of confrontation, and the importance of consistency and commitment and the systematic development of emotional regulation skills and goal-attainment capacity. Transference and countertransference were outlined as major factors in treating the borderline client.

We supplied guidelines for distinguishing between clients with borderline personality disorder and those with narcissistic disorders and discussed the use of empathy in treatment. For narcissistic personalities, empathy is the essential ingredient (Kohut & Wolff, 1978); however, too much empathy may be seen as a sign of weakness by clients with borderline personality disorder. When working with clients with borderline personality disorder (as well as those with other personality disorders, especially narcissism), it is very important that you maintain a strong toehold on reality and constantly monitor the pitfalls of countertransference. Failure to do so will only be used to support the client's distorted perceptions. Establishing explicit short-term and long-term goals is helpful in this regard, and the cognitive behavioral treatment is quite specific about goal setting (Linehan, 1993b). By successfully maintaining your own sense of reality, confronting the client's distorted reality, and providing a constant holding environment where the client can learn trust in self and others are some of the first steps to effectively helping a borderline client change.

CHAPTER 15

Experiential Approach with Mexican-American Males with Acculturation Stress

Fernando J. Galan

In this chapter, Galan shows how to use experiential focusing techniques in work-ing with Hispanic males with identity problems. Galan discusses the development of identity problems in relation to acculturation and biculturation in Hispanic families. In some families, a male child may be placed in the roles of surrogate adult and spouse because he is the only family member who can communicate with the English-speaking outside world. Using Gendlin's (1978) step-by-step method, Galan shows how to define the components of experiential focusing. The very process of developing such protocols helps demonstrate how structure can be applied to work with clients regardless of the theory behind the methods used.

INTRODUCTION

Little has been written about the impact of acculturation on personality development in bilingual/bicultural children, especially in a family in which the mother speaks only Spanish and is culturally traditional and the father speaks only Spanish or is physically absent. Part of the paucity of practice knowledge can be explained by the fact that contemporary research has focused predomi-nantly on generational rather than cultural differences in families. Where cul-tural differences in the Hispanic family have been examined (Thompson & Carter, 1997), bicultural effectiveness interventions have helped practitioners address family conflicts (Szapocznik, Santiesteban, Kurtines, Perez-Vidal, & Hervis, 1984). And although there may be cause to suggest that bilingual chil-dren of monolingual parents perceive their world in broad terms, it remains unclear how developmental issues affect their emerging bicultural identity.

Issues of ethnic identity among indigenous bilingual/bicultural Mexican-American adolescents become more salient in succeeding generations, as thousands of Mexican children become naturalized. For Mexican-born chil-dren who later become citizens of the United States, ethnic identity may not be a serious problem because they were Mexican citizens first and American citizens second. For indigenous native-borns, however, developmental issues of separation and individuation in adolescence may get muddled with inter-generational culture conflict.

This may lead to blurred boundaries in a family and confusion in the definition and implementation of family roles. When children are placed in family roles in which they have no choice, they may develop strong emotions toward parents.

The purpose of this chapter is, first, to discuss the difficulties associated with the stress of acculturation in Mexican-American family functioning. Second, the chapter will define and explore two variations in family roles that may occur during the development of identity formation among Hispanic male children: 1) the adultification of a child, and 2) the spousification of a child. Third, the chapter examines the clinical manifestations or themes of psycho-emotional stress that indigenous, native-born Mexican-American children may face during childhood and adolescence as a result of parental bicultural tension. An appreciation of the influence that acculturation stress has on family dynamics will help social workers understand how children may bear the brunt of a parent's inability or unwillingness to adapt to the larger Anglo society.

When a parent's coping responses in situations outside the family are inappropriate or maladaptive, a child may be called upon to manage family stress. Understanding how a parent's inability to function outside the family can lead to a child's identity problems will help social workers to better appreciate the impact that acculturation stress has on family functioning. Later discussion will focus on directions for a treatment process and specific techniques for treating the emotional consequences created by role confusion.

CONCEPTS OF BICULTURAL FAMILY FUNCTIONING

As bicultural individuals from ethnic minority backgrounds learn the values and behaviors of the majority culture, and as these become part of their world view and coping repertoire in social situations, such individuals are said to become acculturated. Hispanic children are raised with a particular set of family values and behaviors and are exposed to and incorporate a different societal set of values and behaviors as they are socialized in school or work settings.

Mexican-American, Chicano, or Mestizo are terms used to refer to an individual born in the United States of Spanish-Indian-African cultural heritage. For the purposes of this discussion, they refer to individuals whose socialization and childhood and adolescent development have occurred in families residing in the United States. The bicultural socialization has occurred both in the family and in school. A Mexican-American family refers to a family in which the children have been socialized with this dual perspective.

New Americans is a term that refers to foreign-born individuals whose early childhood and adolescent development typically have occurred in another country. Children of new Americans who are exposed to bicultural socialization in human development can also be referred to as Mexican-Americans.

Bicultural conflict occurs when an individual's family values and behaviors are different from those of the society at large; there is a high degree of incongruence, or contrast, between family values and societal values. Although bicultural conflict need not necessarily be a problem, it can lead to bicultural tension. Typically, new Americans who have immigrated to the United States experience bicultural conflict immediately, whereas native-born Mexican-Americans usually experience conflict when they enter child-care or school situations outside the home.

Bicultural tension occurs when an individual's available coping skills are based on only one value system: either that of the family or that of society. The individual therefore is not able to use his or her coping skills in both family and societal situations. For example, if an individual learns coping responses from the family, such responses are used to adapt to family situations. Those same family-prescribed coping responses, however, may be socially problematic and not useful in adapting to situations outside of the family.

When adaptation is difficult, particularly adaptation to the majority culture, issues of adjustment may surface. The pressure to adapt to one's environment is, in part, integral to mastery of situations outside the family. Individuals who are not able to develop coping responses to adapt to societal situations experience stress that can sometimes be displaced on other family members.

STUDIES OF ACCULTURATION STRESS

Research with Cuban immigrants "clearly indicates that the acculturation process in many instances results in the disruption of the traditional closely knit family" (Szapocznik et al., 1984). These changes can lead to behavioral disorders in family members (Scopetta & Alegre, 1975). Szapocznik and Truss (1978) have observed that "since youngsters acculturate more rapidly than their parents, the substantial intergenerational differences in acculturation that develop in the family may either precipitate or exacerbate existing familial, and particularly, intergenerational disruption" (Szapocznik & Truss, 1978). In relation to the functioning of individual family members, Szapocznik and Kurtines (1980) suggest that "the nature of the relationship between the individual's acculturation process (monocultural or bicultural) and the degree of plurality of the cultural context has important implications for the psychosocial adjustment of individuals and families of the migrant culture" (Szapocznik & Truss, 1978, p. 322).

Research on the functioning of individual members in Hispanic families, however, has been scant. Research on mothers of adolescents suggests that acculturation-related disorders in nuclear families are accompanied by intergenerational acculturation gaps in which middle-aged mothers and their adolescent sons tend to be at the acculturational extremes (Szapocznik & Truss, 1978). In pathological families, mothers tend to underacculturate (individual–social context interaction), exhibit rigid and neurotic patterns of behaviors (either a clinical determinant or outcome of the individual–social context interaction), and tend to abuse sedatives and tranquilizers (behavior with biosocial and physiological consequences); sons tend to overacculturate (individual–social context interaction), exhibit acting-out syndromes (either a clinical determinant or outcome of the individual–social context interaction), reject their culture of origin, and abuse illegal drugs such as marijuana, Quaaludes, and cocaine (behavior with biosocial and physiological consequences). The data from these studies reveal that in addition to the normative linear component of the acculturation process, there is another component, which is pathological and nonnormative and which is frequently reflected in severe overacculturation in youngsters and severe underacculturation in parents (pathological individual–social context interactions which are associated with pathological behaviors; Szapocznik & Truss, 1978). Where one parent is culturally traditional (high adherence to family values and low adherence to societal values) and a child is more acculturated (integrated family and societal values) or assimilated (high adherence to societal values to the exclusion of family values and behaviors), the child may be cast in the role of helping a parent relate to society. Interactions with the representatives of social systems can strongly affect the individual's or family's self-esteem (Cohen, 1970). Acculturated or assimilated children who speak Spanish and English usually have the coping skills necessary to adapt to societal situations, whereas their monolingual parents may not. Dual-frame-of-reference children are placed in family roles that correspond to the needs they help their single-frame-of-reference parents meet. "In all, it is very clearly manifested, that the Mexican-American family tends to come into conflict with the dominant society because the value system contrasts sharply with that of the minority, and because no substantial effort has been made to adapt services to the basic difference in consequent diverging needs" (Saenz, 1978). As the children develop coping responses and skills in the majority culture, and as they discover a new power to manage societal situations, they may find themselves in conflict with one or both parents, whose coping repertoire is limited to family situations. Perceived threats to family unity may precipitate crises. There has been little research into the dynamics of strain in families in which individual members are at different levels of acculturation. As mentioned above, children who have the coping skills to adapt to both family and societal situations may find themselves plunged into adult roles in order to help alleviate family stress. The literature is remarkably void of descriptions of the outcomes of these dynamics relative to their influence on the identity formation process in Hispanic children. Consequently, we know little about the choices or consequences that bilingual/bicultural children face when pressured to act in adult roles in behalf of parents. Practice evidence suggests that the tension these children experience often gets displaced as anger in situations outside the home, such as the classroom or church study group.

ADULTIFICATION AND SPOUSIFICATION

Adultification occurs when a child assumes adult roles before adulthood. Spousification occurs when a child becomes adultified and subsequently bonds emotionally as a spouse with a parent. An adultified male child, for example, is one who assumes and carries out adult roles in the family. A spousified male child is one who, as a result of carrying out adult roles in the family, becomes emotionally overinvolved with his mother and in effect replaces his father as his mother's spouse. Adultification becomes spousification when emotional bonds are developed between a parent and a child whose imposed family role is that of the absent adult. When a parent's overinvolvement results in a child perceiving that his or her worth is contingent on taking care of the adult's emotional needs, and when a parent's fear of inadequacy and failure keep the child emotionally bonded as a spouse, a child cannot easily establish personal boundaries and an identity apart from the parent. Identity diffusion results. For example, when a mother develops resentment toward the father and when the child may also have preexisting resentment toward the father, the common emotions that both mother and child experience may contribute to their bonding. In dysfunctional families, role integrity is lost and spousification may provide a creative yet maladaptive antidote to family disintegration.

Bilingual/bicultural children whose independence is stifled by a parent's inability to be independent or responsible become exploited by their circumstances. Their ability to make choices is hampered by role confusion. On the one hand, what they want becomes entangled with what they need to do to maintain family functioning. The pressure on children who feel forced into adult roles in order to compensate for a parent's inability or unwillingness to cope results in tension. The parent's relative powerlessness to manage life in the new language or value system creates stress in a spousified child. Chronic stress results when a spousified child's own fear of inadequacy and failure is not addressed because of the parent's own inability and fears. The failure of a monolingual parent to alleviate the tension the child is experiencing renders the child powerless. An emotionally overburdened child in a spousified role can develop symptoms similar to those of posttraumatic stress disorders. Adultification in itself, without spousification, is less likely to create role confusion than it is to create pressure.

In traditional family cultures or in low socioeconomic family situations, where interdependence and cooperation are operational values, children learn to adapt their roles to fit the needs of the family's limitations. Because children may have coping responses and skills that help them adapt in the majority culture, they may be called upon to be advocates, cultural translators, or problem solvers in a family. This has been observed repeatedly as later generations help traditional parents adapt to the majority culture and thus increase their family's overall adjustment. Bilingual/bicultural children often are called upon to translate and mediate in situations involving their monolingual Spanish-speaking parents and monolingual English-speaking representatives of society. That children respond to these situations and exhibit their bicultural skills to help their parents is not in and of itself a problem. Bilingual/bicultural children who navigate between two languages and two cultures often develop incredible mediation abilities and sophisticated code-switching responses, as well as a high level of social sensitivity and an appreciation of the difficulties encountered by those who speak only Spanish. That they are referred to as "being like two people" is a tribute to an adaptive biculturality.

Thus, bicultural socialization is not inherently pathological. Nor does temporary adultification in itself necessarily create permanent role confusion. The negative circumstances in the environment that surround the acculturation process (in which a family finds itself changing from being solely monolingual/monocultural in the language and culture of origin to becoming bilingual/bicultural in succeeding generations) usually produces the stress attributed to role conflicts in the family. The acculturation stress of a family in transition in an environment of poverty, powerlessness, humiliation, lack of opportunity, and social injustice is sometimes too much for parents to manage. Spousification of children might not occur if negative circumstances in a family's environment were eliminated and appropriate supports were available for families undergoing the intergenerational transitions of acculturation. Many of the difficulties experienced by Mexican-American adolescents result from the inability of schools, media, neighborhood, and community to provide positive bicultural images and the skills with which to master their bicultural environment.

Adultification: The Child as Adult

Adultification affects different children in different ways. Some minority children are not able to make a transition from child to adult early in their lives. Being placed in adult roles can put immense pressure on youngsters and lay the foundation for a series of developmental difficulties, especially with the separation and individuation tasks of adolescence. Rinsley (1971) has observed that a child who develops significant psychopathology, who is "perceived and accordingly dealt with as something or somebody other than what he in fact is may suffer various degrees of distortion of his developing identity."

Bateson discusses the concept of the double bind. He describes this as a learning context in which the growing child is subjected repeatedly to incongruent, mutually exclusive messages for which no resolution is possible and concerning which no further discussion can be developed. This situation exists when a child grows up with family values that are substantially different from societal values at school and gets one set of messages from parents and another set from teachers. Examples include when a parent tells a child cooperation is an important value and a teacher says competition is an important value; when the family extols interdependence and teachers reinforce independence; when the family imprints that respect for people is based on status and age and teachers program that all people should be treated with equal respect. An adultified child may feel cultural pressure to represent family values in social situations and, consequently, experience tension when trying to be loyal to parents and simultaneously act in an adaptive manner. Children who are placed in situations where they are expected to act as adults may experience developmental pressure that could force a denial or postponement of aspects of innocent and carefree childhood in order to protect parents.

Adultification presumes what Rinsley (1971) refers to as adultomorphization, in which the parent

> . . . projects into the child their own reservoir of magic-omnipotence and infantile grandiosity. Such a child becomes, in the parent's mind, a powerful, omniscient being, through identification with whom the parents seek to achieve a proxy sense of mastery and accomplishment. But through the very process of adultomorphization, the parent poses for the child impossibly high standards and expectations of intellectual and emotional achievement, leading to ineluctable failure, which only further infantilizes him. (Rinsley, 1971, p. 11)

Spousification: The Child as Spouse

Where a child, in the role of an adult, becomes emotionally bonded to a parent, the child becomes a symbolic husband or wife. Rinsley (1971) identified two circumstances "in which the parent's depersonification of the child into a symbolic spouse is most likely to occur and have a particularly pathological effect upon the child's psycho-social development."

The first circumstance involves "narcissistic, unemancipated parents who obsessively and repetitively press the child into service as a means of wresting independence from their own parents" (Rinsley, 1971). The second circumstance involves the biological parent who "is bereft of a 'real' spouse as a consequence of abandonment, separation, divorce, or death" (Rinsley, 1971). In the latter circumstance, the parent attaches to the child as a substitute for the departed or emotionally absent husband or wife.

Inferences drawn from experience with Mexican-American adolescent cases suggest that a male child becomes spousified as a result of an emotionally or physically absent father. The clinical subjects were male school dropouts or students who had been identified as at risk, harshly physically disciplined sons, or oldest sons, all of whom had clearly defined bilingual/bicultural coping skills and who perceived their fathers as weak, helpless, sexually distant, or emotionally unavailable in regard to their mothers. The mothers were perceived by their sons as needy, unable to handle crisis alone, unaware, and tolerant of their husband's distance. When the son became emotionally involved in protecting his mother (le tengo que ayudar—I have to help her), a clearly traditional rigid male role expectation, the boy replaced his father. This contributed in part to identity conflict and blurred boundaries between child and adult roles. Additionally, tension in the spousified son created an array of themes of conflict. Experiential social work treatment of the son would later demonstrate the clinical manifestations of psycho-emotional stress associated with spousification.

CLINICAL MANIFESTATIONS

Practitioners need to understand and be sensitive to manifestations of tension experienced by adolescent males who have been spousified. Knowledge of the themes of conflict and tension are essential in formulating a solid assessment. Families under acculturation stress engage in communication styles that influence the dynamics of role definition and role assignment. For native-born Mexican-American males who have been or are in spousified roles, various themes of psycho-emotional stress may be faced during adolescence. In some cases, tension derived from spousification can be observed in childhood.

Self-Judgment and Guilt

The boy who "replaces" his father realizes a sense of power in being able to act in ways in which his father is either unable or unwilling to act. When his mother looks to him to perform roles prescribed for his father, and as she rewards his behavior with loving gestures, a sense of guilt may surface in the boy for "usurping" his father. The guilt may give rise to a need to punish himself because, by stepping in and acting in his father's place, his actions automatically announce that he is in charge, not his father. By taking the role of spouse, the boy relegates his father to an ambiguously defined figurehead. Because the boy's actions, not his intentions, remove the father from a decision-making role, a sense of culpability may be assumed.

Resentment

Spousified sons exhibit enormous rage at their mothers for manipulating them into impossible positions. They become angry because they perceive their mothers as weak and unable to manage for themselves. They may rationalize that if their mothers were socially competent, they (the sons) might not have to assume decision-making roles.

Additionally, spousified sons may feel anger because they perceive their mothers as requiring attention and incapable of being left alone. Spousified sons may get upset at their mothers' need for intimacy and may become angry that they feel pressured to protect them.

Older spousified adolescents may develop distorted views of and repressed rage toward women, whom they perceive as needy. They may become attracted to masculine, assertive women who are perceived as self-sufficient. And although their source of self-validation may be rooted in the need to protect and please women, they may concurrently retreat from intimacy in future relationships because they fear they will be pressured into always having to protect women.

Spousified adolescent males may be angry at their fathers, whom they perceive as being not strong enough to take care of their family responsibilities. Spousified males may see their fathers as weak, helpless, powerless, and indifferent, as talking tough, but not being tough. Because of years of bonding, adolescent males who believe that their fathers are irresponsible have great difficulty in confronting their fathers, much less their own feelings about their fathers. Resentment toward fathers is rampant among spousified males. Its root appears to be a fundamental perception that, "Dad abandoned his role and, in doing so, forced me into it." Integrity, extent of perceived real love of family, and self-respect are areas in which spousified males may have unresolved feelings toward their fathers.

Problems with Separation and Individuation

Spousified adolescent males who work toward their own goals and experience degrees of success may feel that they have abandoned their family. They may believe that they are selfish and that pursuing their own aspirations hurts the family. Questions about whether or not they can or should leave the family, especially the mother, can create anguish. Fear of success may be rooted in fear of separation and individuation, especially if a spousified son believes or knows that without his help his mother's willingness or ability to manage will be severely impaired. Codependent behaviors and exaggerated levels of responsibility have been observed among spousified sons because their own needs do not get met or are repressed.

Blurred Identity and Distorted Role Modeling

Because an adultified or spousified son may not be allowed to express his anger, it may become internalized, and self-hatred may develop. This self-hatred may serve to hide enormous rage and may manifest as a narcissistic personality disorder. With fathers not providing clear directions for what males do and do not do, spousified sons get their structure for behaviors and mannerisms from mothers.

Although they want their fathers to be strong and provide direction, adolescent spousified sons get mixed or no messages about what masculinity is from their absent or seemingly weak parents. Thus spousified sons may become obsessed with images of strong men who are in charge. They also may wonder whether they are adequate as males. Spousified sons may not have a normal frame of reference for male behavior because their fathers have modeled a weak or an absent figure.

Support groups focused on men's issues often provide a context for men to discuss their lack of relationships with their fathers. When men are sad about a father-son relationship that never materialized, they may long for male intimacy and yet struggle through distorted perceptions of what it means to be close to another man, how intimacy can be structured, and whether they can achieve it. Although virtually no research has examined the association between adolescent male spousification and adult capacity for male-to-male intimacy, practice wisdom suggests that spousified adolescents long for male role models.

Shame and Humiliation

Prolonged spousification of adolescent sons inevitably raises the theme of conflict. Separation and individuation may become difficult to accomplish and, as the spousified son reaches the late teen years, shame and humiliation for having trampled on Dad may begin to set in. Where there is evidence of a deteriorated or nonexistent relationship with the father, a spousified son may think that he is to blame for his father's indifference or distance. He also may believe that he can never bond with his father because he has humiliated his father and validated his incompetence. Spousified sons may feel ashamed of and embarrassed by their fathers. Developmental issues relative to autonomy and self-fulfillment may be eclipsed by spousified sons' beliefs that they do not deserve success because of what they have done to their fathers.

ASSESSMENT AND MONITORING

Separation and individuation issues in adolescent human development complicate identity formation. When a child or adolescent in a spousified role is also physically abused, he receives mixed and unclear messages about what he is supposed to do in a family. The Mexican-American child who is adultified and spousified has outstanding roles in the family that may not be brought into a treatment situation until later in life. The following case study provides an example. Ramiro Lopez became acculturated in school, where he learned English while speaking Spanish at home. His mother was culturally traditional, was monolingual in Spanish, and had little understanding of societal institutions. His father also was culturally traditional, spoke little English, and developed a life primarily with other Spanish-speaking workers.

Ramiro's mother was dependent, fearful, and at times hysterical. The only way Ramiro could take care of himself was to take care of her. When Ramiro was 11 years old, his father chose not to involve himself with creditors. Ramiro's mother asked Ramiro to help out. Ramiro's ability to speak English made it possible for him to relay to creditors his mother's plans to catch up on account payments. As Ramiro assumed an adult role, his mother began to applaud his efforts. Ramiro felt both helpful and loved for his actions.

As Ramiro continued to assume adult roles for his mother, she began to confide more in him. She discussed with him money management, plans for home repairs, and the schooling of her two younger daughters. The emotional bonds intensified to the point that Ramiro and his mother discussed every aspect of family life. Even when Ramiro's father could participate in family decisions, both Ramiro and his mother chose to hold discussions when he was away from the house.

Later, when creditors demanded that some financial commitments be made, Ramiro made them on directions from his mother. She believed she would be able to count on her husband's paycheck. When Ramiro's father was laid off temporarily and was home one day, creditors called the house to talk to Mr. Lopez. Even with his limited English, he learned of the commitments he had made. When Mr. Lopez confronted his wife, she told him that Ramiro had spoken to the creditors. When Ramiro got home from school, an angry Mr. Lopez physically abused him for interfering in his business and lying to him. Unable to stand up for himself, Ramiro watched as his mother assumed a "what can I do?" attitude.

The subsequent distancing between Mr. and Mrs. Lopez intensified Ramiro's pressure to act in behalf of his family by helping his mother, even though he was aware of his father's disapproval. Ramiro and his mother both colluded to keep secrets from Mr. Lopez, he to protect his mother from getting yelled at by his father, she to protect him from getting hit by his father.

Comprehensive assessment of acculturation stress in the Lopez family would later reveal spousification of the adolescent male as a factor in precipitating jealous tension in the father. The father's loss of control of family administration, as well as his perceived powerlessness and loss of self-respect, would later surface as enraged envy of his son's abilities. As Mr. Lopez withdrew from intimacy with his wife, Ramiro was blamed. Mrs. Lopez's need for emotional intimacy, coupled with Ramiro's need to protect her in order to protect himself, led to his becoming spousified. With Mr. Lopez clearly relegated out of family decision making, Ramiro became the object of his father's displaced anger. Envy and rage would later be viewed as emotional precipitators for the father's abusive behaviors.

When a child is pressured to do more than he or she is able or willing to do, he or she may develop fears of inadequacy. In part, these fears result from the child being placed in situations in which he or she is inadequate, such as trying to fill the role of an adult spouse or a parent. When a spousified son is constantly expected to fill adult roles, his inability to do so may seem to prove that he is incapable of being a husband or father. This may lead to a deep sense of inadequacy as a male. To be subsequently punished by his father for his attempts to protect the family and ensure its survival may contribute to the son's distorted sense of self and to feeling shame. There are several useful brief assessment tools to measure bicultural identity problems. One customary approach is to assess a client's acculturation. Some good measurement tools are the Short Acculturation Scale for Hispanics (Marin, Sabogal, Van Oss Marin, Otero-Sabogal, & Perez-Stable, 1987) and the Acculturation Rating Scale for Mexican Americans (Cuellar, Arnold, & Maldonado, 1995). In some circumstances, such as when the client's bicultural conflict appears to be a lack of any identity, it may be helpful to assess the client's ethnic identity. One tool for this is the Multigroup Ethnic Identity Measure (Phinney, 1992) or the Simpatia Scale, which ascertains the cultural script of some Hispanics that promotes smooth social interaction (Griffith, Joe, Chatham, & Simpson, 1998). One particularly useful instrument is the Orthogonal Cultural Identification Scale (Oetting & Beauvais, 1990–1991), which is a six-item measure of how much a person identifies with the customs and practices of a number of different cultures. Bicultural problems may be considered in terms of the differences in scores between cultures, such as the Hispanic and Anglo cultures. Other measures of acculturation and cultural identity are reported in Corcoran and Fischer (2000b).

EXPERIENTIAL TREATMENT

The processes of successful treatment of spousification in Mexican-American adolescent males have received little attention in the literature. Consequently, there is little scientific documentation of efforts.

Rinsley (1971) suggests separating the adolescent from the family through admission into full-time residential treatment. The author of this chapter believes such treatment to be excessive, ineffective, and inaccessible to large numbers of Mexican-American families, who do not have insurance coverage and are not likely to appreciate or endorse the rationale of residential treatment.

Szapocznik and others at the Spanish-Speaking Family Guidance Clinic in Florida have experimented successfully with outpatient intervention through the use of one-person family therapy (Szapocznik & Kurtines, 1980) and bicultural effectiveness training (Szapocznik et al., 1984). These are treatment interventions based on helping clients to adapt to biculturality. Interventions based on this philosophy are supported by research that suggests that adjustment to bicultural contexts necessitates an ability to act appropriately in either cultural context. Their work with Cuban families whose individual members are at different levels of acculturation and acculturation stress have realized fascinating results, such as the treatment of related or behavioral disorders through the enhancement of biculturalism in family members, an improved flexibility of family roles, and more openness in family functioning. As of this writing, a literature search disclosed no entries regarding family therapy with Mexican-American families related to the treatment of spousification in adolescents.

In the treatment of the spousified child, it is important to eliminate the rigid role that resulted from the emotional conditioning between parent and child that intensified the triangulation of the child. Appropriate techniques can unravel the web of triangulation and facilitate communication in the marital dyad. Such resolution also temporarily frees the adolescent for important self-liberation and empowerment work. Structural family therapy techniques show promise in helping family members to address the various relationships among members as they affect how decisions in the family are made. The spousified child has a series of tasks to work through as part of treatment intervention:

1. Awareness and education about spousification.
2. Exploration of cognitions (thought forms) and affect (feelings) related to relationship with spousifying parent.
3. Exploration of self-image that has developed as a result of being spousified.
4. Review of situations where parent may have been traumatized, thereby forcing child into adult role.
5. Exploration of complementary behaviors that child learned in order to protect traumatized parent or cope with parent's inability to adapt.
6. Awareness of child's participation with spousifying parent in decision making to the exclusion of other parent.
7. Exploration of child's feelings about replacing other parent.
8. Exploration of child's core survival thinking about his behavior vis-á-vis the spousifying parent's love (examination of codependence).
9. Uncovering of child's deep-seated emotions through a) awareness of the process of spousification; b) how the imposed adult role was a form of emotional manipulation; c) awareness that the child's intense need for nurturance may have led to intense denial of that need; and d) how the child was expected to have the emotions of an adult and spouse.
10. Exploration of child's powerlessness to freely pursue his interests and associated addictive patterns of pain control.
11. Uncovering of child's emotions about himself (self-derogation, self-denial, and self-destruction) and manifested behaviors (anger at self, guilt, and shame).
12. Uncovering of child's emotions toward parents (anger, resentment, bitterness).
13. Uncovering of child's emotions toward life (anger, fear of judgment).

During treatment, the spousified son's work on separation and individuation from parents may become intensified as he staunchly defends his illusory self, which was created by the confusion of roles. Separation and personal integration work using transactional analysis techniques, Gestalt techniques, and self-image modification are usually necessary before any restructuring of new beliefs and clearing of repressed emotions can be effective. Personal leadership building, assertiveness training, and personal problem-solving skill development can later assist the empowerment process toward independence. Social workers should remember that the escape to freedom philosophy may be one of great emotional pain for an adolescent male child, but with the establishment of liberation and empowerment to individuate, termination of short-term treatment comes within reach. Additional posttreatment follow-up may address regret, grief for the loss of self, and guilt for perceived interference with the other parent's role as spouse. These and other associated feelings may suggest that the work of personal integration, separation, and individuation has, in effect, occurred, and that the client may need assistance in releasing the past and forgiving himself.

At the point in the treatment process when repressed emotions surface and are identified, the social worker needs to use techniques to manage and clear the feelings that have surfaced. One set of techniques is experiential focusing. Experiential focusing techniques are structured methods designed to direct the client's attention to his or her physical or internal sensation (bodily) experiences (Gendlin, 1978). These bodily experiences have a profound influence on one's life, one's insights, and one's goals. Focusing is based on the assertion that differences in effectiveness of treatment can be measured not so much by what clients talk about as by how they talk; that is, change seems to occur when the client's discussion reflects change in his or her internal experiences, those internal sensations that are meaningful to the client. Gendlin has labeled these experiences the "felt sense." By focusing on these bodily experiences, clients obtain a special kind of internal experience pertinent to insight and change.

Focusing has been shown to relate to client change (see, e.g., Gendlin, 1973, 1978; Kantor & Zimring, 1976) and clinician's empathy (Corcoran, 1982). Unlike many experiential techniques, focusing is structured in a step-by-step format. Information on focusing is available in book form (Gendlin, 1978) and on audiotape (Olsen, 1978). The focusing techniques that follow have been developed specifically for Hispanic males with identity problems. Used with one or both parents, these techniques are designed to allow the client to disidentify by projecting the emotions and images generated as a result of emotional tension. Through the use of projection, the client becomes involved in an internal dialogue that is nonthreatening and serves 1) to clear the feelings he is having and 2) to dissipate the symbols associated with those feelings.

The first technique is the Affective Release Process. This is used to release any feelings about self, others, or life. The Image Dissipation Process is the second technique. It is used to release the past through an imaging procedure that dissipates the symbols associated with the feelings. As part of the procedure, the client is also directed to make verbal statements of forgiveness.

Emotional Accessing Technique

As preliminary work before using either process, the social worker can ask the client to use his own body to locate where he is experiencing feelings. This is accomplished by using the Emotional Accessing Technique. Successful use of this technique enables the social worker to gain access to an image somewhere in the client's body of the tension being experienced, which can help social worker and client identify the actual feeling producing the tension. This is accomplished by first asking the client, "Where in your body do you feel the tension with your parent?" When the client identifies a specific place in his body where he feels the tension (for example, the stomach), the social worker then asks the client to imagine or make up a picture of what the tension looks like. The client then can describe or draw the image in the specific place in his body where he is experiencing the tension (for example, a thick, dark, heavy black knot in the stomach). In order for the social worker to gain access to the actual feeling the client is experiencing as a result of the tension, the final step of this technique requires the client to enact the image that has just been identified in a specific place in the body. The social worker plays the part of the client in this simple role play. This is accomplished by asking the client, "What is the tension that I am feeling?" The client, playing the part of the dark knot, would respond by identifying the actual feeling being experienced. The dark knot might say, "The tension is because I am scared." The social worker might be able to identify, for example, that the client is experiencing real fear of a parent; that fear was accessed by guiding the client through a projective process. In this way, the social worker can help the client learn to identify his own feelings.

Additional treatment strategies could further identify where in time and space the fear was created; what the client did to protect him- or herself; what interpretations or beliefs he or she made about self, others, or life; what factors kept the fear in place; what kinds of behaviors were developed as a result of the fear and what kinds of behaviors continue; and what skills and behaviors can be developed to address the abatement of the fear. Although further intervention may be necessary and is not delineated here, the three steps of the Emotional Accessing Technique accomplish the identification of the feelings that can eventually be resolved through the use of the experiential techniques described in the next section of this chapter.

Experiential Techniques

Affective Release Process.   The purpose of this process is to address methodically the feelings that the client has just accessed by having the client put into words what he feels and express himself assertively in a manner that helps resolve the issue. Clients often are reticent in expressing their feelings in a session, particularly if they have experienced previous difficulty in personal assertiveness or if their trust of others has eroded over time. Therefore, it is important that the social worker guide this process in a professional, non-judgmental manner that conveys a sense of safety.

The expression of feelings that the client has for a parent can occur in the absence of the parent. In using the Affective Release Process, the social worker asks the client to imagine that the parent with whom he is distressed is sitting across from him. The social worker can ask the client to describe the parent as if he or she were indeed in the room: how the parent is dressed, how his or her hair is combed, how he or she is sitting, etc. Carefully describing the person with whom one is distressed creates a more vivid image and helps feelings come to the surface more easily. The actual steps of the Affective Release Process follow.

Step 1. Have the client state, as if the person with whom there is distress were actually present, all of the things he does not appreciate about him or her. The social worker asks the client to express all of the feelings he is experiencing to the image he has described of the person. Specifically, the social worker guides the process by explaining that the client needs to begin expression with the following phrase: "[Actual name of person with whom client is distressed], what I don't appreciate about you is . . ." (For example, "Mom, what I don't appreciate about you is that you didn't stand up for me when . . .") As the client feels freer to express all the things about which he feels tension, the social worker provides support by quietly echoing what the client has just said and by asking the client, "What else do you not appreciate about Mom?" Additionally, the social worker can not only help the client express his feelings about the person with whom he is distressed, but also unravel feelings the client may have about what the person did. The practitioner can support the expression of more feelings by asking, "What else do you not appreciate about what Mom did?" or "What else do you not appreciate about what happened to you?"

This step continues until the client has completely expressed all the feelings he has about the person. This single step should not be time limited; social workers should not interfere with the free flow of feelings once the client begins to express them. Notes from practice reveal that clients may use an entire counseling session for this one step. Additionally, as social workers allow clients the freedom to direct their own work, clients may end sessions with a greater sense of trust in the social workers.

Step 2. Have the client state, as if the person with whom there is distress were actually present, all of the things he does appreciate about him or her. In this step, the client is asked to focus on the things that he does appreciate about the other person. This step provides the client with an opportunity to acknowledge positive feelings he has for the person and a perspective for those feelings. It recognizes that although clients can have negative feelings about a significant other relative to specific negative experiences, they may also have overall positive feelings about their relationship with that person. As clients have the opportunity to express their general feelings about the relationship, this step brings a sense of balance to an otherwise difficult review of an experience.

It is important to note, however, that some clients may bring to their treatment a historical perspective that is not positive because of a turbulent and distrustful relationship with a significant other. This has been observed in clients who have been abused, neglected, or who have suffered chronic tension as a result of multiple traumatic experiences. These clients may choose not to express what they appreciate about people with whom they are distressed because positive feelings do not exist.

Step 3.   Ask the client whether there is anything else he would like to say to the person with whom there is distress. This step provides an ending to this structured manner of self-expression and an opportunity for the client to acknowledge his general feelings toward the person. The social worker can guide the client by asking, "Is there anything else you would like to say to Mom?" or "Is there any final thing you would like to say now to close?"

Clients may seem quiet at the conclusion of this technique. This may suggest that the client is tired after having expressed deep feelings; it may suggest that the client is reflective about his realization of how he really felt; or it may be a natural response to the completion of the process. As the client is provided with the structure in which to express all of his feelings relative to the discomfort that caused the tension, the resolving of affect becomes an empowering tool.

Image Dissipation Process.   People create symbolic images of their experiences with themselves, others, and life. Symbolic images convey meaning and feeling. Clients who experience difficult and traumatic events in their lives may suppress feelings associated with the tension of those events. Because defense mechanisms allow people to postpone or deny feelings about difficult events, they may not have complete awareness of the underlying emotions that influence their motives and behaviors. Based on this understanding, the Emotional Accessing Technique described earlier provides the social worker with a structured way in which to achieve consciousness of underlying feelings through the identification of a symbolic image.

Having completed a process that has cleared the affect identified through the symbolic image, it is now desirable to structure for the client a way in which to dissipate the symbolic image. The rationale for dissipating or dissolving the symbolic image of the client's tension is the connection between images and emotions. Although emotions represent one system of communication and images represent another, their connection occurs when the messages of emotions become converted as a body of information to symbolic images. Symbolic images become encoded with the information of emotions. A whole-person approach to clearing tension would necessarily suggest not only the clearing of affect, but the clearing of images as well. Because individuals' feelings about themselves, others, and life are encoded in their symbolic images, the dissipation of the mental picture created to identify the tension accomplishes an important therapeutic task. This is the release of the body of information from the emotions of the tension through the dissipation of the sensory agent that carries them.

The Image Dissipation Process accomplishes a second important task, namely, the forgiveness of self. This is important when the client makes a connection between the image of what happened and his own culpability. As symbolic images act as sensory agents of emotions and become internalized in the client, they can serve as springboards for the development of negative or illusionary thinking about the self. In clients who bring to their treatment sessions strong internalized negative feelings or beliefs about themselves, the release of feelings and the dissipation of symbolic images from role tension may not be enough. Observations from practice have shown that clients who use negative experiences to judge themselves suffer relentless stress. The symbolic images become not only the sensory agents of the emotions of the difficult experience, but also register the emotions the client had about himself in that experience. Where internalized judgment of self occurs as a result of a difficult experience, it becomes additionally important to dissipate the symbolic image because it also acts as the sensory agent of nonforgiveness.

The preliminary client preparation work the practitioner does before using the Image Dissipation Process involves bringing the client's attention back to the symbolic image that was accessed earlier. The practitioner can explain to the client how mentally dissolving or destroying the symbol of the tension can help remove the sensory push that would bring the emotions to the surface all over again. Additionally, the practitioner can explain that the faculty of the imagination is used to complete this process. Successful outcomes of the therapeutic use of the imagination in practice have been observed to result in client perceptions of peacefulness and empowerment.

Step 1.   Ask the client to focus his thinking on the symbolic image. The social worker asks the client to identify the image and what it looks like. (For example, the client describes the tension as being like a dark, heavy black knot in the stomach area.)

Step 2.   Ask the client to use his imagination to expand the symbolic image, making it larger and larger until it dissipates (changes or explodes) and then tell what he sees afterwards, if anything. The social worker is helping the client to mentally dissolve the symbolic image. Additionally, the social worker is interested in the next symbolic image that surfaces, because it determines whether this step will need to be repeated.

Step 2-A.   Ask the client to repeat aloud a set of positive affirmations and a statement of forgiveness of self. This step is led by the social worker, who models for the client self-talk that acknowledges the release of any judgment the client has of himself. (For example, the social worker may say, "Repeat with me . . . with all of my power, with all of my protection, with all of my love, I forgive you, John, for the image of the dark, heavy knot.") With the completion of both parts of this step, the client has dissolved the symbolic image and cleared himself of any self-judgment that was or could have been derived from the tension of the negative experience.

If the client imagines a new symbol after dissolving the original one, repeat steps 2 and 2-A. This process continues until the client no longer imagines any symbols or until the client imagines a symbol with which he is comfortable and that he wishes to keep.

Step 3.   Ask the client to reimage the area in the body where the original symbolic image was experienced. The purpose of this step is to determine whether the symbolic image has completely dissipated. (For example, the social worker says, "John, go back and reimage your stomach and tell me what you see.") Successful outcome of this step results when the client reports that the symbolic image is gone, that the sensory agent identified with the tension has been eliminated. When the client reports that the symbolic image is cleared, the process ends.

As a part of this step, a client may report that another symbolic image exists. The social worker should determine whether the client is comfortable with the new symbolic image. If the client wishes to dissolve this and any new symbolic images, the social worker should guide the client through the process again until the client is comfortable. If the client wishes to keep a new symbolic image because of a positive association made with it, the social worker ends the process by acknowledging the value of the positive outcome of the creative process.

If a client has difficulty with the concept of dissipation, the practitioner can ask the client to imagine a procedure through which the symbolic image can be dissolved or eliminated. It has been observed in practice that clients have imagined the symbols being erased, painted over, torn, and covered, all with the same result of eliminating the sensory agent, which is the goal of this technique.

GENERALIZING THE INTERVENTION TO RELATED PROBLEMS

The evaluation of the impact of experiential treatment techniques limited to Mexican-Americans has been encouraging. In terms of the special population of Mexican-American males with identity problems, clinical trials are currently being conducted to study the effects of these specific experiential techniques. Practice experience and evaluations of treatment suggest that the techniques are successful with ethnic minority clients and overburdened adolescents experiencing role tension from acculturation stress. Additionally, the use of these techniques has been successfully evaluated with treatment of war veterans experiencing symptoms of posttraumatic stress disorders; treatment of high-risk antepartum obstetrical patients experiencing symptoms of pregnancy-induced hypertension, diabetes, and hyperemesis gravidarum; and treatment of adults who were molested as children and who are experiencing intimacy dysfunction in marriage. In some cases, clinical analysis of high-risk antepartum obstetrical patients who are adolescents and of ethnic minority background has revealed preexisting role tension from acculturation stress.

No empirical data have been set forth in the literature that support the validity or reliability of these specific techniques, although research on other Gestalt techniques has been encouraging (see Simkin & Yontef, 1984). Clinical case studies suggest that these techniques have application in helping to address not only the role of tension associated with acculturation stress, but also tension associated with posttraumatic stress. Gerber posits that "the most powerful of all healing modalities is the patient's own mind. Positive, spiritually uplifting verbal affirmations may be used to change negative message tapes that may be playing through the subconscious mind. Transformational healing images are also of benefit, especially when visual imagery is combined with the use of affirmations" (Gerber, 1988). Recent works by professionals in the helping professions suggest that, although empirical data are incomplete and many of the methods that address affective and self-image modification work have validation only in observations from practice, the direction in which these techniques are developing shows much promise.

CONCLUSION

Much work has been completed in the past few years in building knowledge of the treatment of behavioral disorders related to acculturation stress in families. Although biculturality and generational conflict can contribute to acting out and disengagement, both can also lead to a higher-level integration of the personality. As practice-based research reveals the intricacies of identity formation in bicultural males, more in-depth analysis may support biculturality as a phenomenon that is dynamic and self-affirming.

CHAPTER 16

Mediation Techniques for Persons in Disputes

William R. Nugent

In this chapter, Nugent discusses interpersonal, nonviolent conflicts and shows how to use mediation to resolve such disputes. The fact that these disputes exclude violent conflicts illustrates the important principle of defining what specific problem to use with an appropriate intervention. Mediation itself has several well-defined components that help to arrive at mutually agreeable outcomes in a dispute. The components of mediation include establishing rapport, ventilating feelings, caucusing, defining the problem, generating solutions, and implementation. Drawing from a variety of theoretical perspectives, Nugent also shows how to use techniques such as reframing. The importance of client participation in problem solving and contracting is also illustrated.

INTRODUCTION

Numerous practice settings can present the social worker with interpersonal conflict and the practice-related problem of how to resolve it. Examples include the following:

1. You are a school social worker who is asked to intervene with two students who are about to come to blows over some issue.
2. You are a social worker in a residential program for adolescents, such as a runaway shelter. The mother of a client, during a visit to see her daughter in the shelter, suddenly becomes very angry, grabs her daughter, and threatens to "knock her block off."
3. You are doing community organization work and are faced with a dispute between a group of residents in a neighborhood and a minority family that recently moved to the area.
4. You are working as a community mediator for a county court system. You are asked to help resolve a dispute between two neighbors over a barking dog.
5. You are working as a therapist and are asked to help a divorcing couple work out a divorce settlement that includes child custody issues.

In each of these situations, the social worker is faced with a dispute and the task of helping resolve interpersonal conflict.

Conflict is an inevitable aspect of life and interpersonal relationships. Strayhorn (1977, p. 1) writes, "Conflict is the rule, not the exception, in human relationships." In and of itself, conflict is neither good nor bad, neither adaptive nor maladaptive. What is of critical importance is the manner in which individuals involved in a dispute attempt to resolve the conflict. Properly handled, conflict situations present a wonderful opportunity for the enrichment of interpersonal relationships and the growth of individuals and society. Improperly managed, conflict can lead to a wide range of destructive outcomes, such as the deterioration or destruction of relationships, families, and in some cases, human beings, as in the case of physical violence and war.

Some all too commonly used procedures for resolving conflict are adversarial and have win/lose outcomes. With such approaches, one party in a dispute wins (i.e., is "right" or is the last person standing after a fistfight) and the other loses (i.e., is "wrong" or sustains the most physical damage in a fistfight). Unfortunately, regardless of who wins or loses in an adversarial approach to conflict resolution, the relationship loses. Thus, if the disputants are involved in some type of ongoing relationship, whatever it might be, it is of great importance to avoid win/lose approaches to conflict resolution.

A far more desirable approach to resolving conflict is a cooperative one in which outcomes are win/win. Such an approach leaves all persons with the sense that their needs have been met. More importantly, the relationship wins in that it continues and becomes stronger, deeper, and richer than before the conflict was worked through.

This chapter presents a win/win approach to conflict resolution called mediation. You will learn a strategy, an overall plan, for doing mediation. This strategy is essentially a problem-solving approach to conflict resolution. You will also learn several specific intervention procedures that help implement this win/win strategy. These interventions are drawn from a number of areas, including methods of community conflict resolution, the work of Milton H. Erickson, cognitive behavior therapy, a number of systems of marriage and family therapy, and the writings of those who do mediation. The role that you will have in helping resolve disputes will be that of a *mediator*, and the process itself will be called *dispute resolution* or *mediation*.

PROBLEM IDENTIFICATION

Disputes, Conflicts, and Their Manifestations

Conflict arises any time people involved in relationships, such as friends, family members, coworkers, or neighbors, have differing needs, wants, desires, expectations, goals, or means of achieving certain ends (Chetkow-Yanoov, 1997; Kruk, 1997; Leviton & Greenstone, 1997; Weeks, 1977). The aspects of conflict that the social worker will want to observe are not only the content (i.e., the issues over which persons differ) of the conflict, but also the means being used to attempt to resolve the conflict. Indeed, the conflict itself may not be the real problem. Rather, the methods being used to attempt to resolve the conflict may be the central problem to be worked on. This is an example of a principle of problem formation and resolution developed by Watzlawick, Weakland, and Fisch (1974): the *attempted solution* to a difficulty (such as conflicting goals, desires, expectations, etc.) can lead to a problem. When this happens, it is the attempted solution that becomes the target of change, not the difficulty that spawned the attempted solution. Thus, the social worker in the role of mediator will work to interrupt the ongoing problematic attempts at conflict resolution that disputants have been using and involve them in a cooperative, win/win dispute resolution process.

There are a number of common indicators of ineffective and adversarial methods of conflict resolution. They are the indicators of attempt solutions to conflict that have created a problem for those involved and include the following:

1. Anger that increases in intensity over the course of the attempted resolution.
2. Movement toward more aggressive, hostile, forceful, destructive, and nonpeaceful resolution tactics.
3. Mistrust that increases in intensity.
4. Increased polarization of persons in the dispute, who become more firmly entrenched in rigid positions, demands for particular "solutions," and perceptions of one another.
5. Movement away from negotiation tactics.
6. Blaming stances and message styles.
7. Increased use of obstructive message styles, such as overgeneralizing and blaming.
8. Misunderstanding of other people's views, positions, needs, etc.
9. A "tunnel vision" negative view of other persons (Beck, 1988).
10. A negative bias in attribution of motives to other persons involved in the dispute (Beck, 1988).

The greater the number and intensity of these indicators in any dispute, the more problematic the methods being used by disputants in an attempt to resolve the conflict.

Assessment and Monitoring

As the social worker helps people resolve disputes, he or she may want to evaluate objectively any intervention used as part of the process. There are a number of objective assessment tools available. The particular measurement instrumentation used will depend in part upon the relational context in which the conflict occurs, such as marriage, family, professional, business, peer-relationship, and so forth. For example, the State portion of the State-Trait Anger Scale (Spielberger, Jacobson, Russell, & Crane, 1983) or the Anger Axiom Scale (Malgady, Rogler, & Cortes, 1996) might be used to monitor the level of anger felt by disputants. The Anger Axiom Scale is especially useful in practice with Puerto Ricans. There are other anger scales available for consideration (Corcoran & Fisher, 2000). The social worker might work with the disputants to develop an individual rating scale to measure specific aspects of the conflict (Bloom, Fischer, & Orme, 1999). Individualized rating scales are easy to construct and are client and problem specific, and some research has suggested that they can have psychometric characteristics comparable to those of standardized Likert-type scales (Nugent, 1992a). "Thought listing" procedures may be used to assess and monitor cognitive aspects of conflict (Caccioppo & Petty, 1981). The following are excellent sources of measurement instrumentation: Hudson (1982); Corcoran and Fischer, (2000a, 2000b); Chun, Cobb, and French (1975); Comery et al. (1973); Goldman and Sanders (1974); and Goldman and Busch (1978, 1982).

The social worker can use data gathered from his or her measurement procedures and single-case design methodology to monitor graphically how the dispute resolution process is progressing, as discussed in chapter 5 of this book. At the simplest level, the social worker may make repeated measures of aspects of the dispute (such as levels of disputants' anger) during the dispute resolution process, plot the resulting measurements on a graph, and thereby monitor progress (or lack thereof) using a simple intervention-only design. More complex evaluation procedures may also be used (Bloom et al., 1999).

Doing Mediation: The Dispute Resolution Strategy

The dispute resolution strategy may be described as a five-phase problem-solving process:

1. Establishing rapport with all disputants and altering nonfacilitative or negative feelings.
2. Defining the conflict issues in behavioral, solvable, and win/win terms.
3. Generating as many alternative solution options as possible.
4. Choosing from the alternative solution options and creating a composite plan for resolving the dispute.
5. Implementing the composite plan and evaluating its effectiveness.

This process, although modeled in five sequential and distinct phases, should not be taken as linear. This means that you will not necessarily move sequentially through each step, completing one before you move on to the next. You may need to return to a previous phase one or more times during the course of helping to resolve a dispute. Indeed, the first step, establishing rapport, is a continuous process that must be maintained throughout the entire mediation process (Leviton & Greenstone, 1997).

Specific Intervention Tactics

Several specific intervention procedures that can help the social worker to implement the mediation process will be described in this section. Specific intervention techniques to be discussed and the phases of the mediation process in which they are useful are shown in Table 16-1.

Establishing rapport and changing feelings. The mediator must first establish rapport with each person involved in the dispute. Rapport may be defined as a warm, empathic relationship within which the disputants have a sense of trust in the mediator (Welton, Pruitt, & McGillicuddy, 1988). According to Welton et al. (1988), rapport serves a critical function:

> Rapport contributes to successful mediation in several ways. It facilitates media-
> tor influence over the disputants and makes the disputants more committed to the
> mediation process. . . . Rapport may even contribute to one disputant's taking the
> needs of the other disputant more seriously, since the mediator, who is trusted, is
> seen to take these needs seriously. . . . (p. 182)

The mediator also must facilitate the change, as much as possible, of strong nonfacilitative feelings. A nonfacilitative emotion is one that hinders the creation of a cooperative, mutually satisfying resolution to a dispute. Examples of such feelings are anger, resentment, hate, fear, and confusion. Anger especially must be safely and effectively managed. When disputants are in the grip of such feelings they are unlikely to work to understand other disputants, consider alternative definitions of the dispute, or negotiate win/win solutions (Zillman, 1993). Indeed, disputants in the grip of strong feelings may to some extent be hindered in any attempts to cooperatively resolve a dispute because of "mood congruent recall." This term refers to the apparent inability of people to bring to mind memories that are inconsistent with a specific mood, such as hostility or depression (Barlow, 1988). For example, a husband who is feeling hostile toward his wife will have a difficult time remembering incidents in which his wife did something that left him feeling warm and affectionate toward her. This will remain true until his hostile mood has either lessened in intensity or gone through a qualitative change.

Four specific intervention procedures that are useful for establishing rapport and changing strong feelings are 1) imposing structure and defining roles (Levi & Benjamin, 1977); 2) active, or empathic, listening (Gordon, 1970; Hepworth & Larsen, 1986); 3) caucusing (Welton et al., 1988); and 4) reframing (Watzlawick, 1978; Watzlawick et al., 1974). The primary goal

TABLE 16-1 Intervention Procedures for Dispute Resolution Phases

Phase I: Establishing Rapport and Dissipating Feelings
  A. Establishing rules for interactions
  B. Establishing psychological contracts
  C. Defining participants' role behaviors
  D. Active listening
  E. Caucusing
  F. Refraining

Phase II: Defining the Conflict
  A. Use of behaviorally specific language
  B. Reframing
  C. Listening for implied definitions of the dispute

Phase III: Generating Alternative Solutions
  A. Caucusing
  B. Brainstorming
  C. Refraining

Phase IV: Choosing Alternatives and Creating a Plan
  A. Rating alternatives
  B. Causcusing
  C. Quid pro quo contract negotiations
  D. Reframing

Phase V: Implementing the Plan and Evaluating Its Effectiveness
  A. Quid pro quo contract
  B. Agreeing upon follow-up meetings

---

of mediation is the production of a solution that resolves the dispute. Consequently, it involves both task and process components (Kruk, 1997). An intervention that helps to achieve both process and outcome goals is the imposition of structure on the interactions between disputants (Levi & Benjamin, 1977). This can be achieved through several techniques that are described below.

Establishing ground rules for the mediation process. The mediator can impose structure by describing rules governing participants' behavior during the mediation process. The rules used, such as no interruptions while another is speaking, can be designed so as to help facilitate the development of rapport and hinder the escalation of nonfacilitative emotions and behavior (Leviton & Greenstone, 1997).

Establishing a psychological contract with all participants involved in the conflict resolution process. This contract calls for each participant to adopt, as much as possible, a problem-solving orientation during the conflict resolution process. It also calls for each participant to express his or her feelings and views openly and honestly, but in a manner that follows the structure of the mediation process and behavioral ground rules for participation that were laid out by the mediator.

Defining the role behaviors for all participants. This is done, in part, through the psychological contract already discussed. Role behaviors are further prescribed by the mediator, who describes her or his own functions in the process. It often is useful to define one of the roles as that of translator. This role requires the mediator to work to alleviate misunderstandings between the disputants that seem to result from misperceptions and misinterpretations of what others are saying. It also is useful to frame the role of the mediator as one of helping each participant get, as much as possible, what he or she needs during the conflict resolution process. In other words, the process is framed as a cooperative win/win procedure from the beginning of the mediation.

The opening statement. Each of the above procedures can be implemented in an opening statement made by the mediator at the beginning of a mediation. The mediator takes a few minutes in a joint meeting of the disputants to clearly verbalize ground rules, get all parties to agree to the psychological contracts, and define the role behaviors of participants. The first few minutes of a mediation session can be very important to the ultimate success of the mediation (Leviton & Greenstone, 1997).

Active listening. Hepworth and Larsen (1986) and Gordon (1970) give in-depth discussion on what active or empathic listening is and how it is done, so I will not spend a lot of time on the "how to's" of this procedure. The reader probably has already encountered this interpersonal communication method and has a sense of its value. There is both practice wisdom and research evidence that suggest that this technique is helpful in facilitating change (Nugent, 1992b; Nugent & Halvorson, 1995).

It is important to remember when using active listening in mediation to consider the effects that a paraphrase of one disputant's statements might have on another disputant. It is possible for the mediator to create a problem with one of the disputants by paraphrasing a statement in such a way that it angers or offends the disputant. You must construct your active-listening paraphrases in such a way that they are acceptable to all persons who hear them. For example, suppose that disputant A says, "He is so inconsiderate of people's feelings. He makes me so mad!" The mediator responds with the following paraphrase, "So you're angry at him over the insensitive behavior." Disputant B hears the mediator refer to his "insensitive behavior" and now becomes angry at the mediator and begins to feel that the mediator is siding with disputant A. Nugent and Halvorson (1995) discuss some of the ways in which active listening can lead to negative outcomes.

It is almost impossible for a social worker (or anyone else) to be too proficient at active listening. It is important in conflict resolution work to listen not only for feelings but also for how disputants interpret events, behaviors, and situations.

Numerous writers have pointed out that it is not the events, behaviors, or situations that cause people distress, but rather the symbolic meanings they attribute to these things (Beck, 1976, 1988; Burns, 1980; Watzlawick et al., 1974; Watzlawick, 1978). Frequently, conflict is exacerbated, if not caused by, the symbolic meanings disputants attribute to certain behaviors or actions (Zillman, 1993).

Disputants often will confuse a possible solution to a conflict situation with the needs or wants that are at the heart of the dispute. For example, a young woman in a residential program for adolescents who was in a dispute with a young man over a missing radio said, "I want him arrested! I know he stole it and I am sick of having things stolen! There have been a bunch of my things stolen! There have been a bunch of my things stolen and no one cares. No one has done anything about my things." The mediator, using active listening, noted to the young woman, "It sounds like you're really sick of things disappearing and no one paying attention to your complaints. It also sounds like the most important thing to you is that you find a way to get people in the shelter to respect your belongings. You need to feel that your things are safe in the shelter, to feel that you have some space of your own and a sense of security for your stuff." This statement by the mediator apparently functioned to separate the potential solution of arresting the young man (which, it turns out, meant in the young woman's mind that others in the shelter would be frightened and therefore leave her things alone) from the more fundamental issue of the young woman wanting to feel that her belongings were secure. Up until this point, the young woman had been rigidly focused on having the young man arrested as the only possible solution. Subsequent to the active-listening statement, the young woman became open to a number of alternative possibilities.

Caucusing.   Caucusing refers to the intervention tactic of meeting separately with each person (or group) involved in a dispute (Welton et al. 1988). This is to be distinguished from joint, or conjoint, meetings, in which all persons involved in the conflict are present. There are a number of potential outcomes from caucusing that facilitate cooperative dispute resolution:

1. Reductions in levels of anger, tension, and defensiveness.
2. Acquisition of information about interests, assumptions, and interpretations underlying the conflict.
3. Increased levels of rapport between mediator and disputant as a result of the mediator's ability to focus on the individual (or individual group).
4. Increased effectiveness of brainstorming for alternative solutions and increased willingness to consider alternative resolutions to the conflict.
5. Increased ability of the mediator to focus responsibility for coming up with creative alternative solutions on the individual or individual group.
6. Increased ability of the mediator to influence the behavior of individual disputants.

Most of these advantages accrue because of the absence of the other persons involved in the dispute. Blades (1984), Evarts, Greenstone, Kirkpatrick, and Leviton (1983), Kolb (1983), and Witty (1980) discuss the theoretical reasons for using caucusing. Welton et al. (1988) present experimental evidence demonstrating the facilitative effects of caucusing. Taylor, Barry, and Block (1958), Dunnette, Campbell, and Joasted (1963), and Bouchard (1972) give research evidence of the superiority of individual brainstorming over that done in a group setting.

There are a few disadvantages to caucusing. Welton et al. (1988) note that disputant statements in caucus sessions are likely to be less accurate than those in joint sessions. Also, occasionally a disputant may be able to coopt the mediator. Marriage and family therapists have warned about the dangers of being told something by a spouse or family member in an individual meeting session that the person wants kept confidential, a situation that may interrupt joint problem-solving discussions between disputants. Finally, problems may arise if the disputants who are not involved in the caucus sessions talk with friends, relatives, or other supporters and are influenced by input from these sources.

Reframing.   Reframing is a useful and versatile intervention technique (Watzlawick et al., 1974; Watzlawick, 1978; Bandler & Grinder, 1982). This procedure also is called relabeling (Weeks & L'Abate, 1982) or redefining (Hepworth & Larsen, 1986). Watzlawick et al. (1974, p. 95) write that to reframe means ". . . to change the conceptual and/or emotional setting or viewpoint in relation to which a situation is experienced and to place it in another frame which fits the 'facts' of the same concrete situation equally well or even better, and thereby changes its entire meaning." To reframe some event, behavior, or situation means to change how it is interpreted, which changes the meaning that the event, behavior, or situation has for the individual. The person's worldview, perception, understanding—in a sense their "truth"—has been altered (Watzlawick, 1978). By changing the interpretation, the person's emotional response also changes. Thus, reframing can be used as an intervention to alter intense emotions and problematic behavioral expressions of emotion (Nugent, 1991). Reframing also can be used to break up the rigid, limited view of a situation that persons involved in a dispute may hold. It can be used as a means of changing disputants' perceptions so that they may become more open to considering alternative solutions to a dispute. Indeed, sometimes simply reframing how something is interpreted can eliminate a problem, with no other intervention needed (Zillman, 1993).

One of the clearest, and perhaps most creative, examples of reframing comes from the clinical work of Milton Erickson. Erickson was approached by the mother of a fourteen-year-old girl who had become obsessed with the idea that her feet were too large. The mother told Erickson that the girl had become more and more withdrawn over the past three months and that all the mother's efforts to reassure her daughter had failed. The girl had become very reclusive.

Erickson, being a medical doctor, arranged to give the mother a physical exam at her home with the daughter in attendance. In Haley (1973), Erickson recounts:

> When I arrived at the home, the mother was in bed. I did a careful examination. . . . The girl was present. I sent her for a towel, and I asked that she stand beside me in case I needed something. . . . This gave me an opportunity to look her over. She was rather stoutly built and her feet were not large.
>
> Studying the girl, I wondered what I could do to get her over this problem. Finally, I hit upon a plan. As I finished my examination of the mother, I maneuvered the girl into position directly behind me. I was sitting on the bed talking to the mother, and I got up slowly and carefully and then stepped back awkwardly. I put my heel down squarely on the girl's toes. The girl, of course, squawked with pain. I turned to her and in a tone of absolute fury said, "If you would grow those things large enough for a man to see, I would not be in this sort of situation!" The girl looked at me, puzzled, while I wrote out a prescription and called the drug store. That day the girl asked he mother if she could go to a show, which she hadn't done in months. She went to school and church, and that was the end of three months' seclusiveness. (p. 198)

Erickson managed to change this girl's view of her feet, and put an end to an increasingly rigid pattern of behavior, with this one intervention. Other specific examples of reframing can be found in Haley (1973), Bandler and Grinder (1982), Weeks and L'Abate (1982), Watzlawick et al. (1974), Watzlawick (1978), and Hepworth and Larsen (1986).

There are two general ways in which a person's interpretation of events, behaviors, or situations may be reframed: the "systematic" procedure and the "finesse" procedure. The cognitive restructuring methods such as "thought catching," "the triple column method," and "identifying the distortion," described by writers such as Burns (1980), Beck (1976, 1988), Williams (1984), and Deschner (1984), are excellent examples of the "systematic" approach to reframing, as is the problem definition procedure described below. The cognitive restructuring approach has clinical and experimental evidence supporting its effectiveness. (Barlow, 1988; DeRubeis & Feeley, 1990; Deschner, 1984; Nugent, 1991; Williams, 1984).

The following steps might be followed in applying the clinical restructuring techniques to reframing:

1. Frame part of the dispute between the involved parties as resulting from possibly erroneous perceptions. Explain how feelings and behavior appear to result, at least to some extent, from how a person thinks. For example, in families, disputes can arise from individuals incorrectly mind reading the intentions and feeling of another family member.

2. Inform the person about any of a number of distorted thinking patterns, called "cognitive distortions" and described by Burns (1980), Williams (1984), and Beck (1988), that seem relevant to the conflict. A list of some of these distorted patterns is provided in Table 16-2.

TABLE 16-2   Several Cognitive Distortions and Their Definitions

Mind Reading: Assuming that one knows the thoughts, feelings, motives, intentions, etc., of another without him or her explicitly communicating them.
Example: Jane sees Bob frowning and thinks he is angry at her.

Fortune-Telling Error: Imagining some event in the future and then acting (i.e., basing one's subsequent behavior) as if this event had already occurred.
Example: Joe imagines asking Sue out on a date and in his imagination sees her turn down his request. So because he knows she will turn him down, he does not ask her out.

Overgeneralization: Thinking that a particular behavior, event, or situation represents a never-ending exclusive pattern. This pattern may be involved with a phenomenon called mood congruent recall described by Barlow (1988).*
Example: A traffic light turns red as Jim is driving across town. While sitting at the light, Jim thinks to himself, "These lights always turn red for me."

Personalization: Imagining that 1) the behavior of others is directed at oneself; and/or 2) that one is responsible for events, the behavior of others, or situations that one actually has little or no influence over.
Example 1: Jackie sees two people laughing at a table next to hers and thinks they are laughing at her.
Example 2: Joe's son is arrested for smoking marijuana, and Joe thinks that it is all his fault (because he was a "bad parent") that his son got involved with drugs.

Magnification: Blowing the significance of an event, behavior, or situation out of proportion.
Example: Betty gets a B on an exam and feels that she is a failure as a person.

Minimization: Belittling or minimizing the importance of some event, behavior, or situation.
Example: Eric goes through a master's degree program with all As and thinks, "It really means nothing; anyone could have done it."

Clairvoyance Error: Assuming that others can read you well enough to know what you need or want without your actually letting them know (sometimes this assumption is turned into an expectation or demand of another person).
Example: Kim gets home from work needing some comforting from Ed. She expects him to "know" she needs comforting without her telling him (and becomes resentful when he does not comfort her).

Biased Attributions: Attributing only negative (or positive) motives or interpretations to the behavior of another person. This distortion may also be related to the phenomenon of mood congruent recall.*
Example: Over time Jane comes to interpret all of Bill's behavior as coming from his "lack of concern for me."

Selective Focus: Noticing only a particular type of event, behavior, or situation consistent with a particular belief, and ignoring (or failing to notice) those that are inconsistent with the belief.
Example: Bob has come to "believe" that his son "has no respect" for him. He notices behaviors that his son engages in that fit this belief but fails to note times when his son behaves in ways that are inconsistent with this interpretation.

*Mood congruent recall refers to the phenomenon that human beings, when in a particular mood (such as feeling angry or depressed), will have an easy time remembering events that fit this mood and will have a very difficult time remembering events that do not fit this mood. See Barlow (1988) for a discussion.

3. Have the disputant relive in his or her imagination a relevant part, or parts, of a conflict situation. During this revivification, have the person be alert for and identify "automatic thoughts" that seem to just pop up in the person's mind and are assigned the value of "truth" without any reality testing. Beck (1988) gives a description of this technique, which he calls the "instant replay," while Williams (1984) refers to it as "thought catching."

4. Help the disputant to identify distortions in his or her automatic thoughts and challenge their validity by reality testing. This can be done by having the person write down accurate, distortion-free alternatives to the automatic thoughts. Reality testing also can be done by helping a disputant come up with some means of determining which of his or her views of an event, behavior, or situation are valid (Burns, 1980; Williams, 1984; Beck, 1988).

This systematic approach to reframing has been used most often in clinical contexts. However, you can adapt this reframing approach to any context in which you have good rapport and in which you will have multiple contacts with the disputants.

The following method of defining the problem to be resolved in mediation is a second example of a systematic approach to reframing. I am indebted to a colleague of mine, Ms. Elaine Wynn, for my knowledge of this approach to reframing. This problem definition method involves three steps: 1) listing aspects of the current undesirable state, 2) listing aspects of the future desired state, and 3) framing a "What do we do to get from the current, undesired state to the desired state?" question that becomes the "problem to be resolved" in the mediation. These steps are written on a flip chart or blackboard by the mediator so all persons involved in the mediation can see them.

The current undesired state is the way things currently are; it is the conflict situation that has brought the disputants into meditation but is framed in terms of the needs of the disputants as opposed to their positions. The disputants' positions are the solutions or demands with which they come into mediation. In contrast, their needs are the emotional desires that underlie the conflict situation and on which their positions are based. The desired state is the state of affairs that the disputants would like to have exist as a result of resolving their conflict. The listing of aspects of this desired state should be connected with the current undesired state by addressing the disputants needs listed in the current undesired state. Finally, the "What do we do to get from the current, undesired state to the desired state?" question forms a link between the undesired state and the desired state of affairs. If all disputants agree with the definitions of both the current undesired state and the desired state, and if needs as opposed to positions are listed on the flip charts, then the "What do we do to get from the current, undesired state to the desired state?" question redefines the problem from one in which the disputants attack each other in a win/lose manner into one in which they work collaboratively on a mutually agreed upon goal that involves a win/win outcome.

This process can be better understood by considering the following example. Betty has threatened to take Joe to court over a noise problem. The houses in which Betty (a single mom) and Joe live are next to each other in a residential neighborhood. Joe's garage faces the side of Betty's house on which both her and her seven-year-old daughter Edna's bedrooms are located. Joe is a talented auto mechanic who supplements his income by working on cars after his daytime job. He often works on cars until 11:00 P.M. or even midnight, and he uses air tools to do some of his work. These tools make a good deal of noise and keep both Betty and Edna awake at night until Joe has completed his work. Edna has been suffering from a lack of sleep, and this problem has led to friction between her and her mom and to problems at school. Betty has complained to Joe about the noise, but she does not feel that her concerns have been addressed because Joe has continued to work on cars until late at night. She has threatened to sue him in an effort to get him to stop. This situation has led them to try using a community mediation center to resolve this problem before taking it to court. Betty enters mediation saying, "He has to stop working on cars at all hours of the night or I will take him to court." Joe enters mediation saying, "I am tired of her complaining. I have tried everything I know how to do to pacify her, nothing works."

In the mediation session the mediator has Joe and Betty list the aspects of the current, undesired state on a flip chart. Betty lists the following things:

1. Edna is not getting enough sleep.
2. Betty is not getting enough sleep.
3. Edna is frequently cranky because of a lack of sleep.
4. Edna and Betty are frequently angry with one another over problems that appear to stem from a lack of sleep.
5. Edna is having problems at school that appear to be related to a lack of sleep.

Betty sums up her listing by saying, "We need to be able to sleep through the night without being awakened by the noises made by Joe's tools." Notice that none of these listed aspects of the undesired state of affairs contain positions taken by Betty in regards to the dispute. Compare this list and her summary statement with her statement at the beginning of the mediation: "He has to stop working on cars at all hours of the night or I will take him to court." This is a position statement, not a statement of underlying needs. The mediator must make sure that underlying needs, and not positions, are placed onto this list.

1. Edna would be sleeping through the night without being awakened by noise from Joe's work.
2. Betty would be sleeping through the night without being awakened by noise from Joe's work.

3. Betty and Edna would feel more rested and would be less irritable with one another.
4. Edna would not be having problems at school.
5. Betty would feel that Joe has done what needs to be done to resolve the dispute.

Joe lists the following things:

1. He would be working on cars without having Betty complain about it.
2. He would be using whatever tools he needs to use to do the work that needs to be done on a car he is working on.
3. He would feel that he could do his work without worrying about what Betty is going to say.

Both Betty and Joe agree that his listing captures the way they would both like for things to be after they have resolved their dispute. They then create, with the assistance of the mediator, the following "What do we do to get from the current, undesired state to the desired state?" question:

"What do we do to get from the situation in which Betty and Edna are being awakened by noise from Joe's tools, and in which Joe feels limited as to what he can do and worried about what Betty is going to say about his work, to a situation in which Betty and Edna are sleeping without being awakened by noise from Joe's work on cars and in which Joe can use the tools necessary to get the work done that needs to be done on a car?"

Both Betty and Joe agree that his problem statement captures what they want to accomplish. This question now becomes the "problem to be worked on" through the remainder of mediation.

Notice how this process has transformed the dispute from one in which the problem lies with the other person into one in which they are collaboratively working to resolve a mutually agreed upon problem that is external to both persons. This transformation is a reframing, and the procedure that is used to arrive at this transformation is an example of a systematic approach to reframing.

The finesse approach is exemplified by the reframing done by Erickson described above. In this approach, the mediator creates in his or her own mind an alternative interpretation of events, behaviors, or situations and attempts to communicate this alternate meaning to the disputant in such a way that he or she accepts it in lieu of the interpretation he or she has been holding. I call this the finesse approach because it is less obvious and less direct and takes more creativity and flexibility on the part of the mediator.

The finesse approach to reframing has two fundamental steps:

1. The mediator creates an alternative interpretation, or framing, of an event, behavior, or situation that is different from that held by the dis-

putant. This interpretation must fit the event, behavior, or situation the disputant is focusing on as well as the framing the disputant is currently using, but also must entail different meanings and imply alternative solutions to those attempted by the disputant.

2. The mediator then must communicate this alternative interpretation to the disputant in such a way as to maximize the probability that he or she will drop the old interpretation and accept this new one.

There are a number of ways to create an alternative interpretation. You may directly change the meaning ascribed to the stimulus. For example, verbal labels such as "insensitive" might be redefined as "defending oneself from being hurt." The label "submissive" might be redefined as "seeking authority and direction." Weeks (1977) and Weeks and L'Abate (1982) give numerous other examples.

Time may be used as an element in reframing. For example, a disputant said, in an earlier example, "I want him arrested! I know he stole it and I am sick of having things stolen! There have been a bunch of my things stolen and no one cares. No one has done anything about my things." This person's perception of the situation and her proposed solution (having the other person arrested) might be reframed by the response, "Yes, you are angry at having your things turn up missing and *up to this point you have not thought of another way of getting what you want* besides having him arrested." The italicized portion of this statement (if accepted by the disputant) essentially puts the conflict into a frame of reference in which other solutions are possible but not imagined or thought of up to this point in time. The implication is that, as time goes on, other solutions may be found that are satisfactory.

Another way in which reframing can be done is context reframing (Bandler & Grinder, 1982). This form of reframing is based on the assumption that all behavior can be viewed as appropriate, given a relevant context. Thus, the practitioner finds a context in which a behavior, currently being rigidly framed in an all-or-nothing manner as problematic, would likely be viewed as positive. When done successfully, the rigid cognitive frame created by the disputant is disrupted, opening up the possibility of alternate solutions. Emotional responses can also be affected, both in intensity and in type of response. For example, consider a situation in which a single mother whose son has been arrested for selling marijuana is upset and angry. This situation has caused substantial conflict at home between the mother and son. Imagine further that the boy had developed a small network of friends who have been helping him sell. The mother has framed the situation, in part, as the boy being "totally bad," a problem that has resulted from her "being a failure as a mother." This view is very rigid. The situation might be reframed by having the woman imagine what the young man would need to do in order to establish a successful automobile dealership. She might be asked to describe business-oriented tasks such as marketing, advertising, and public relations. This could allow the social worker to reframe the situation to show that she actually has done quite a good job as a parent. Her son obviously has the ability to do all these business-related activities because he had to have done them to establish his marijuana-selling network. She might be told that while it is unfortunate that he has chosen to sell an illegal product, she might imagine how successful he might be if he were to choose to market something that is legal and more socially acceptable. If the woman accepts this reframing, she might develop different feelings and views of herself and her son. There are some exercises at the end of this chapter that will help you to gain some skills at finesse reframing.

How a reframed interpretation is communicated to a disputant is critical to the success of this technique. You can increase the likelihood of acceptance by "pacing" the client prior to verbalizing the reframed interpretation (Bandler & Grinder, 1975; Lankston & Lankston, 1983). Pacing refers to meeting the client at his or her frame of reference prior to leading him or her into a new one. This can be done in the following manner:

1. Summarizing, via an active-listening type of paraphrase, the disputant's perceptions.

2. Using the disputant's language in this paraphrase. For example, if the disputant is an adolescent, you will not want to use words that are unlikely to be in his or her vocabulary.

3. Bridging from this pacing over into a delivery of the new (reframed) interpretation. For example, let us return to the statements by the disputant, "I want him arrested! I know he stole it and I am sick of having things stolen! There have been a bunch of my things stolen and no one cares. No one has done anything about my things." In this situation, no one knew where the radio was or whether or not it had been stolen. The young woman's insistence that the young man be arrested inflamed him and inhibited the consideration and adoption of alternative solutions. The young woman's view, framed in her statements above, might be paced and then reframed in the following manner:

   a. "Yes, you are very sick of your things disappearing"

   b. "You are also sick of seeing other people around here react to your complaints in ways that seem uncaring."

   c. "You also sound very angry that no one has yet responded to your complaints in a way that you see as caring."

   d. "It sounds like one of the most important things for you is to know that your things are respected and that you have some private space."

Items 1 and 2 are pacing statements that utilize the woman's words "sick" and "cares." Item 3 is a pacing statement that bridges into a reframing. Item 4 is a reframing statement that may alter the young woman's focus from aggressive retribution (throwing the accused young man into jail) to meeting the needs of privacy, respect, and security. If the young woman accepts this reframing, a plethora of alternatives becomes available.

Historical evidence provides some anecdotal evidence concerning the effectiveness of finesse reframing from the context of international politics. One example is that of King Christian X of Denmark, who reframed a request from a special Nazi emissary for a solution to Denmark's "Jewish problem" by replying, "We do not have a Jewish problem; we don't feel inferior." Later, after the Germans issued an order that all Jews had to wear the Star of David, the king again reframed the situation by announcing that, because there were no differences between one Dane and another, the German order applied to all Danes and that he would be the first to wear the Star of David. The Danish population responded overwhelmingly to the king by wearing the Star of David, and the Germans ended up canceling the order (Watzlawick et al., 1974, pp. 105–6). Fogg (1985) gives other approaches to, and examples of, reframing conflict.

Defining the conflict. Reframing is an intervention that not only can be used to help change strong negative feelings, it also is useful during the problem definition phase. Most often disputants have unknowingly defined a dispute in such a manner that it cannot be resolved without one of the persons involved losing in some way, if it can be resolved at all. For example, when people argue over exactly how some past event occurred, there is little chance that the dispute can ever be satisfactorily settled. Reframing the dispute into something that can be settled is a very useful intervention tactic in such cases.

Consider again the young woman who says, "I want him arrested! I know he stole it, and I am sick of having things stolen! There have been a bunch of my things stolen and no one cares. No one has done anything about my things." It would be very easy in this case to become involved in a no-win game of trying to determine whether or not the young man really did steal the woman's radio. With the dispute defined as, at least in part, "did he or did he not steal the radio," the mediator can rest assured that the young man will fight to prove he did not, while the young woman will fight to prove he did. This is a win/lose definition of the conflict. Reframing the dispute into one in which the young woman finds a satisfactory means of feeling that her belongings are safe in the shelter changes the problem from one with essentially one solution (a verdict about the young man's guilt or innocence) into one with many alternative paths to resolution. Always listen carefully to how disputants are implicitly defining the conflict. Many times you will hear alternative definitions of a conflict implied by what disputants say, even though the exact content of their words may clearly define a dispute in win/lose terms. Once you hear such an implied alternative definition, you can reframe the dispute in these new terms, often with great success.

The three-step approach to systematic reframing described above is an excellent way to get disputants actively involved in problem definition. In fact, this systematic reframing approach can be used as a specific problem definition process. As disputants work their way through this process they will create a new frame within which to view the problem to be solved. This new frame is one in which the "problem" is no longer the other disputant but rather is a "thing" external to all disputants and is a "thing" that the disputants are cooperatively working on to solve.

Another useful intervention during this phase of the conflict resolution strategy is the use of open-ended questions to elicit behaviorally specific definitions of behaviors that are being interpreted in "problem" terms. For example, a father complains that his son "needs to show more respect for authority." The mediator might ask, "How would you like for him to show you respect?" as a means of eliciting behaviorally specific descriptions of "respectful" behavior. Strayhorn (1977) refers to this procedure as "asking for more specific criticism." It is also useful to ask for specific examples of desired (or undesired) behaviors.

Generating alternative solutions.   In this phase, a useful intervention is brainstorming (Levi & Benjamin, 1977). This can be done in a caucus session, or by having disputants in a joint session write down alternatives (Levi & Benjamin, 1977). In brainstorming, the mediator has the disputants create as many alternatives solutions (including wild, creative ones) as they can without evaluating the feasibility of the alternatives. Premature evaluation of alternatives tends to inhibit the creative process.

Choosing alternatives and devising a plan.   Useful procedures during this phase are rating alternatives and using a quid pro quo contract. Rating alternatives involves having disputants rate their level of satisfaction with a given alternative (Levi & Benjamin, 1977). This can be done by having each person rate his or her satisfaction on a scale from −10 (totally dissatisfied) to +10 (totally satisfied). The disparity between scores can serve as an index of the degree of disagreement between disputants, and the sum of all ratings for a given alternative can serve as a useful index of "total satisfaction" with an alternative. This procedure can be used by the mediator to operationalize the ideas of "maximal mutual satisfaction with a solution" and "a win/win solution." The mediator works with disputants to develop a planned resolution that has the highest sum of all ratings and the smallest discrepancy between ratings among a set of possible solution plans. The plan with the highest sum of all ratings and smallest difference between ratings will be the one that entails the greatest mutual satisfaction among disputants.

A quid pro quo contract is essentially an agreement between disputants that says, "I will do this, if you will do that," with the "this" and "that" spelled out in clear, behaviorally specific terms. There are a number of studies demonstrating the effectiveness of negotiating and contracting as a behavioral change procedure (e.g., Jacobson, 1978). The contract, which is best written and signed by all disputants, should specify who will do what, with whom, in what manner, and when or in what situations or contexts. For example, a mediator might write the quid pro quo contract shown in Table 16-3 for two neighbors involved in a dispute. Each disputant, along with the mediator, gets a copy of this written agreement.

There are several important things in this written agreement. First, it clearly specifies who will do what, when, and in what manner. Second, the agreement alternates listing what different disputants will do. It has been found that having a number of actions to be carried out by one disputant listed in their entirety prior to listing the actions to be performed by a second disputant can sometimes lead to an agreement being rejected. A disputant seeing a long list of things that he or she agrees to do, without the list being broken up by things the other disputant agrees to do, can get the feeling that he or she has lost. Finally, the agreement does not contain professional or technical language or jargon. It is best to write an agreement in language that disputants will understand.

Implementing and evaluating the plan.   After an agreement has been reached, it is implemented by the disputants. It is important to evaluate

---

TABLE 16-3   Sample Quid Pro Quo Contract

Dispute Resolution Agreement

Joe Jones agrees to keep his dog out of John Smith's flower bed.

John Smith agrees to call Joe Jones on the phone and discuss any incidents involving Joe Jones's dog on John Smith's property before calling the animal control center.

Joe Jones agrees to have his dog, Growler, complete a dog obedience class within six months from today, July 19, 1999.

John Smith agrees to construct a fence around his flower bed within six months from today, July 19, 1999.

Signed: _____
             Complainant

Signed: _____
             Defendant

Signed: _____
             Mediator

Date: _____

---

the effectiveness of the agreed-upon settlement. This can be done by agreeing to a future meeting in which the agreement is once again discussed. Many times unforeseen difficulties in satisfactorily carrying out an agreement can threaten to rekindle a conflict. By having an agreed-upon future meeting to discuss such possible difficulties, the mediator can head off a renewal of the conflict.

Generalizing the Dispute Resolution Strategy

The role of mediator is useful in many practice situations, several examples of which were given in the beginning of this chapter. The mediator role is generic in the sense that it can be used across a very broad range of settings and contexts. You need not be a marriage and family therapist in order to find yourself in the midst of an interpersonal dispute. Regardless of the practice setting, you will find the techniques discussed in this chapter appropriate and effective.

Especially exciting from a community practice perspective is the growing trend in many states to establish citizen dispute resolution centers. These practice settings entail invaluable community service and work. Persons involved in disputes with others in the community, whether they be neighbors, people in business, friends, or family members, come to these centers in order to peacefully and productively resolve their conflicts. Many such centers provide alternatives to the court system. Social workers who serve in such centers will find the techniques in this chapter especially useful.

CONCLUSION

The problem-solving strategy described in this chapter provides an overall plan for the dispute resolution process. The listing of interventions in Table 16-1 provides a possible sequencing of intervention procedures that you can use as you work through this process. These interventions have been matched with the strategy step in which you may find them most useful. However, as noted earlier, the dispute resolution process is not linear. You may find yourself moving to and from any one of the problem-solving steps more than once during the mediation process. More important than trying to fit the dispute resolution process into a neat and invariant sequence of steps is becoming skilled at using all of the intervention procedures as well as a creative flexibility in sequencing (and even combining) these interventions.

The cognitive behavioral approach to reframing is less useful in contexts in which you have limited contact with disputants. For example, in some county court mediation settings the mediator will meet with disputants for at most an hour or an hour and half. In this setting, the cognitive behavioral approach to reframing is not as useful as the finesse approach. In contexts in which you will have more prolonged contact with disputants, say, several meetings over several days or even weeks, you may find this reframing approach useful.

Finally, keep in mind that the interventions presented in this chapter are like tools. Tools can be used in a variety of ways and need to be used to fit the job at hand. Some of the procedures discussed in this chapter may be more useful in some contexts than in others. Given the practice wisdom and research evidence about the tools described earlier, it would seem that the creative and thoughtful use of these tools can lead to productive, win/win resolutions to interpersonal conflict across a broad range of practice settings.

REFRAMING EXERCISES

1. For each of the following "negative labels" come up with one or more interpretations that are "positive." For example, for the label "nosy," as in "he is really nosy," you might reframe it to mean, "a person who is very curious and inquisitive." In each of the phases below, the negative label is italicized.

   a. He is *nerdy*. She is *stubborn*. He is *ornery*.
   b. She is *reclusive*. He is *passive*. She is *submissive*.
   c. He is too *self-critical*. She is too *seductive*.
   d. She is *insensitive*. He is *impulsive*. She is *oppositional*.
   e. He is a *crybaby*. She is too *withdrawn*. He is a *dumb jock*.
   f. She is *stuck-up*. He is *wandering*. She is too *controlling*.
   g. He is *oversensitive*. She is a *nymphomaniac*. He is *manipulative*.

2. For each of the situations below, find one or more contexts in which the italicized behavior would be considered appropriate, even desirable. Then, write out a statement you might use to do a context reframing of the behavior. You may reframe the meaning of the behavior as well as do a context reframing.

   a. A mother complains to you that her daughter, "*sleeps with every guy she meets*. She meets some new boy, and the next thing you know she is in bed with him."

   b. A father complains that his son, "*never does any work around the house*. All he does is watch TV. He's a lazy bum."

   c. A supervisor complains about a subordinate, "*She never does things the same way twice*. She always wants to do *things some new-fangled way* rather than standardize them as the agency's regulations require."

   d. A son complains about his father, "He is always on my back. *He is always telling me what to do*. I can't stand him."

CHAPTER 17

Engaging Nonresident Fathers in Social Work with Fragile Families

Waldo E. Johnson, Jr.

In this chapter, Johnson broadens the traditional scope of social work practice with families to include a discussion on a critical contemporary social theme: How to involve or engage unmarried, nonresident fathers in the care of the child and family. Johnson examines the barriers to paternal involvement and highlights the best practice wisdom regarding paternal involvement, the relevance of the paternal and maternal family of origins, and the institutional supports needed to encourage paternal involvement. This chapter includes a discussion about the concept of unmarried and nonresident fatherhood as a basis for social work practice. This discussion provides the reader the historical context and significance of fatherhood and social work practice. The reader is presented with the challenges, conditions, and limitations involved with nonresident fatherhood, as well as the factors influencing paternal involvement and nonresident fatherhood. Information about the early beginnings of programs for nonresident fathers is provided, as well as a detailed discussion on the importance of knowing the family systems and family-of-origin factors involved with nonresident fatherhood. The chapter includes a discussion about the role of finances in father involvement from conception onward as a basis for using the strengths perspective with this population. Johnson stresses that being informed about paternal involvement is of fundamental importance for ensuring successful practice. The reader is also provided with information and ways of thinking about the critical issue of access to family support services for unmarried, nonresident fathers. Providing practice support to nonresident fathers from fragile families and in at-risk circumstances is emphasized

INTRODUCTION

Traditional notions about American family life conjure up nostalgic images of father, mother, and children residing in a nuclear household. Such notions also presume that the family unit operates independent of extended kin and friend networks. In these depictions, the father is the designated and often the only provider, the breadwinner, while the mother assumes primary responsibility for maintaining the household and child rearing, virtually limiting or restricting her labor force participation outside the home. This autonomous family unit is also presumed to be totally self-sufficient, in financial and nonfinancial matters, one that operates without government intervention or financial/nonfinancial support from the extended family. However, such depictions of the American family structure and its intended function are becoming increasingly rare. Both the structure and function of the American family have evolved over time as it endeavors to adapt to both structural and social changes in the world order.

Family historian Stephanie Coontz (1997) examined the variety of family types that have successfully and unsuccessfully existed throughout American history. She contended that "when families succeeded, it was often for reasons quite different than the stereotypes about the past suggested—because they were flexible in their living arrangements, assistance or support. And when families failed, the results were often devastating. There was never a golden age of family life, a time when all families were capable of meeting the needs of their members and protecting them from poverty, violence and sexual exploitation" (p. 2).

Coontz's findings not only called into question the sustained romanticism that permeates contemporary dialogue about the demise of the family, middle class family values, and a desire to return to the traditional family bemoaned by some social scientists and politicians, but also redefined the family historically as a resilient American institution that is anything but normative. The historical context in which Coontz described the American family acknowledges that various family structures and configurations are indeed responses to racial, socioeconomic, technological, and demographic shifts imposed upon the extensive array of racial, ethnic, and cultural groups that compose American society. American families, as Coontz suggested, have been anything but passive reactors. Resilience notwithstanding, these various family structures and configurations often require external support to sustain themselves and to promote the highest individual functioning. This chapter examines paternal role involvement among poor nonresident unmarried fathers in fragile families (in which children are born out of wedlock to low-income and poorly skilled parents) and how family-sensitive social work practice can support both paternal and maternal efforts aimed at improving family functioning and child well-being.

Going against the Wind: The Social Construction of Unmarried, Nonresident Fatherhood

Men, in their roles as husbands and fathers, irrespective of their racial, socioeconomic statuses and preparation, have overwhelmingly embraced and undertaken the provider role. Cazenave (1979) contended that African-American men have fully embraced the provider role as an "interface phenomenon" (p. 67) by which provider role success validates their undertaking nurturing and other supportive roles. Cazenave's contention raised concern about this paternal involvement framework given that African-American husbands and fathers are less likely than their white counterparts to enjoy provider role success because of the confounding structural barriers of race and socioeconomic status. These structural barriers, combined with educational, vocational, and, among young fathers, developmental unpreparedness, are linked to psychological role strain, which is common among African-American fathers and is induced by their inability to uphold their own paternal expectations (Bowman, 1989).

Provider role failure among fathers and male heads of households that results in father absenteeism and irregular or nonfinancial and other material support may appear as noncommitment to parenthood and family headship (Johnson, 1995; Ehrenreich, 1983). Clearly, some fathers reject their paternal responsibilities, which are strongly associated with the financial and psychological well-being of their children. Provider role failure among poor urban nonresident and unmarried fathers may more accurately reflect the influence of evolving structural and demographic societal changes on family formation patterns and paternal role behaviors (Johnson, 1998). While some fathers shirk their paternal responsibilities without just cause, the extent to which the fathers described above encounter difficulty in shielding their families from hunger and lack of clothing and shelter may be explained in terms of their increasing unpreparedness to qualify for jobs that sustain families. These unmarried fathers often assume paternal obligations subsequent to making poor choices regarding formal and vocational education. Their efforts to gain employment are occurring during a period of labor force development when the skill level necessary to assume and sustain family headship and paternity has increased. Men in intact married families are often better prepared educationally and vocationally for entering and sustaining themselves in the labor force chiefly due to their advanced age. Their labor force participation is more likely to yield wages that will sustain a family, thus making them attractive as husbands and fathers. In contrast, adolescent and young adult men who become fathers before they are fully prepared educationally, vocationally, and developmentally to assume the economic as well as the noneconomic expectations and challenges of family life and parenthood are less likely to sustain themselves in intact families (Johnson, under review).

The increase in young fatherhood among adolescent and often poorly educated young adult males has occurred concomitantly with the heightened expectation that persons entering the labor force possess increased formal education and technical work skills. This heightened labor force expectation, given many young fathers' lack of educational and occupational preparation, renders them virtually ineffective as family providers, protectors, and guardians. As a result, poor young fathers often resist committing to marriage and traditional familial and paternal roles. They comprise the growing number of inner-city men excluded from "the male marriageable pool" to which Wilsonian theory partially attributes the declining marriage rates among the inner city poor (Wilson, 1996).

The importance of economic security cannot be minimized as a basis for couple and family formation. Given the male dominance in the labor force and in social leadership, it is plausible the economic security and development of the American family is hinged largely on the success of husbands and fathers. Paternal involvement, however, encompasses far more than providing financial support. When examined solely from an instrumental perspective, our understanding of paternal involvement is limited in terms of the multiple, interactive roles which fathers play in their paternal development and the effects of paternal involvement on child well-being. The assumption of multiple, interactive paternal roles is particularly crucial when framing paternal involvement among poor unmarried, nonresident fathers, given that their developmental and socioeconomic statuses often truncate their effectiveness as financial providers.

Boyd-Franklin (1989) contended that cultural issues, including racism, extended family patterns and informal adoptions, role flexibility and boundary confusion, religion and spirituality, and the socioeconomic differences between poor inner-city single parents and middle-class families, highlight the broad diversity among these African-American families. Without needed parenting supports, poor fathers, like poor mothers, experience great difficulty in meeting the needs of their children. Efforts undertaken by these young fathers to assume traditional head-of-household and paternal responsibilities are often unsuccessful because of the lack of preparation and formal social supports to assist them.

American social welfare policy encompasses a long-standing recognition but fluctuating commitment to providing public support to families in need. This recognition and commitment is punctuated by the persistent need to distinguish those deserving of public support from those viewed as undeserving (Patterson, 1994). Men fall into the category of "undeserving poor," meaning that their poverty is attributable to their unwillingness to take responsibility for themselves. It is largely believed that work opportunities for men are boundless and only those who are given to laziness and sloth find themselves in need of help. Traditional public support for men has been uneven and sensitive to the waves of political change. While the number of acceptable roles for men has increased historically since social Darwinism was formally embraced in American thought (Hofstader, 1944), public support for aiding men has generally waned. It has remained small in scale in comparison with the public financial support for women and children, who are generally considered as the "deserving poor," even as members of the same impoverished families.

Contemporary responses to the deserving poor, however, have not escaped critique. Conservative interpretations suggest that women and children originally targeted for public support were victims of unfortunate life circumstances, for example, widows and children who were orphaned as a result of military service or accidental work-related deaths (Mead, 1986; Murray, 1984). According to these interpretations, nonmarital parenthood that results in public dependency raises a social concern of whether it is worthy for public financial support. This intersection depicts the failure of American social welfare policy to fully reflect how the economic and structural changes in American social life have affected individual and family functioning.

Social work responses have generally embraced the provision of support to the deserving poor via efforts to meet maternal and child needs to families in distress. With the exception of social work intervention practices framed from a systems orientation, these poor families are often presumed to function in the total absence of fathers and male members (Anderson-Smith, 1988). The findings of Danziger and Radin (1990) suggest that fathers' absence does not necessarily mean uninvolvement. When residing in the household, their impoverished presence has made some social work interventions more contentious and difficult to justify, often resulting in their becoming invisible or deserting their families in order that their families may qualify for public, poverty-level support. Effective social work intervention aimed at fragile families supports the presence and involvement of fathers, and under circumstances where fathers appear absent, encourages their return and active engagement (Johnson, 1998).

FACTORS INFLUENCING PATERNAL INVOLVEMENT AMONG UNMARRIED, NONRESIDENT FATHERS

As stated earlier, the contemporary American family encompasses a broad range of structures. The two-parent, nuclear family, long idealized as the family structure of choice, continues to decline in number as divorce and cohabitation rates steadily rise. The legal and nonlegal statuses of couple formation have important consequences not only for relationship dissolution, but also for child and family development, and these consequences also determine the survival of the traditional nuclear family unit (Johnson, 2000). Unmarried parenthood has evolved into a major family structure among all racial and socioeconomic groups in the United States, but it has had a uniquely different impact on poor, young couples. While some of these couples never cohabit, many of the cohabiting relationships end before the pregnancies come to full term or within a year of the birth.

Social work interventions aimed at engaging unmarried, nonresident fathers in family support and development must consider and integrate factors that influence as well as facilitate paternal involvement. Becoming a father prematurely (chronologically and developmentally) and having a child out of wedlock means that many of the ways in which fathers become involved in their children's lives are truncated (Johnson, 1998). Given their usual impoverished status, due in part to their truncated developmental statuses, unmarried, nonresident fathers, like their partners, are in need of formal and informal social supports to lessen their otherwise difficult transitions into parenthood. Fathers in general often face difficulties in gaining access to parenting support services. Because parenting support services are generally tied to child custody, unmarried, nonresident fathers seldom have full or partial custody. If they have not established legal paternity, they are at risk of being ignored and unserved by both the legal and social service systems.

Fatherhood programs have evolved in response to the needs of low-income, noncustodial parents. The existing fatherhood programs are geared to tackle many of the issues facing nonmarital parents among nonresident parents, but the family support field has not given sufficient attention to the needs of fathers as parents. Organizational efforts and service provision among fatherhood programs is inconsistent. Efforts to identify paternal role issues and best practices for addressing these issues remain in the early stages of development. The small number of fatherhood programs and their geographic concentration also complicate efforts to assess their effectiveness in promoting paternal involvement among nonresident parents.

The following facts should be considered and integrated into social work interventions aimed at engaging unmarried, nonresident fathers and their families of procreation. The nature of the couple's relationship with the father's and the mother's family of origin, paternal contributions during pregnancy, and paternal access to parenting support services for fathers are important factors for integrating unmarried, nonresident fathers into social work interventions with fragile families. These factors are based on both field- and practice-based empirical research examining the paternal perceptions, pattern of involvement, and life course trajectories of unmarried young fathers.

Couple Relationships before and during Pregnancy

The formation of couple relationships among unmarried people suggests that young males are indeed capable of forming bonding relationships. Although earlier studies depict expectant unmarried mothers as victims of "hit-and-run" victimizers, Florsheim, Moore, and Suth (1997) report that the quality of the relationship among expectant mothers and fathers is of primary importance in understanding the couple's commitment to one another. Novotny (1998) reports that young expectant fathers are prone to express a mix of positive and negative emotions about their partners. His research explores how these fathers sustain the mixed emotions and how they impact relationship quality in light of the developmental changes they experience. Moore (1997), using data from the National Survey of Family Growth and complementary data from the National Survey of Adolescent Males, found that among females who describe their first sex as voluntary, 73 percent indicate that their first partner is someone they had been "going steady" with; another 20 percent were friends with their first partner or dated him occasionally.

In contrast to perceptions that many nonmarital births occur between young parents who barely know one another, these studies suggest that couple relationships do indeed precede nonmarital parenting. These and other research findings suggest that the relationship between the unmarried fathers and mothers both prior to and immediately following the birth is a critical factor in predicting paternal involvement (Florsheim et al., 1997; Cochran, 1997; Danziger & Radin, 1990; Marsiglio, 1989; Westney, Cole, & Munford, 1986; Lamb & Elster, 1986; Hendricks & Montgomery, 1983; Hendricks, Howard, & Caesar, 1981). In particular, fathers who took part in decision making (especially pregnancy resolution) were highly involved in parenting (Miller, 1994). However, it is unclear to what degree the relationship between the young parents varies by race and ethnicity and the cause(s) for such differences (Florsheim et. al., 1997; Danziger & Radin, 1990). For example, young Hispanic couples are more likely to maintain their relationships than young African-American couples. The higher rate of marriage among young Hispanic couples might explain this, but there is no real clear explanation.

As stated earlier, the relationship between the unmarried father and mother both prior to and immediately following the birth is a critical factor in predicting and sustaining paternal involvement. Miller (1994) found that those fathers who took an active role in decision making (especially pregnancy resolution) were highly involved in parenting. Many young unmarried prospective fathers tend to view pregnancy resolution decisions as resting with the expectant mother (Johnson, 1993) and tend to abide by her wishes. Maternal decisions regarding pregnancy resolution, however, do not prevent unmarried expectant fathers from resisting paternal involvement subsequent to the birth of the child. Pregnancy resolution decisions that do not allow input from the young father may deteriorate an already fragile couple relationship (Johnson, 1993; Marsiglio, 1989).

Discussion about pregnancy resolution is much more likely to occur when the couple has a long-standing, monogamous relationship. Among adolescents and young adults, the relationship duration is generally short in time, often less than one year (Marsiglio, 1989) as compared with traditional adult relationships that result in an out-of-wedlock pregnancy. Yet, in examining the factors that contribute to the young unmarried father's involvement with the child, the evolution of his relationship with the young mother may provide some insight into predicting his subsequent paternal involvement. Paternal identity among poor, young males often foreshadows their parental behavior as fathers (Johnson, 1995). Some young unmarried fathers are willing to assume paternal responsibility, although they often lack the necessary education, skills, and development for paternal role success. Marsiglio (1988) examined racial differences in paternal readiness among adolescent fathers. His findings suggest that poor, African-American adolescent fathers often embrace normative paternal expectations more strongly than their white counterparts. In the Marsiglio sample, the inability of the young African-

American fathers to undertake these paternal role expectations (primarily instrumental obligations shaped by prevailing normative expectations) contributed to paternal role strain (Bowman, 1989) that often incapacitated their efforts to engage in other paternal role functions.

Father's Family of Origin Influence on Paternal Involvement

The reaction of the father's family of origin to an out-of-wedlock pregnancy and/or his paternity often impacts his paternal involvement (Miller, 1994; Johnson, under review, 1993; Christmon, 1990a; Rivera, Sweeney, & Henderson, 1987, 1996; Sullivan, 1986). Social support (both emotional and practical) offered to the young unmarried father by his family of origin for his assumption of paternity is a critical factor in determining his engagement with the child. Miller (1994) found that paternal grandmothers' provision of social support to their sons in their roles as fathers was particularly influential in shaping paternal behavior. In Miller's research study, 36 percent of the respondents reported that their mothers played important roles in assisting them in child-rearing activities, as well as in teaching them about fatherhood. Miller defined social support in terms of both emotional support, which included offering advice, counseling, or just listening to the father's concerns, and practical support, which included offering financial resources and actual assistance in child-care activities provided by the baby's paternal grandmother. He further states

> The emotional support these young fathers received from their mother is associated with improved parenting behavior in that the father perceives that he can obtain the necessary guidance within the environment in order to perform his responsibilities. Through this type of support, the young father is able to gain an understanding of what is expected of him as a father. (Miller, 1994, p.372)

Although conventional wisdom attributes nonresident fatherhood among poor urban males to premature adolescent forays into sexual activity, empirical research linking this societal belief to such outcomes remains elusive. Given the large number of urban, impoverished young males residing in single, female-headed households, there is urgency in identifying how various family structures and compositions affect the young males' subsequent sexual and parenting perceptions and behaviors. Clearly, there is much to learn about the influence of parents and other family members in shaping paternal role development.

Earlier studies suggest that the response of the father's family of origin to the pregnancy and his paternity positively influences his paternal involvement (Miller, 1994; Johnson, 1993; Christmon, 1990a; Rivera et al., 1987, 1996; Sullivan, 1986). In contrast, other studies question the impact of the father's family of origin on his paternal role development (Christmon, 1990b; Anderson, 1989). Variations in study samples and differences in variables and factors examined and methods employed possibly explain these contrasting findings, but in the absence of analyses that can be examined across studies, these findings remain unclear. For example, Miller found that mothers are particularly influential in shaping their sons' paternal behavior as unmarried young fathers. This contention potentially offsets concern raised about the unfulfilled role of absent fathers in shaping their sons' paternal behavior. Anderson, in contrast, found that street culture in poor urban communities often exerts a stronger influence on young men's paternal identity and role performance than parents and family, often resulting in a rejection of paternal role development. These differences in research findings raise important questions about the circumstances of family relationships and environment as facilitating and/or buffering young men's perceptions and behavior toward paternity.

Some young fathers in the Johnson (1993) study reported that their mothers and grandmothers were the determining factors in their becoming involved with their out-of-wedlock children. They depicted these parents not only as encouraging them to become involved fathers, but also as facilitators of paternal involvement. They gave money to the young father so he could provide regular financial support to his child when he was unable to earn money and gave money or gifts directly to the children on holidays and special occasions. Thus, as stated above, such social support (both emotional and practical) offered to the young unmarried father by his family of origin for his assumption of paternity is critical factor in determining his engagement with the child.

Empirical studies examining how the father's family of origin acts as a barrier to paternal involvement are yet to be undertaken. Young fathers who resided with their families of origin frequently reported pressure, both perceived and real, to provide financial support for their residence. This expectation, while not unrealistic, often diminished the level of support they could provide for their children and families of procreation. Given their limited earning potential, these expectations and demands weakened the paternal role with which they were most likely to identify and subsequently weakened the couple and parenting relationship (Johnson, 1993).

Mother's Family of Origin Influence on Paternal Involvement

Even fewer studies have documented the maternal family of origin's influence on paternal involvement among young unmarried fathers (Cervera, 1991; Danziger & Radin, 1990; Sullivan, 1986). These studies examined the maternal family of origin's receptivity to a young unmarried father's engagement with the young mother and child as a major determinant of his paternal involvement. These findings, along with anecdotal information, contribute to the depiction the maternal family of origin as gatekeepers, who prevent unmarried, nonresident fathers from sustaining contact and involvement with expectant young mothers following the acknowledgment of the pregnancy, during the pregnancy, and subsequent to the child's birth (Johnston, 1993; Sullivan, 1985). This is unfortunate, since, as Danziger and Radin (1990) report, unmarried, nonresident fathers are often a source of emotional support to their expectant and parenting partners. Although the extent to which and the circumstances under which father involvement among unmarried, nonresident fathers affects child development remains unclear, it is clear that positive father involvement contributes to the child's emotional and financial well-being and development (Lamb, 1997).

The research studies cited previously are unidimensional in their examination of the influence of the maternal family of origin on paternal involvement among unmarried, nonresident fathers; thus, they describe or assess the family constellation as a barrier to paternal involvement. No empirical studies have examined how and the extent to which the maternal family of origin facilitates paternal involvement among unmarried, nonresident fathers. The prevailing traditional research usually depicts paternal involvement among African-American unmarried parents, which is less likely to result in marriage than is white and Latino out-of-wedlock parenting. In addition, the ethnic and cultural identities and socioeconomic statuses of both the maternal and paternal families of origins may influence on how these out-of-wedlock pregnancies are handled. Anecdotal information suggests that among young Latino and white couples, who have higher marriage rates than their African-American counterparts, the maternal family of origin is more likely to support the involvement of the young unmarried father in his family of procreation, especially if his involvement leads to his undertaking a responsible parenting role (Coontz, 1997).

The extent to which the prevailing research tradition offers a racial perspective for examining paternal involvement among unmarried fathers heightens concern about resulting policy and intervention practice because the pervasiveness of this problem crosses racial boundaries. Yet, this racial depiction ultimately affects how policy and practice intervention practitioners frame the problem and the range of possible solutions available toward its eradication. This uneven research tradition has contributed to intervention practice that fails to undertake a system approach in family therapy and support activities. In a family systems approach, the maternal family of origin, as an active participant in the father's procreative family's support system, is encouraged to acknowledge and legitimize other potential sources of support for mothers and their children. In this approach, nonresident fathers are acknowledged.

Father's Financial Contributions during Pregnancy

Providing financial support is virtually synonymous with fatherhood and is regarded as the prime paternal role and responsibility among many unmarried, nonresident fathers. Much of the research on unmarried fathers has examined some aspect of instrumental or financial paternal support, generally as an indicator of paternal commitment and involvement. Some research findings document that many unmarried, nonresident fathers provide financial and other material support to their children (Miller, 1994; Danziger & Radin, 1990; Sullivan, 1986). These findings also suggest that many fathers sustain a level of paternal involvement in spite of their failure to provide financial support to their children.

Paternal involvement during pregnancy is a strong indicator of the quality of the relationship between the unmarried couple. Paternal provision of financial support and other forms of material and emotional support are often crucial to the physical and psychological well-being of poor unmarried mothers during pregnancy. It is an indication of the future commitment to the child. Although the nature of unmarried parenting relationships is such that they are extremely fragile, paternal involvement during pregnancy establishes a baseline of fathering commitment that might increase subsequent to the birth of the child. In addition, many unmarried, nonresident fathers traditionally do not establish legal paternity immediately following the birth of their children, so paternal involvement during pregnancy establishes a critical link to their children that is negotiated based on social determinations of child visitation (Johnson, 1993; Sullivan, 1985).

When preparation and readiness for becoming involved is predicated on the prospective unmarried father's success in providing financial support, even during pregnancy, those fathers with truncated formal and vocational education will likely experience difficulty in living up to such a unidimensional perspective of paternal involvement. The resulting quality of the relationship between the unmarried couple may be irreparably damaged, causing an estranged relationship between the father and his unborn child that continues throughout the child's life.

Access to Parenting Support Services for Unmarried, Nonresident Fathers

The availability of parenting support services for unmarried, nonresident fathers has been examined and cited as an equally critical factor affecting paternal involvement (Johnson, 1998; Allen-Meares, 1984). While many of these studies explored access to parental support services in the context of traditional maternal and child services, these examinations include a mixed bag of programs with varying service qualifications and provisions.

Fatherhood programs have emerged as the primary mechanisms designed to assist noncustodial fathers (or noncustodial parents, who are most often fathers) in their paternal development (Johnson, 1998). Although an emerging literature describes these programs as crucial to supporting paternal involvement among unmarried fathers, their results and benefits are mixed at best. The fatherhood programs chronicled or assessed to date tend to be either small, community-based programs with a broad range of foci and services or large demonstration projects that provide a range of support services but seldom survive beyond the pilot phase (Johnson, Levine, & Doolittle, 1999; Salter & Johnson, 1997; McLaughlin, 1995; Achatz & MacAllum, 1994; Klinman, Sander, Rosen, & Longo, 1986). In addition, fatherhood programs are extremely limited in number, thereby raising concern about their capacity to serve the escalating number of fathers in need.

This raises a continuing criticism of traditional social work and welfare services aimed at unmarried mothers. The maternal and child focus has operated primarily at the exclusion of the unmarried, nonresident father. It is unlikely that the proliferation of fatherhood programs will and can adequately serve all the unmarried, nonresident fathers. While these programs fill a huge void by serving a large population who are otherwise unserved, a systems approach to family support addresses the needs of all members of the family system, irrespective of their legal and/or residential statuses.

SOCIAL WORK PRACTICE WITH UNMARRIED, NONRESIDENT FATHERS IN FRAGILE FAMILIES

Identification of the factors that promote and inhibit paternal involvement among unmarried, nonresident fathers and the role that intervention strategies like fatherhood programs and enhanced social work practice with fragile families play are important for improving their paternal role and partner functioning and ultimately child well-being. These breakthroughs in service provision will guide researchers, policy makers, and social work practitioners in improving paternal role and partner functioning and child well-being outcomes. The benefits of these enhanced efforts aimed at improving paternal role functioning will be shared by the targets—unmarried fathers, unmarried mothers, and their children—and society in general.

Becoming a father prematurely (which is often the case with unmarried fathers) and out of wedlock means that many of the ways in which fathers become involved in their children's lives are at a minimum truncated (Johnson, 1998). Given the impoverished statuses that are descriptive of many unmarried, nonresident fathers, these fathers, like poor unmarried mothers, are in need of formal and informal social supports to lessen the difficult transition into parenthood. Fathers in general often face difficulty in gaining access to parenting support services. Because parenting support services are generally tied to child custody, unmarried, nonresident fathers who neither reside with their children nor have established legal paternity (which is the usual pathway to gaining legal custodial rights) are at risk of being ignored and unserved (Salter & Johnson, 1997). The family support field, in which fatherhood programs operate and which is closely related to social work practice with families, has not given sufficient attention to these unique needs of unmarried fathers and mothers and children in fragile families.

Paternal involvement among unmarried, nonresident fathers is affected by the type of relationship between the unmarried parents. Preliminary findings from the Fragile Families and Child Well-Being Study suggest that poor, unmarried couples who remain in romantic cohabiting or noncohabiting relationships subsequent to the birth of a child are more likely to negotiate paternal visitation and child-care arrangements (Johnson, 1999). Many of these fathers neither resided with nor established legal paternity for their children. Parental connections to their children were based on the maintenance of a minimally friendly relationship with the child's mother, the custodial parent. Even when child visitation arrangements for nonresident fathers permit regular visitation, the arrangements are fragile and extremely sensitive to changes in the couples' relationships (Johnson, 1998). These socially constructed parenting relationships often erode when either parent becomes romantically involved with another person or when family and friends interfere in the couple's affairs.

Strategies for Engaging Unmarried, Nonresident Fathers

Meyer (1987) called for "a unifying perspective to provide greater cohesiveness to social work practice" (p. 414). Such a perspective reflects the person-in-environment focus that has become central to the purpose of social work practice, captures the multiple strands of practice without espousing any particular approach or theory, and addresses the complexity that characterizes the case situations. This framework offers the best strategy for aiding the cause of poor, unmarried, nonresident fathers in fragile families.

In assessing the individual and familial needs of poor, unmarried, nonresident fathers, numerous issues emerge. The first is the need for broader, integrative perspectives of paternal involvement that include and value affective or nurturing contributions of parents (especially fathers) in addition to instrumental or financial contributions. Social work practitioners who work with poor nonresident fathers can ultimately empower them by helping these men to enlarge their conception of fatherhood and paternal involvement. Given these fathers' limited labor force participation, recognizing and embracing affective as well as instrumental paternal roles are crucial to a realization of more fulfilling paternal relationships with their children. Early findings from both the Paternal Involvement Project in Chicago and the Father Resource Center at Wishard Memorial Hospital in Indianapolis, both innovative programs aimed at low-income noncustodial fathers, support the contention that one resource that many of these fathers have in great abundance is time that can be spent building a nurturing relationship with their children. These programs promote this contention by assisting fathers in establishing legal paternity and negotiating visitation rights, believing that once sustaining relationships are fostered, these fathers will financially support their children when possible.

Gender-based parenting roles are rapidly becoming obsolete, and if family formation is an ultimate goal, real flexibility in parenting roles is necessary to accommodate mothers who enter the formal labor force and fathers whose stronger parental involvement may lie in their ability to engage in full-time child rearing and socialization. Such arrangements have yet to be fully explored but clearly highlight that there are gaps in strengthening family support and income security among fragile families. Child and family development courses offered to fathers enrolled in the above-mentioned programs also support this contention. In addition, promoting early attachment to their children increases more consistent father involvement over time (Lamb & Oppenheim, 1989). Given the rising divorce rates and the vast array of family structures that represent the American family, helping unmarried, nonresident fathers bond with their infants not only improves infant development, but also connects the father to his child in ways that potentially will sustain their relationship during marital dissolutions as well as the bouts of unemployment that are unique to these men.

Intervention efforts should first support father-child involvement even before employment preparation in order to increase fathers' motivation and initiative to address other individual needs. Many low-income nonresident fathers also had limited involvement with their own fathers, often due to similar circumstances in the relationship between their parents. They desire to become more involved with their own children, but their unemployed and nonresidential statuses tend to minimize their chances to form developmental relationships with their own children. The proposed approach is a reversal of the traditional method for engaging fathers, who have generally pursued alternative trajectories in family formation and participation. Some fathers may require substantial preparation before they can acquire jobs and financially support their children. Forming such an attachment and commitment to their children may provide the motivation needed to work toward improving their individual preparation for work and problems with sustaining relationships.

There must also be improved education and training to ensure stronger labor force attachment and retention. Most fathers, regardless of their poor preparation or limited ability to financially support their children, believe that providing financial support is crucial to becoming a responsible father. Although institutionalized racism continues to plague their endeavors, inadequate work preparation that inhibits adaptation to technological advances also hampers their potential success in gaining employment. Fathers, regardless of their marital or residential status, should be afforded the best opportunities to parent their children, and the quality of fatherhood is enhanced with advanced education and training. Fathers, spouses or partners, and children alike will all benefit. Work readiness skills, job-seeking and retention skills, and high school, GED, vocational, technical, college, and military service are among the educational services that social workers can provide or facilitate in their clinical interventions with these fathers.

There is a need for individual and innovative, client-centered family therapies aimed at strengthening the unmarried, nonresident father's capacity for relationship building and improving parenting experiences. Prior life experiences often shape the manner in which future relationships are formed. Broken or unfulfilling parenting and family relationships can constrain the conception and formation of future ones. Unmarried fathers and mothers in these fragile families often need assistance in relationship building. The absence of a legal bond like marriage often implies that the couple can maintain loose commitments to each other. This posture is maladaptive for sustaining families.

Parental commitment and consistency are especially crucial if nonresident parenting arrangements are expected to prevail. The fathers may require individual therapy focusing on paternal status in general and its relationship to the multiplicity of roles that men in families are expected to undertake. They may also require family therapy involving not only their partners and children, but also their own families of origin and their partners' families of origin. These family constellations can be sources of strife and conflict. Effective social work practice with fragile families mandates that thorough assessments be taken to identify the range of potential problems that may impede acceptable paternal development and family functioning. It also mandates that the social worker address contextually all related issues that affect the presenting problem.

These recommendations represent individual interventions appropriate for consideration with unmarried, nonresident fathers in the social worker's effort to support paternal involvement. Potential structural interventions are equally broad and extensive, from advocating for more paternal developmental policies that encourage stronger father-child attachment, to supporting legislation that strengthens this attachment by improving unmarried, nonresident fathers' labor force attachment and addressing institutional barriers to paternal involvement like racial discrimination. Social work practice in group therapy may evolve into the support of father networks that advocate for improvements in paternal status among unmarried, nonresident fathers. The combined individual and structural interventions represent the ecological perspective that is pervasive in the profession of social work advocated by Meyer (1987). This unifying perspective represents the range of social work theoretical and conceptual orientations, practice models, and populations that clinical social work practice seeks to, and ultimately can, address.

CONCLUSION

Impending changes in the public support of children born into fragile families present a mixed bag of possible results. Change is imminent, and the process does not promise to be always humane. Social workers are the leading intervention professionals charged with achieving the desired outcomes. However, the methods of and high expectations placed on clinical social work to achieve these outcomes may be at odds with the profession's goals and ethics. As a result, the profession is forced to employ strategies that, at best, straddle the line between professional commitments to society and to the individual.

CHAPTER 18

A Family Eco-Behavioral Approach for Elders with Mental Illness

Elsie M. Pinkston

Glenn R. Green

Nathan L. Linsk

Rosemary Nelson Young

In this chapter, Pinkston and colleagues examine the use of applied behavioral analysis as a practice technology for training and supporting family caregivers of the elderly with mental illness. Operant conditioning and social learning theories are provided as a guide for training caregivers in popular approaches for increasing new behaviors, decreasing undesirable behaviors, and establishing new behavioral skills. The chapter captures the interests of the reader who wants to know more about effective social work practice. The authors present a detailed discussion about the procedures used to teach social workers who work with families of the elderly with mental illness. This chapter provides the reader with knowledge of the empirical supports that govern the reliability and validity of the methods used in working with family caregivers of the elderly. Pinkston and colleagues give the reader the conceptual foundation for developing scientific practice methods in gerontology. Because family caregiving is one humane and culturally supportive environment, the reader is given the basis of the treatment approaches used to prepare family caregivers for their roles as change agents and case managers linking their relatives to community resources. The chapter provides a very rich discussion of the intervention procedures and guidelines for assisting family members in their roles as caregivers. The goals and specific procedures associated with particular objectives are described in detail with very rich examples. The chapter describes the ways and means practitioners use to educate family caregivers and methods for maintaining the behavior change established by the family caregiver during treatment. The chapter describes for the reader the methods that social work practitioners will need to use to discontinue professional involvement and the best ways to transfer the treatment program to the control of the family. It describes the way in which the practitioner experimentally prepares and assigns treatment conditions necessary to maintain the gains achieved during the treatment phases.

PROBLEM STATEMENT

A major achievement of the twentieth century is long life (Neugarten, 1990). As we enter the twenty-first century we assume that this trend will continue and that issues of family care will increase as the number of aging people increases. This achievement brings with it a series of new mental health problems and family responsibilities associated with the very elderly. This chapter is designed to address those problems and to offer assistance to family and community caregivers and service providers. Three assumptions guide this work: 1) Families are the primary unit of care for elderly people; 2) behavioral family training methods are effective; and 3) a broader ecological approach that includes the community will be effective.

This chapter contains specific procedures designed to aid practitioners who teach family caregivers the skills that promote high-quality care for declining elderly people. The training procedures include modeling, corrective feedback, rehearsal, and reinforcement. The explicit intervention techniques use behavioral interventions and specific community service linkages to improve home care. An analysis of how individuals interact with their environment and a combination of behavioral techniques such as contracting, stimulus cues, and reinforcement-based interventions comprise the most highly developed and evaluated interventions. For the most common problems, such as urinary incontinence, low-rate activities, bizarre verbal behavior, and self-care deficits, step-by-step instructions are presented that include procedures for evaluation and revision of each intervention. These procedures represent an application of parent-training techniques derived from operant theory and adapted to elderly people and their families. When applied to the elderly, these explicit procedures are generally effective and show lasting change (Linsk, Pinkston, & Green, 1982; Pinkston & Linsk, 1984a, 1984b; Pinkston, 1994, 1997).

This is a tested service model, which is based on social learning, operant, and case-management approaches. By following the training procedures, practitioners teach caregivers to specify desirable and undesirable behaviors. Caregivers then learn to use behavioral procedures, such as stimulus cueing and reinforcement, to increase the frequency of desired behavior of older people as well as the opportunity for gratifying experiences. Practitioners also teach families how to obtain appropriate community services that provide additional resources for the enrichment of clients' quality of life. Assessment and intervention efforts by practitioners are scheduled in clients' homes for ten or fifteen sessions per client. Additional procedures are introduced to enhance maintenance and for necessary program modifications in the initial plan. A follow-up assessment is conducted to determine the effectiveness of these procedures in achieving maintenance.

These methods emphasize 1) the utility of an individualized measured approach, 2) the efficacy of informal support in treating behavior problems associated with institutionalization, 3) the value of integrating behavioral training procedures and community-linkage procedures for increasing social involvement and decreasing psychiatric complaints, and 4) the importance of ongoing assessment to determine program effectiveness and the appropriateness of modifications.

The program method is divided into seven steps: 1) referral, 2) assessment, 3) definition of behaviors and recording of baseline data, 4) behavioral education of support persons, 5) design of intervention, 6) termination and maintenance, and 7) follow-up. All of the steps are important, but the acquisition and maintenance of positive behavioral effects are essential and are integrated into all parts of the program.

The client, the caregiver, and the practitioner use assessment, an integral part of treatment, to design and revise the intervention. Each client's program is assessed daily, using standardized and individualized instruments. Progress is measured by comparing records of the client's postintervention behavior with baseline data. Preintervention and postintervention questionnaires are used to assess the client's ability to perform daily life tasks and to interact with others at home and in the community. Direct observation measures, recorded by the caregiver and, at times, the client, and indirect measures of functioning and attitudes also aid in evaluation and revision of intervention procedures. Evaluation throughout all aspects of the program helps to establish valid treatment methods.

The procedures in this chapter are based on the findings of a research and service project conducted by the staff of the Elderly Support Project (ESP) and funded by state and federal grants. These particular procedures are supported by two research articles (Pinkston & Linsk, 1984b; Pinkston, Linsk, & Young, 1988).

The broader purpose of this chapter is to present a model for assisting older people who are no longer able to meet their own personal and social needs because of age-related physical and psychological changes. Clients appropriate for these services are age 60 or more, tend to be socially isolated, and exhibit diminished capacity for personal care and other daily life tasks. Many have limited mobility due to physical disabilities such as arthritis and cardiovascular problems. They also have intellectual or emotional difficulties or disorders, including clinical diagnoses of organic brain syndromes, depression, and paranoia, as well as a range of physical impairments. Behavioral deficits and excesses take the form of low rates of socialization, limited regular activities, eating disorders, exercise deficiencies, wandering, destructive acts, excessive smoking, argumentative or bizarre speech or excessive complaining, deficient self-care behaviors, or any combination of these traits. These behaviors often result in an increased risk of relocation or institutionalization. Moreover, they decrease rates of interaction with the community. This further reduces pleasurable activities by limiting access to stimulating situations where social intercourse and friendship might be found, that is, access to reinforcers is decreased.

This program was tested with clients and caregivers who met the criteria just discussed. The procedures improved long-term functioning and decreased the likelihood of institutional care for many of the clients. This was particularly true with older people whose behavioral deficits were in excess of their physical disabilities. These procedures successfully improved the support systems of both the clients and their caregivers, thus decreasing family stress. Generally, the behavioral improvements were maintained over time, as shown by six-month and yearly assessments.

Families usually regarded the program as helpful, viewed the data recording and corrective feedback as important, and found their participation in the design and implementation of the intervention procedures rewarding.

In summary, this behavioral treatment program employs families to enhance the informal client supports, to implement linkage procedures to formal support services, and to improve service coordination. Treatment and linkage procedures facilitate joint planning among older persons, their families and other support persons, and practitioners, to build sustaining systems for older people.

BEHAVIORAL GERONTOLOGY

The problems of the mentally and physically impaired elderly have been analyzed from a behavioral perspective. Lindsley (1964) specified the interrelationship between deficit behaviors of aging persons and environmental shortcomings in terms of appropriate discriminate stimuli and opportunities for reinforcement. This analysis calls for the provision of therapeutic consequences and prosthetic approaches to the problems of the elderly. Hoyer and his colleagues also described the behavioral context of problems of the elderly in terms of the physical and social environment. The more recent behavioral gerontology literature includes reports of the analysis and design of living environments for the elderly (Pinkston, 1997; DeRoos & Pinkston, 1997) and discussions of the advantages of a behavioral approach to treatment of the impaired elderly (Bourgeois, Schulz, & Burgio, 1996; Burgio & Burgio, 1986; Carstensen, 1988).

Fortunately, a wide range of behaviors of older people have been analyzed, treated, and evaluated, and they provide a bank of treatment procedures. In this chapter, behaviors of older persons are classified into categories of self-care, negative activities and verbalizations, positive behaviors, and social contacts. Programs to treat problems in these behavior categories have been developed, particularly in residential institutions.

Programs have been formulated to improve self-care behaviors including eating, dressing, elimination, and walking. Eating problems were treated using positive reinforcement and modeling and feedback (Baltes & Zerbe, 1976; Blackman, Gehle, & Pinkston, 1979). Self-dressing was enhanced by providing materials, prompts, and cues. A number of techniques using schedules and reinforcement procedures were developed to intervene with incontinent elderly people (Pinkston, Howe, & Blackman, 1987). Additional personal care behaviors that have been treated or investigated include brushing teeth, bathing, and sleeping (Pinkston & Linsk, 1984a).

A number of programs were developed that focus on reducing negative behaviors such as self-injurious actions (Mishara, Robertson, & Kastenbaum,

1974) and repetitive movements. Tardive dyskinetic movements were effectively reduced using differential reinforcement of incompatible activities (Albanese & Gardner, 1977; Jackson, 1980).

Programs that increase positive activities included adherence to medical regimen, physical exercise, and activity programs. Participation in activities in long-term care or hospital settings was the objective of several interventions. For instance, by comparing a number of motivating procedures, McClannahan & Risley (1974) found that a combination of discriminative cues and reinforcement most effectively increased participation in structured activities and that program materials were effective stimuli that encouraged such participation. Hoyer and his colleagues also examined participation as a component of studies of specific verbal response increases (Hoyer, Kafer, Simpson, & Hoyer, 1974). Blackman, Howe, and Pinkston (1976) made access to food a reinforcing consequence for participation in proximal social behavior. Linsk, Howe, and Pinkston (1975) demonstrated how teaching a practitioner to ask more questions could increase attending and talking by impaired elders in social group work programs. Levendusky (1978) demonstrated the need for corrective feedback to improve task behaviors of those attending a sheltered workshop for the elderly. All of these techniques may be useful to families concerned about increasing the social participation of the community-residing elderly.

Social and verbal behaviors have been treated to improve quality of life within geriatric institutions (Baltes & Barton, 1977; Hoyer, 1973). Inappropriate verbalizations have been decreased through the use of differential attention techniques. Linsk et al. (1975) successfully developed methods to increase verbal participation with extremely withdrawn and impaired elderly people in a home for the aged. In addition, interpersonal skill-training procedures, including behavioral components, have been used to teach communication, negotiation, and social skills to nursing home residents. Strategies have been suggested to enhance memory, improve orientation, and reduce confusion (Bourgeois, 1990, 1994; Bourgeois, Burgio, Schulz, Beach, & Palmer, 1997).

In summary, a diverse array of behavioral techniques were developed and evaluated for use with older persons. Since 1968, most of this work has occurred within psychiatric hospitals or long-term nursing facilities. Application of these methods to community settings is incomplete. Whereas institutional staff have generally been the primary engineers of behavioral change, application to home settings requires that families be trained to successfully apply behavioral techniques.

FAMILY TRAINING OF CAREGIVERS

As treatment of developmental and behavioral disorders is shifting from the mental health or long-term care institution to community agencies and persons within the immediate environment, families are emerging as a primary resource for extending home care. Although self-management programs have been used successfully with older clients, many older people are unable to act as their own caregivers or support persons. In such cases the family becomes the focus.

Family eco-behavioral methods use reinforcement techniques and environmental management procedures to achieve and maintain improvement (Burgio & Burgio, 1986; Carstensen, 1988). Research has resulted in families being widely accepted by behaviorists as active participants in their elders' therapy (Bourgeois et al., 1996).

Behavioral family treatment includes several aspects of treatment and experimentation that are relevant to family-based care of older people: 1) use of currently accepted behavioral treatment procedures and their effects, 2) use of the home setting for family education and intervention, 3) treatment of a wide range of behavior and socialization problems concerning diverse family members, 4) specific procedures for training caregivers, and 5) a well-developed evaluation methodology (Pinkston, Levitt, Green, Linsk, & Rzepnicki, 1982).

These research and practice findings demonstrate that family members can be taught through instructions, contracts, modeling, rehearsal, and corrective feedback to alter their relatives' behaviors using contingency management procedures. We extend these procedures to relatives of older people with behavior problems and teach caregivers to be more effective in the care they give. Techniques can be used to decrease inappropriate behaviors and to increase desirable behaviors of elderly people and their support persons, thus providing a positive alternative to institutionalization.

LINKAGE WITH COMMUNITY SERVICES

Linking the client to the correct available resources in the community is of great concern for social welfare and for society at large. This is a particularly important behavioral perspective because such linkage is a major way to increase the client's access to reinforcing consequences that will maintain appropriate behaviors. Assessing the need for and providing appropriate service delivery of community services to the elderly is an ongoing problem that requires the further development and evaluation of procedures. While many referrals for service are made, clients may or may not pursue them. Attempts to obtain service are often discouraged by unreceptive or overworked staff, or a mismatch between clients and available resources may occur. Specific methods to monitor linkage activity and resource availability are necessary to provide good service. Weissman (1976) designed a task-centered model of linkage that contained 1) problem identification, 2) resource location, 3) option exploration, 4) resource selection, 5) resource connection, and 6) verification of resource assistance. The linkage to service is central to the maintenance both of elderly persons within the community and of their caregivers' support systems.

HOME-BASED INTERVENTION

We have developed effective procedures to be used with the seriously impaired elderly living at home (Green, Linsk, & Pinkston, 1986; Linsk et al., 1982; Pinkston & Linsk, 1984a, 1984b). We have found that family caregivers of the elderly can implement behavioral methods; that stimulus control and reinforcement are particularly useful; that behavioral family interventions reduce excesses and deficits for the impaired elderly; that caregivers improve their skills, as institutional staff have in previous research; and that single-case methods help to plan and implement interventions as well as evaluate results.

Home-based intervention ensures that family members will be likely to cooperate and comply with treatment goals because they have learned to treat them in the setting where they occur. This removes the necessity to develop a complicated transfer of learning methods from the clinical setting to the home. It also decreases the number of missed sessions during treatment.

In our initial study (Pinkston & Linsk, 1984b), there were twenty-one caregivers and their mentally and physically impaired elderly patients. The median age of the clients was 70, and the caregivers' average age was 59. Caregivers were primarily female and spouses (58 percent) or adult children (42 percent). The sample of clients was 50 percent white and 50 percent African-American. The behavioral interventions used to increase positive behaviors of caregiver and patient dyads and to decrease noxious patient behaviors included didactic lessons, role play, corrective feedback, and data collection. The very encouraging outcome of this research led us to conduct a larger study.

Our second test of the model with sixty-six clients and their caregivers allowed us to replicate our behavioral family research (Pinkston et al., 1988). Our clients were at least 60, had physical or psychological problems, showed "excess disability" (Kahn, 1965; Kahn, Goldfarb, Pollock, & Peck, 1960), behaved badly, and used very little of the community. They had a family member or significant other able to participate in behavioral change efforts.

More important, the caregivers had time for the program, were motivated (adversely affected by the client's behavior), had access to the client's important consequences, had adequate skills or ability to learn skills, and were in good mental and physical health.

ELDERLY SUPPORT PROJECT (ESP)

As stated above, the ESP was implemented in seven steps: 1) referral, 2) assessment, 3) definition of excesses and deficits and recording of baseline data, 4) education of support persons, 5) development of intervention plan using contracting, modeling, cueing, and reinforcement, 6) development of a plan for maintenance of intervention effects, 7) follow-up. (For a detailed description of the program, see Pinkston & Linsk, 1984a.)

Research Designs

Single-case designs (Baer, Wolf, & Risley, 1968, 1987) were used to evaluate the effects of intervention, by comparing baseline observations with intervention observations. Clinical multiple-baseline (Pinkston et al., 1982), multiple-baseline, and AB (baseline, treatment) designs were used most frequently, if the behavior problems under study were not life threatening. These designs showed caregivers the power of their interventions. Pre- and posttests determined the mental status and other demographic characteristics of the clients and their caregivers.

We used direct observations by clients, families, and research staff. The primary observers were usually family members; reliability observations were made by staff members other than the practitioner. These observations were recorded by time sampling (Baer et al., 1968; Pinkston et al., 1982) and checklists (Pinkston & Linsk, 1984a).

Research Support

Our sixty-six clients had serious impairments: Mental status averaged 54 of 100; physical health rated a mean of 5.57 (6 = most negative); mental health, 4.12; activities of daily living, 4.77; social resources, 3.00; and economic resources, 2.36 (Pfeiffer, 1978). The average age of the clients was 73; the male-to-female ratio was 45/55; 66 percent were white, and 34 percent were black (see McGadney, Goldberg-Glen, & Pinkston, 1987 on the issue of working with black elderly clients). The clients' marital status was 58 percent married, 36 percent widowed, and the rest divorced or single. Their mean annual income was $13,020, with 56 percent of them living in their own homes.

The mean age of the caregivers was 64; 75 percent of them were female. Their relationships were 45 percent spouse, 28 percent child, and the rest spread evenly between siblings, friends, or other relatives.

In keeping with the behavioral clinical approach, 86 percent of the interventions were to increase desirable behaviors. Behavioral improvements occurred in 76 percent of the cases; they were sometimes small but were valued by these caregivers. The negative behaviors were so extreme they had to change if the clients were to improve at all.

Failures to improve were associated with poor health of the caregiver, a nonreversible physical condition of the client, and, in a few cases, refusal by the caregiver to record data and implement the program. Caregivers reported a greater degree of personal competence following training; they said they felt more able to cope with their problems. They also reported positive consequences of caregiving (Washington & Pinkston, 1986). Even so, they did not show a significant decrease in score on the Zarit Burden Scale (Zarit, Reever, & Bachman-Peterson, 1980).

These procedures fulfilled the promise shown in earlier research with depressed and demented elderly clients at home. This added to the literature conducted in nursing homes with a similarly impaired population of elderly people. It is apparent that caregivers can be taught to use behavioral procedures, including contracting, cueing (verbal and physical), modeling, and differential reinforcement, and thereby can provide a more prosthetic environment for maintaining elderly people at home.

INTERVENTION PROCEDURES AND GUIDELINES

Assisting family members and elderly clients to alter problem interactions, to provide tangible and needed services, and to increase the occasions and opportunities for stimulation are the goals of any intervention promoting change or maintenance of change. Home-based behavioral interventions build upon an existing and tested model of family intervention and adapt the model's various components to the needs, abilities, and disabilities of an elderly population. As with most structured efforts to modify behavior, this program establishes its particular components according to the individual characteristics of each client, the people that the client interacts with, and the environmental contingencies. It provides realistic and important documentation as different problems are modified, diverse techniques are attempted, and the successes and failures of those efforts are revealed.

Assessment accomplishes a number of tasks: a thorough familiarization with the general circumstances surrounding the identified client, a specification of target problems and their relative importance, a contingency analysis depicting the antecedents and consequences of those target problems, and daily observations by trained family members or other observers. After assessment, emphasis is shifted from gathering information to using that information to formulate and implement efficient and effective behavioral interventions.

Contacts with family members have centered on the practitioner's gathering information and using it to formulate ideas about possible interventions. The information collected during the assessment is used to teach family members new methods of interacting with the client that produce meaningful and socially relevant change.

The Caregiver

Behavioral interventions require a person at home who assumes responsibility for using the behavioral techniques that the practitioner teaches. This person is referred to as the caregiver. The practitioner teaches the agent of change to alter his or her own behavior or to reorganize household tasks and other schedules to reduce the problem behavior of the identified client.

The practitioner is not the ideal person to be the caregiver because of his or her limited interaction with the client. A two-hour interview represents less than 3 percent of the time the client spends each week with family members, friends, and professionals. Employing this support network to the fullest possible extent, therefore, vastly increases the opportunities to modify the client's behavior. The caregiver is selected from family members and friends and taught requisite skills. The tasks of the caregiver are detailed elsewhere (Pinkston & Linsk, 1984a), but they include consistently using the techniques developed, reporting difficulties, noting successes, providing reinforcement opportunities, and assisting the practitioner in problem assessment.

Guidelines for selecting caregivers for older people have not been clearly tested. The caregiver must be someone who has important interactions with the elderly client and who is willing to assume the tasks of the change agent. The caregiver checklist (Pinkston & Linsk, 1984a) may be useful in evaluating potential caregivers. Choice in selecting the caregiver is often limited. Most likely, the caregiver will be the spouse, if the client is married to a capable person. Otherwise the caregiver is likely to be a friend or one of the client's children. Although one person will usually serve as the main caregiver, attempts should be made to involve as many of the people who regularly interact with the client as possible in the overall change effort.

Excellent opportunities to describe the probable course of the intervention arise in the process of selecting the change agent. In describing the tasks of the caregiver, typical situations and anecdotes from previous cases can be included. The practitioner can reemphasize the fact that the caregiver will be making systematic changes in his or her own behavior to affect the behaviors of the client. Finally, the selection of a caregiver allows the family members reasonable opportunities to withdraw from the intervention if they decide that the tasks involved are too much for them to undertake at the time. It also allows practitioners to negotiate reasonable alternatives to the required tasks with family members.

It is advantageous to consider using the person trained to be the observer, if a family member, as the caregiver. Many of the traits that make for excellent observers also make for excellent caregivers. Among them are the ability to discriminate the occurrence and nonoccurrence of a target behavior, the ability to engage in a task contingent on the occurrence of the behavior (act or record), and the necessary time and commitment. Although the roles of caregiver and observer are different, many of the necessary skills overlap and complement each other.

Goals

The practitioner, after a thorough and complete assessment and the collection of baseline data, develops with the client, family members, institutional staff personnel, and other significant individuals a comprehensive statement of the desired effects of intervention, or how things will be different after successful treatment. The practitioner assists the clients, the caregiver, and significant others in the development of time-limited, achievable goals. This process is begun by eliciting from the family members and the client their perceptions of the current problems, including their frequency and typical family responses to them. From this summary, the practitioner presents detailed information on what will be different following intervention. An increase in self-care skills as a goal, for instance, is inadequate. The practitioner can use this general and vague goal to define explicit behavioral goals. Components of appropriate goals include 1) the exact nature of the problem, 2) how the problem will be different as a result of treatment, 3) where that change will occur, and 4) whose behavior will change.

The development of goals necessitates the involvement of significant others, including the caregiver and service providers. Because of the unique nature of the interactions between a client and significant family members, a common statement of goals must often be negotiated. It is important to spend the time and effort before intervention to develop an agreed-upon common statement of goals. This avoids the possibility of involving an individual who has the potential for sabotaging successful behavior change.

Goals for an impaired elderly person are highly individualized. They are directly related to the target problem and should be formulated in concise, short, specific statements. In the process of generating goals, the practitioner should attempt to involve the client. If the client has intellectual limitations, the practitioner should explain the goals in simple and understandable terms and attempt to get the client to restate them in his or her own words, to increase identification and agreement with the goals.

Behavior Change Strategies

The practitioner begins each program design by using the functional analysis presented earlier, the observational data, and the anecdotal reports, selecting one of three directions that guide intervention efforts. If the data reveal overt deficiencies in behaviors, a behavioral program is developed that increases opportunities for stimulation and reinforcement or increases contingent reinforcement. If data reveal an excess in behavioral frequency, efforts are directed toward reducing those excessive behaviors while increasing positive adaptive behaviors that are incompatible with the undesired activities.

Increasing Opportunities for Reinforcement

Practitioner efforts attempt to increase the frequency and quality of opportunities for reinforcement. Reinforcement is a primary focus when assessment and baseline information reveal that contingent family responses are given for appropriate behaviors but that there are barriers or other stimuli that interfere with opportunities for the client to engage in reinforcing behaviors. Opportunities to engage in behavior are lost when others take over many of the day-to-day tasks the client formerly engaged in, often as a result of the client's illness. For example, an elderly client who lives alone may never relearn to shop for groceries following recovery from a stroke because the daughter has taken over this task. A client may never have an opportunity to cook again because family members removed the gas control on the stove after the client was burnt once. Limitations on opportunities for reinforcement often result from the reactions of family members to a previous problem situation. Family members remove the responsibility for specific behaviors, and the concomitant opportunity to receive reinforcement through their successful performance, because of past client failures to adequately perform the task.

Family members are not the only individuals with the power to remove or limit behavioral opportunities for reinforcement. Medical personnel frequently make recommendations that inadvertently limit behavioral opportunities. A physician may recommend that an ambulatory patient be restricted to a wheelchair because of falling incidents. Once in the wheelchair, the client can never be reinforced for attempting to walk even though the physiological ability exists. Or a physician may prescribe major tranquilizers because of overt displays of verbal aggression. The medication effectively reduces the verbal aggression, but it also reduces the overall level of verbalizations, thereby reducing opportunities for the client to be reinforced for appropriate verbal behaviors. Other examples are elderly clients who refuse to leave home because of fear of crime. Staying inside effectively eliminates major opportunities for interpersonal socializing.

Intervention strategies develop programs that teach family members to increase the naturally occurring cues and prompts in the home environment. Ogden Lindsley (1964) was among the first to propose that increasing these cues is an effective technique for expanding the opportunities for, and thus the reinforcement of, deficit behaviors. The practitioner teaches family members to set the client up for reinforcement and to assure that the client is reinforced for the target behavior. These behavioral programs necessitate that the client has the physiological abilities and skills to perform the behavior and that, if the behavior were to occur, it would normally be reinforced.

The environmental cues taught to family members do not have to be complex. Linsk taught a social worker in a reorientation group for impaired elderly clients simply to ask more questions (Linsk et al., 1975). This research demonstrated that increasing questions resulted in more task-oriented verbalizations by the elderly clients. Blackman (1981) has shown that asking clients to dress increases those clients' independent dressing abilities. Blackman's research is important because the staff in the residential facility where the study was undertaken indicated that the clients involved did not have the ability to dress themselves. These studies point to the promising ability that simple cues, questions, and requests all have in increasing environmental opportunities and subsequent reinforcement of target behaviors.

Socialization deficits of the impaired elderly are frequently targets for change. Clients often lack social contacts because there is no one to interact with at home, because family members find those interactions punishing, because clients fear leaving the home, or because clients experience mobility difficulties. Increasing the opportunities for reinforcement is a viable method of increasing socialization. Depending on the level of impairment, suitable services are often available in the community. These services include nutrition sites, meals-on-wheels programs, adult day treatment (see DeRoos & Pinkston, 1997, for behavioral programming in day care), in-home housekeeping or nursing care, and respite care. As Weissman has illustrated (1976), arranging these services is more complex than just giving the family the name and phone number of a service agency. It is typical for practitioners to arrange transportation, find the closest or most appropriate service, handle financial agreements with service providers, quell family fears, and educate service providers on behavioral techniques appropriate to their relationship with the client.

Teaching family members to use environmental cues and community or home help services has two functions. One is to increase the opportunities for client reinforcement. The second is to reduce the amount of care family members need to provide. As clients become more impaired, the stress increases for family members. Family members often find their own lives restricted because of their care-taking responsibilities. Clients who increase skills and behaviors that are deficient are likely to reduce the quantity of needed care provided by relatives. Increasing environmental opportunities provide clients and their family members with increased opportunities to engage in reinforcing activities.

Increasing Behaviors

Deficit behaviors are targeted for increase when caregivers learn to use contingent reinforcement techniques to increase the frequency or duration of low-frequency behaviors. Among the techniques family members can be taught to use are more frequent praise, social attention, touch, special activities, enjoyable activities, and tangible reinforcers like food, cigarettes, or physical stimulation.

Practitioners should avoid complex reinforcers when possible. The elderly are frequently in such a state of deprivation that simple reinforcers like touch and attention are sufficiently powerful to accomplish desired changes. It is impossible for practitioners to know in advance which reward will actually reinforce and increase a desired behavior. Attention may be reinforcing to one client but not to another. Only a functional analysis can establish a reward as a reinforcer. The following are guidelines for selecting potential reinforcers: 1) select those activities that are already enjoyed and that occur naturally, 2) select simple reinforcers such as touch, smiles, and attention, 3) select reinforcers that are compatible with the family values, and 4) avoid tangible reinforcers when possible.

The contingency analysis is used to determine reinforcers with a potential for increasing a deficit behavior. What can maintain one behavior can frequently be used to increase another. In addition, to reinforce a deficit behavior, practitioners can select an activity or behavior that occurs frequently (Premack, 1959). A client who often telephones, for example, can be asked to keep the activity of telephoning contingent upon the occurrence of a target deficit behavior. Daily walks can be made contingent upon bathing. Smoking cigarettes can be made contingent upon out-of-bed activities.

Once the practitioner and the client select a behavior or activity for use as a reinforcer, it should be ascertained whether the activity or behavior can be used contingently. Change agents and clients often resist using certain activities contingently, and, if this occurs, the practitioner should select an alternative activity. Asking family members and the client if they can use the activity or behavior as a contingent reinforcer is essential.

Deficit behaviors often have to be broken down into simple components, that is, the desired behavior is broken into its successive tasks. Dressing is a complex task involving numerous skills and components. Skills include gross and fine motor coordination, eye-hand coordination, ability to discriminate shapes and colors, and grasping abilities. The components of washing a dish, for example, include scraping excess food into the garbage, filling the sink with hot water, soaking the dish in the hot water, washing the dish with a dishcloth, rinsing the dish with clean water, placing the dish in a dish rack, drying the dish, and placing the dish in the cupboard. Each component is a step toward the completion of the task. Self-care skills with impaired elderly clients can be successfully increased when the behavior is broken down into its simple parts and contingent reinforcement is given for successful performance of each step.

When the physiological impairment is severe, practitioners should develop alternative behaviors for reinforcement. If an increase in dressing is the target behavior, loafers might be substituted for shoes that tie. Pullover shirts can be substituted for shirts that button. The practitioner then shifts to training the caregiver to increase the overall behavior rather than attempting to increase components of the behaviors.

Once the appropriate behavior is targeted and the potential reinforcers are established, the practitioner teaches the caregiver to use the reinforcer contingent on the occurrence of the desired behavior. Family members are taught basic guidelines of reinforcement: that it be given after the behavior has occurred, given immediately by the caregiver, accompanied by social and physical attention, and given in a positive manner.

The use of contingent reinforcement by caregivers is a simple procedure, although effective use may require focused training and practice. Initial attempts of caregivers to alter their responses to a specified behavior are often uneven. It is frequently quite hard not to lapse into the prior behavioral pattern that maintained the undesired behaviors. Old behavior patterns are formed from persistent habits, and alternative habits must be taught and conscientiously practiced. The practitioner assures adequate use of contingent reinforcement by monitoring data reports, using reliability checks, and providing initial and subsequent instructions. The practitioner uses caregivers' actual performances as analytic tools to determine the successful use of interventions, rather than accepting verbal descriptions of performance.

Increasing contingent reinforcement has two purposes. One is to increase the frequency of positive behaviors through the caregiver's contingent praise, touch, social attention, or tangible rewards. A second purpose is to increase the overall amount of stimulation available to the client at home. Impaired elderly people, because of their physical disabilities or dependence on others, are often deprived of social excitement or physical contact. They may not talk to anyone for hours and enjoy only minimal tactile stimulation or physical affection. The only social stimulation may be the television. To increase the physical, verbal, and auditory stimulation of a deprived individual is often a major intervention objective.

Decreasing Behaviors

Family members frequently cite negative behaviors as their primary concern regarding an aging relative. The client cries too much, is too dependent on others for assistance, does not use the toilet, or does not leave home. These negative behaviors are appropriate for behavioral programming efforts.

The goal of any behavioral program is to maximize reinforcing opportunities. Punishment procedures that diminish reinforcement, either through the presentation of an aversive stimulus or the removal of a reinforcer, are avoided. Programming goals are to decrease the excessive behavior while increasing a positive adaptive, yet incompatible, behavior. Incompatible behaviors are behaviors and activities that cannot occur at the same time as target negative behavior. Pleasant talk and accusations are incompatible because it is impossible for both to occur simultaneously. Programming efforts are devoted to increasing social activities, as opposed to reducing isolation. If out-of-home activity increases, excessive time in bed will be reduced.

This technique, increasing incompatible behaviors, is often the initial programming effort. Practitioners teach the family caregiver to use reinforcement, or shaping, to increase incompatible behavior. Selecting the incompatible counterpart of a negative behavior is a difficult but creative task for the practitioner. First, the practitioner develops lists of behaviors targeted for increase that, by their occurrence, prevent problem behavior from occurring. The practitioner then teaches the family caregiver to reinforce a positive component of the target behavior that needs strengthening. Every behavior can be stated as an excess or deficit. When stated as a deficit, this component of the behavior is the target for increase. Instead of programming for a decrease in sloppy eating, a more appropriate method is to program for an increase in the deficit positive component—neat dining habits.

A client who complains about tension, nervousness, and anxiety may find relaxation training a helpful incompatible behavior. A structured procedure, often recorded on an audiotape, may direct the client to relax and tense specific muscles or breathe in a systematic way. The client is given a tape recorder and asked to listen to the tape and practice relaxing once or twice a day. In a later phase, the client may be taught to pair the exercise with a specific situation. Finally, the client may be instructed to use the procedure independently, without the tape. The procedure has been used with identified clients as well as support people.

Family members, when presented with these positive intervention strategies, often assert that the primary problem is being avoided. Practitioners should explain the connection between the deficit and the excess behaviors and the fact that the frequency, duration, or intensity of the negative behavior will be decreased as a consequence of promoting positive behaviors. They should then explain the connection between increasing positive behaviors and eliminating problem behaviors. Occasionally caregivers should be told that aversive or punishment techniques may be harmful, ineffective, or even likely to increase the negative behavior.

Difficulties may arise with reinforcing incompatible behaviors. If those difficulties continue or the technique is ineffective, the practitioner can teach an alternative intervention technique. This technique, differential attention, reinforces the positive component of a behavior while systematically ignoring the negative component of the behavior. Differential attention has received mixed evaluations of effectiveness (Herbert et al., 1973; Wahler, 1969), but initial reports suggest that it may be a powerful tool with older families (Green et al., 1986).

Family members are taught to ignore constant nagging by an older relative and reinforce pleasant conversations, or to ignore repetitive actions and reinforce the single performance of a positive behavior. It is critical to teach family members that the reinforcement component of the technique is as important as the ignoring component and that *ignoring is never used alone.*

Differential attention gives the family caregiver something to do when negative components of the behaviors occur: Ignore the behavior. Structured methods and monitoring procedures are available to assist in avoiding overuse of ignoring. The frequency of ignoring can be monitored by attending to the data recorded by the client. Excessive ignoring is usually indicated by an overall decrease in the client's positive behaviors. If this occurs, the practitioner helps the family increase the positive reinforcers associated with positive behaviors or increase cues to signal the desirability of positive activity. By the use of strong reinforcement techniques, contingent and effective reinforcers, and detailed guidelines for using these procedures, the practitioner is able to effectively teach the family caregiver what to do to improve behaviors, as opposed to paying undue attention to the client's negative behaviors.

Intervention techniques are taught to caregivers, emphasizing the behavioral conditions surrounding the problem and family responses to the problem. Practitioners frequently intervene relative to more than one problem and teach family members more than one of the behavioral techniques.

Training and Delivery Systems

Training family caregivers to contingently alter their responses to their relatives' target behavior requires a structured educational approach. The goal of this training is to teach caregivers the skills and knowledge necessary to use the technique independently of the practitioner, practitioner feedback, and clinical sessions. Delivery systems, contingency contracts, individualized attention programs, and token economies supplement practitioner efforts in training family caregivers to alter their contingent responses.

Educating the Caregiver

A didactic approach is used to teach a change agent the behavioral techniques. The practitioner first presents each technique verbally. The practitioner describes the technique, when it is used, and when it is not used. For instance, the practitioner tells the family caregiver to touch the elderly relative every time the relative uses the bathroom independently. The particulars of touching are described. Explanations of when not to touch the relative, when assistance is unnecessary, are also included in the description.

Informing a caregiver of how to perform a behavioral technique is often insufficient. The change agents might not understand the technique and its uses and timing, or might state that he or she can perform the technique, when, in reality, he or she cannot. It is advantageous to accompany verbal descriptions with demonstrations and role plays. The technique is demonstrated or modeled for the caregiver by the practitioner. The practitioner's modeling of the technique demonstrates to the caregiver how and when to use the technique and also demonstrates to the client that target behaviors will be reinforced. After the practitioner has modeled the technique for the family caregiver, the practitioner has the caregiver demonstrate the technique in role plays. This demonstration by the caregiver can use either real situations that arise in the clinical interviews or hypothetical situations.

These demonstrations by the caregiver provide the practitioner with opportunities to offer feedback and reinforcement for the correct use of the technique. If difficulties arise, the practitioner can cue the family when to use the technique. This might include spending time at the home of the elderly client specifically to monitor and cue the change agent when to use the technique.

Training of caregivers then shifts focus from in-session training of caregivers to outside-of-session performance of the behavioral technique. This shift occurs only after the family caregivers have successfully demonstrated the technique in session. Once caregivers use the technique outside of the sessions, the practitioner should observe family interactions, alone or with a trained observer, to assure accurate use of the technique. If difficulties arise, these problems can be ameliorated in the clinical sessions.

The absolute effectiveness of different training components, of course, will not be demonstrated until desired behavior changes can be documented. However, using a variety of techniques, assuring that they are individualized for a family, and providing frequent and contingent reinforcement and feedback make it likely that the caregiver will use the developed technique correctly in day-to-day interactions with the client.

Delivery Systems

If problems arise when the caregiver implements the behavioral techniques or if the practitioner believes that the caregiver's ability to alter contingent responses is limited, the practitioner can structure the intervention technique through several methods including contingency contracts, individualized programs, and token economies. Contingency contracts include a specification of what reinforcer will be provided when a particular behavior occurs. Contracts are feasible with the elderly provided they have the capacity to negotiate the provisions. Dimensions relevant to contracts are the provisions for the "if . . . then" relationship. If a client takes a daily walk, then a specific consequence, a special dessert, is provided. Among the problems altered by use of contracts are phobias, low rate social interactions, high-rate complaining, cigarette use, and excessive amounts of time in bed. When the elderly person is involved in the negotiation of the terms of the contracts, the caregiver is often reminded by the elderly relative to deliver agreed-upon reinforcers. This involvement of the client serves to give feedback to the caregiver that the negotiated terms have been met.

An individualized attention and feedback program is developed to increase the frequency of contingent reinforcement provided by the caregiver. Practitioners often find that the caregiver has the skills and knowledge to provide reinforcement but delivers those reinforcers at low rates. This program provides an account and a cue to give individual and social reinforcement. One method involves giving the caregiver a checklist that requires recording the effects of reinforcement efforts twenty times a day. The responsibility for recording prompts the caregiver to reinforce the client twenty times. An important component of the change program is to involve the caregiver in setting the criteria for change. Another is that the criteria start out low and gradually increase. The more family involvement there is, the higher the likelihood of an effective outcome. The program increases the probability that the reinforcement techniques are properly implemented by the family change agent.

The most structured intervention is the token economy. Token economies should only be used when family caregivers experience considerable difficulty in implementing a behavioral technique. The token economy includes points or other "tokens" such as chips or coupons, which can later be exchanged for tangible reinforcers. This system provides tangible evidence of delivery of reinforcers. In addition, it provides systematic protocols for the delivery of reinforcers, the methods of delivery, and the value of the reinforcer. Token economies may be viable for the impaired elderly residing at home, but research has only begun to evaluate their effectiveness with this population. Nevertheless, when there is family involvement and motivation, token economies may well be effective methods of delivering reinforcers.

PLANNING FOR MAINTENANCE OF CHANGE

After interventions have been introduced, training has been completed, and it has been ascertained that the caregiver is carrying out the program, two tasks are left. First, the effects of the programs are evaluated, and then the necessary changes and additions are made. Once it is assured that the program changes have been effective, it is necessary to ensure that they will continue to operate in the client's environment. Planning for maintenance of change in effect begins long before planning for case closure. The need for maintenance is a part of the initial assessment. Maintainable procedures must be incorporated into intervention planning and implementation. After maintenance procedures are effectively established, case termination can be planned.

The major task in the maintenance phase is to ensure that the appropriate and necessary supports are available for the client to continue achieving an adequate level of reinforcement to live a positive lifestyle. Maintenance is achieved through systematic fading of components of the intervention rather than abrupt ending of contact, through environmental reprogramming procedures, through ensuring that the responsibility for the ongoing interventions is in the hands of the clients or caregivers, and through ensuring that required community services are available and used. Nay (1979) has outlined maintenance procedures as 1) follow-up, 2) retraining, 3) systematic fading of practitioner, and 4) environmental reprogramming.

Each procedure is evaluated to determine the need for maintenance plans and consequent retraining of support persons. Maintenance needs are most clearly evaluated by withdrawing the treatment and observing whether gains are continued. For example, a family who has been using a visitation and telephone schedule to structure their interaction could discontinue weekly scheduling and continue to monitor contacts. If these do not deteriorate, a schedule may no longer be necessary. Very often, however, although the training procedure may no longer be needed, a less intense procedure is necessary to maintain gains.

Fading

A frequent component of maintenance procedures is fading. Fading refers to gradual reduction of the frequency or intensity of a procedure to a level that will nevertheless still maintain the behavior change. In the example just used, the family might no longer need to make a daily schedule of contacts but could fade the scheduling to a weekly basis. If successful, the interval between scheduling is faded to alternate weeks or months. The initial fading procedure is taught as part of the treatment completion phase. Families can independently initiate further fading following intervention.

Fading may include decreasing client-practitioner contact, decreasing data collection tasks, or decreasing a component of a specific procedure (as illustrated earlier). Fading of data collection has been feasible with ESP clients and helpful as a method of decreasing expected activities of clients or support people as intervention goals are met. Data collection forms may be simplified over time. For example, forms may be reduced from a comprehensive activity checklist to focus on more limited targets. Similarly, data collection in later phases may be reduced from daily to fewer times per week. When behavior change is maintained, collection may be cut to once per week and later eliminated. Data collection may be resumed for follow-up verification. In work to date, however, clients have occasionally persisted in collecting behavioral data after the contract for data collection has expired or been renegotiated.

Fading of intervention may require special consideration. A working principle is that fading of intervention should not decrease the overall amount of reinforcement available to the clients or support persons. One must therefore be hesitant to ask families to decrease reinforcement, positive attention, or reward-related cues, as the availability was so limited and implementing simple praise often required considerable training. It is not the reinforcement that is the target of fading, but the delivery system for the reinforcement. For example, a contract to thank an elderly father each time he makes a telephone call may be faded or dropped; the appreciation for the call has not decreased. If calls decrease subsequently, however, the procedure (or a part of it) may need to be reinstated.

Fading of practitioner contact is an inherent part of termination or case transition procedures. Whereas the client may see the practitioner daily or several times a week in early phases, by middle phases this might be limited to every week or so. In later phases the frequency of contact can be faded to every three or four weeks, then systematically to every six or eight weeks. By continuing contact, the practitioner ascertains if the behavior change has been maintained and provides additional support or training as needed. A criterion often used for case termination is two months of successful goal achievement, followed by monthly follow-up telephone calls.

Environmental Reprogramming

Environmental reprogramming refers to the modification of the client's environment so that it continues to foster behavior change after intervention. Environmental reprogramming can be achieved in several ways. The major method used in this approach is the training of support persons in behavioral techniques so they can continue to monitor behavior and implement changes. Because the training occurs in the client's home, and responsibility for implementing procedures is taught to client and support persons on an ongoing basis, the need for programming the transfer of learning of treatment effects may be minimized.

Baer and Wolf (1970) described the procedure of setting a behavioral trap, where contingencies are rearranged to ensure continued reinforcement of appropriate behavior, assuring behavioral maintenance. Several kinds of environmental arrangements can be programmed. Physical changes include changes in furniture to promote more self-initiated behavior. For example, with a man who had difficulty with falling, practitioners observed that falls occurred often when he got out of his chair. The family agreed to provide a higher chair with pillows on it, enabling him to get out of the chair more safely. Consequently he was able to transfer from the chair independently.

Similarly, efforts to relocate the individual to another setting, either for a few hours or permanently, are forms of environmental reprogramming. Social changes in the environment may include introducing new people into the setting, increasing the frequency of visiting, and introducing access to outside services or agencies through community service linkages.

Note that most of these suggestions are often viewed as intervention procedures. In effect, maintenance occurs throughout intervention and is a criterion in selecting interventions.

Program Transfer

Program transfer refers to transferring responsibility for program design to clients or to support persons. Transferring the program is in effect reprogramming the environment. During the maintenance phase the practitioner takes less active responsibility for treatment development and monitoring the training of clients to increase their involvement in this regard.

It is often possible to transfer program responsibility from the practitioner to the support person. One method of doing this is through formally instructing the client of the behavior principles. A portion of contact may include teaching the client the function and techniques of using reinforcement, shaping, and cues.

More often, family members assume program responsibility through formal and informal contracting. Whereas the practitioner initially collects data, the caregivers take over implementation. Whereas the practitioner initially contracts with the older person directly for activity, in later phases the practitioner instructs the caregiver to renegotiate contracts. Whereas the practitioner initially calls to remind the client of an agreement to go to an activity center, the family may assume this responsibility when the habit becomes established. Ideally, all responsibilities are initially taught to family members and the practitioner then functions in an advisory capacity. With individualized clients, however, the amount of program responsibility given to the clients is often varied according to their interest, performance, and reinforcement levels.

The older individual may learn to take program responsibility also, even though behavior problems may be evident. In many cases caregivers began as primary data collectors, only to be replaced or supplemented by clients directly recording data later on. Clients' participatory abilities are often underestimated. Similarly, the clients are often the best sources of the terms of specific contracts.

COMMUNITY SERVICE LINKAGE

Community service linkages refer to any ongoing participation or contact with a service agency outside the home. Often, however, clients need assistance in learning about service linkages. Community service linkages are defined as strategies for increasing the amount of reinforcement available to an older person on an ongoing basis. Linkages may include increased family contact or medical care, as well as community service agencies. Although they may often be implemented as initial or preliminary interventions, or even as primary interventions, linkages are included as part of maintenance procedures to stress the need to ascertain ongoing reinforcement after the practitioner leaves the scene.

When to Link

A number of criteria are important in determining when to foster community linkages. First, services available to the client are assessed in initial interviews. A formal assessment can emphasize identifying service supports, or this information can be conveyed informally. Second, the necessary services are assessed. As goals and desirable outcomes are formulated, the practitioner considers what outside sources of help may foster increased activity or happiness. Third, the practitioner assesses what behaviors are required for service participation. Will an individual need to learn to negotiate a bus system in order to get to a doctor or an educational program? Will a client need to be continent to participate in a day center or sheltered workshop? Will the client need to be able to answer the telephone to use a telephone reassurance program or answer the door to let in a home health aide?

The fourth criterion related to needed behaviors regards what services are necessary to maintain behavior change. If a person has learned to increase his or her social conversation, what service will be required to maintain this increase in conversation? Put differently, how can the practitioner and the family assure that people will be around to talk to the person and thereby reinforce his or her need for conversation (and intellectual stimulation)? Is there a social club or senior activity group that could be joined? Is transportation available? How does the relationship to such services need to be monitored to assure continued involvement?

A major consideration is the impact of service changes on intervention evaluation. If the homemaker who has been assisting Mrs. Jones changes, the practitioner needs to consider this in evaluating the client's self-care activities. If the physician changes medications, the practitioner may notice more or less independent care or even provide data to document side effects.

In fact, evaluation is an important component of service linkages. A service linkage requires the same careful monitoring as a behavioral intervention to ensure successful implementation and effectiveness. Each service should serve a behavioral function—to increase or maintain something needed by the client. Home health services can maintain self-care skills, social interaction, and physical needs. Transportation can maintain out-of-home activity. Evaluation designs applied to other behaviors can be applied to service evaluation as well (although the services may in effect be intervention packages that are somewhat complex to assess). The collection of baseline data on a problem for which community service is sought can precede service initiation. AB designs can be used to evaluate the success of a service on some specific behavior. For example, one client, Mrs. White, complained constantly, particularly about physical symptoms. Her husband learned to record her complaining daily. After she began in a day care program, her husband's data collection confirmed that her complaining was less of a problem.

Linkage Procedures

In the ESP, a seven-step linkage procedure was adapted from Weissman's work (1976). Linkage steps include problem identification, resource location, option exploration, resource selection, resource connection, verification or resource assistance, and follow-up/evaluation.

Sources of Service Linkage Information

Work with the elderly requires the development and constant updating of files on individual and community resources. Networking is an essential source of current and qualitative information about resources.

Certainly, community information programs include information about services for senior citizens. Area Agency on Aging offices often provide useful referral information. Often, however, clients need assistance in a personalized resource search. Clients themselves often are good sources of information about what is available to them. Clients or family members may or may not be able to pay for services—a factor that must be taken into account. Often family and friends are available to provide services. Churches and community contacts may be of help as well.

More than occasionally, the required service cannot be located for the client. At these times, the practitioner, the client, and the family think together about temporary or longer-term methods for providing the service and attempt to design an alternative.

Termination and Follow-Up

When intervention is successful, service to the client is not actually terminated. Visitation ceases, but training has produced learning and habit changes that assure that services will continue to be used. The goal of interventions is to structure ongoing sources of reinforcement for the clients and to do what is possible to see that clients retain these after contact with the practitioner is discontinued.

As contact is discontinued with clients, a method to assure systematic follow-up is put in place. Telephone follow-up begins on a monthly basis and then is faded to semimonthly and, finally, quarterly. Follow-up continues for at least one year following termination.

Follow-ups include some reassessment of client and support person functioning, perhaps using posttest instruments or consumer satisfaction interviews. Presence of target behaviors is reassessed, and retraining is provided as needed.

A second kind of follow-up involves the availability of practitioners to answer questions and receive program reports following termination. Because the clients are elderly, and often deprived socially, provision for ongoing social contact is an essential part of this approach.

SPECIFIC APPLICATION OF BEHAVIORAL PROCEDURES

Because family concerns about older relatives encompass many needs and problems, including specific behavior problems, we have outlined a method that families can use to ameliorate behavior problems in order to maximize use of existing resources, improve interaction, and, it is hoped, increase family satisfaction. More complete examples are delineated for the practitioner to use to teach families to increase rates of social contacts, self-care routines, meaningful activities, and positive verbal behaviors.

Increasing Social Contacts

Isolation and withdrawal from community and family living are problems that beset older citizens. Social isolation may occur because of too few opportunities for socialization. Low rates of social skills may be related to physical or social losses, too few sufficient reinforcers following social participation to sustain further socialization, or both. Older persons and their families may require assistance to determine reasonable levels of social engagement. For some, who previously had many social contacts, physical changes related to aging may mean that simple involvement in daily activities is so taxing that social efforts need to be reduced. For others, who have retired and are still able to meet their daily social and physical needs, old age may be a time of emptiness, and social activities may need to be increased. Although the need for social contact is crucial for all ages, the amount and kind can change over time. Often it is as sumed that contacts with friends and family are satisfying, when in reality the visits are unpleasant to family members. In Table 18-1 specific steps are listed to aid the practitioner in teaching families to stimulate and reinforce social behavior.

Improving Self-Care

Self-care deficits among the elderly include losses in ability to dress, to eat independently, to maintain hygiene behaviors, and to use toilet facilities appropriately. Self-care deficits can be related to physical changes such as ambulation problems, tremors, and coordination difficulties. Often, however, self-care deficiencies arise when memory or cognitive organization declines. Then the cause is an inability to remember the time and procedural steps required to complete the task, rather than physical disability. A person may be able to go to the washroom adequately, but may not respond to bodily or temporal cues and therefore becomes incontinent. In long-term care facilities, an individual may be denied opportunity for adequate self-care through restraints or lack of resources. Families may learn to provide appropriate cues, reinforce, and attend appropriately to self-care efforts.

A general self-care procedure is illustrated in Table 18-2. For each activity a specific desired behavior is defined and broken down into necessary substeps. A time schedule specifies both the frequency and the duration of the desired activities. Actual interventions provide an opportunity for the activity to occur, prompting correct attempts to engage in the activity, praising gradual achievement of each step, and using primary rewards, touch, and assisting when necessary. As highlighted in Table 18-3, inappropriate behaviors are ignored, and the results of each trial are recorded, so that success can be evaluated and procedures changed if need be.

Improving Verbal Behavior

Family caregivers experience communication difficulties as exceedingly frustrating to manage. These verbal problems increase the difficulty of providing care. Conversations between older people and others are sometimes quite limited; families frequently complain that they do not know what to talk about with older, impaired relatives, and they report that they avoid potential encounters. Communication problems often include excessive talking by the older person, including chronic complaints or repetitive statements. Some caregiving spouses complain that they have heard the same story every day of

TABLE 18-1 Intervention Procedures: Increasing Social Contacts

Step	Implementation
1. Defining desired behavior	1. Select a specific behavioral outcome using baseline data assessment data to determine low-frequency activities involving others. Check the behavior with family and client to verify its social and clinical relevance. Define the desired outcome in operational terms.
2. Evaluating resources required to achieve desired social contacts	2. Resources required may include transportation from relatives or agencies, funds, and cues to elicit necessary behaviors.
3. Selecting desired time, place, and components of the social contact	3. Discuss possible times and places when the social contacts may occur and steps the client will need to engage in (i.e., getting dressed, arranging for transport, going to activity).
4. Eliciting agreement to engage in activity	4. Present one or more possible target activities to the client, along with discussion and explanation of the time, place, and resources available and the behavioral components. Ask the client if he or she is willing to participate. Enlist involved relatives in providing resources, participating, and reinforcing client's agreement to participate.
5. Specifying the contract in writing	5. Once agreed upon, formalize the contract in verbal and written form. Use either a task assignment contract or an individualized contract to state the specific activity agreed upon, who will do what to achieve it, and when this will occur. Give a copy to each participant.
6. Rehearsing components of the social contacts	6. Have the family practice the required steps to achieve the social contacts.
7. Prompting social contacts	7. Incorporate a variety of possible reminders or prompts including 1) calendar notes/appointment books, 2) reminder telephone calls from practictioner or family members, and 3) verbal prompts from those living with clients.

TABLE 18-1   Intervention Procedures: Increasing Social Contacts *(continued)*

Step	Implementation
8. Reinforcing social contacts immediately	8. Teach available caregivers to notice, call attention to, and praise social contacts when these occur and to avoid complaining about the client's not engaging in desired contacts.
9. Recording	9. Have caregivers note social contacts on recording forms.
10. Monitoring and providing feedback	10. Review the data at least once a week and provide verbal praise for task adherence.
11. Renegotiating the contract	11. If task adherence does not occur, review each step of the procedure and suggest and recontract for necessary changes.
12. Recontracting	12. When adherence does occur, consider the need to recontract to achieve additional outcomes.

SOURCE: Pinkson & Linsk, 1984a.

their married lives. Even more upsetting may be the client who perseveres with negative statements that are threatening, embarrassing, or sad such as, "I want to die," "my wife has another man," or "nobody does anything for me." What are commonly referred to as hallucinations or memory deficits are viewed as verbal excesses. When persons with Alzheimer's disease or other mental disorders complain, question, accuse, or hallucinate, families could conclude that they can do nothing except try to reassure the clients or convince them that their claims are not so. Research and practice suggest that the reinforcing quality of this response can actually increase both the frequency and intensity of the disorder. Similarly, individuals who are depressed, deficient in activities or stimulation, and sensorially and socially deprived do not improve as a result of caregiver rationalizations regarding their pain or fear, particularly when those rationalizations are their main source of attention.

An alternative approach for analyzing verbal deficits includes determination of antecedents, consequences, and alternatives to be reinforced. Socially deprived older people often respond to questions such as "How are you?" or "What did you do today?" with a detailed description of their medical conditions and physical or social complaints. The questions stimulate negative or

TABLE 18-2   Intervention Procedures: Self-Care Behavior

Step	Implementation
1. Defining desired behavior	1. Select a specific behavioral outcome (i.e., client will dress in underwear, slacks, shirt, shoes, etc.; client will wash face three times a day; client will use washroom four times a day).
2. Setting and using a schedule	2. Designate a time to begin and end each occurence of self-care.
3. Providing response opportunity	3. Arrange or ask client to arrange materials (e.g., clothing, soap, and towel) so that they are usable and within easy reach.
4. Prompting correct behavior	4. Have the support person prompt the client to go through each step of the task in the correct order. If there is no response, the prompt is repeated once or twice, then two minutes later if necessary.
5. Allowing time for behavior to occur	5. If the client is attempting to complete a self-care task, instruct the caregiver to wait until the task is completed. This should occur within five minutes.
6. Praising appropriate behavior	6. If the client is able to complete the task, the caregiver offers praise or touching (food, token, or point on the recording form may also be used) and then prompts the client to go on to the next step.
7. Assisting if the behavior does not occur	7. If the client does not respond to the prompt within thirty seconds, the caregiver guides the older person through the various steps required. The caregiver provides help with any items the client is unable to complete because of physical impairment or pain.
8. Ignoring inappropriate behavior	8. If the client engages in inappropriate behavior such as complaining, arguing, or any behaviors that serve to bring about an unnecessary delay in the process, the caregiver should remove attention from the client until the behavior ceases. Caregiver then returns to step 4.
9. Recording	9. Behavior is recorded on recording form.

TABLE 18-3   Intervention Procedures: Elimination Program for Incontinence and Bowel Accidents

Step	Implementation
1. Defining desired behavior	1. Select a specific behavioral outcome.
2. Setting and using a schedule	2. Using baseline data to select frequency, determine a schedule of intervention. Begin with a frequency that ensures *successful* washroom use, usually one-half hour more frequently than reported incontinence or accidents. Often a one-hour or one and a half–hour schedule is used initially. If baseline is inconclusive, begin with a one and a half–hour interval and adjust to meet client's needs. Often the schedule can be modified after a few days, based on client performance.
3. Providing response opportunity	3. Provide access to toilet, urinal, or bedpan. May consist of asking if client wants to use washroom, wheeling or walking person to washroom, or giving client urinal or bedpan.
4. Prompting correct behavior	4. Have support person ask client if he or she wishes to use washroom. If response is negative, the prompt is repeated ten minutes later.
5. Allowing time for behavior to occur	5. If the client is ambulatory or mobile without help and able to self-toilet, instruct caregiver to wait at least five minutes for response to occur.
6. Praising appropriate behavior	6. If client goes to washroom appropriately, tell caregiver to praise him or her, either verbally or with a material reinforcer (food, token, a point on the recording form). Self-initiated appropriate toilet use is *always* reinforced.
7. Assisting if behavior does not occur	7. If behavior does not occur within thirty minutes or client is incontinent, have caregiver ask client if help is required and provide it (dressing, location, cleaning, etc.). If behavior still does not occur, caregiver waits until next interval and returns to Step 3.

TABLE 18-3   Intervention Procedures: Elimination Program for Incontinence and Bowel Accidents *(continued)*

Step	Implementation
8. Ignoring inappropriate behavior	8. If incontinence or soiling occurs, client instructs caregiver to assist in cleaning up or dressing (or give instructions if client can do so independently). Minimal conversation or physical touch occurs. The change agent should *never* engage in criticism, solicitous conversation, praise, or intense physical contact. Both should ignore the behavior as much as possible.
9. Recording	9. Have the caregiver record behavior on recording form.

repetitive responses. Somewhat different questions or cues may elicit more positive responses, such as "What would you like to do today?" "You are looking good today," or "Shall we go for a walk?"

Many older adults with behavior problems are bereft of opportunities to give their opinions, choices, or reports on experiences, and allowing more opportunity for them to do so may elicit more interesting responses. Also, clients may not receive adequate consequences for their appropriate attempts to socialize. A daughter who ignores all attempts of her mother to engage socially may notice that her mother begins to complain, fantasize, verbalize, or escalate positive conversation to an excessive level in a demand for social attention. Or a spouse that punishes conversation by saying, "Don't talk to me now. Can't you see that I am busy?" should expect the usual response to punishment, that is, anger, frustration, fight, or flight. Finally, the presence of problem verbalizations may imply insufficient activities. Programming alternative activities and reinforcing appropriate behavior while ignoring negative behavior have been supported by the findings of the ESP. The procedures have been associated with decreases in hallucinations, pain, and complaining.

General procedures for decreasing negative verbalizations are presented in Table 18-4. Family caregivers are taught to monitor verbal behaviors, usually for one hour twice a day for high-frequency behaviors and continuously and frequently for low rate behaviors. A desirable alternative behavior is defined, and a criterion for reduction of excessive behavior is selected. In almost all cases alternative behavior is selected to be increased and maintained. Attention is never withdrawn from negative behaviors.

TABLE 18-4   Intervention Procedures: Decreasing Negative Verbalizations

Step	Implementation
1. Defining desired behavior	1. Select a specific behavioral outcome, using baseline assessment data to define realistic improvements. Include expected frequency of negative verbalizations and frequency of alternative positive verbalizations (i.e., complaints to be decreased to less than one per hour; positive statements increased to two per hour).
2. Specifying intervention to be used (differential attention or reinforcement)	2. Adapt the specific procedure and write it down for use in training caregivers. Delineate exactly which behaviors are to be ignored and which are to be attended to or reinforced. Define and illustrate these behaviors. Specify when the procedure is used, by whom, and under what conditions.
3. Training caregivers in use of procedures	3. Introduce caregivers to procedures first through oral and written instructions. Demonstrate how the procedure is used through modeling, illustrating both praise and ignoring. Give family members an opportunity to rehearse the procedure, first acting as the client while the practitioner models and then acting as themselves while practitioner acts as client. Caregivers then practice the procedure with the client while practitioner monitors, giving cues or feedback as needed.
4. Explaining procedure to client and eliciting consent	4. Inform the client of the procedure and give him or her opportunities to ask questions and to agree to participate. If the client objects to the procedure, introduce necessary changes.
5. Setting criteria for ignoring and praising, if needed	5. Specify criteria for use of the intervention; negotiate if necessary.

TABLE 18-4   Intervention Procedures: Decreasing Negative Verbalizations
(continued)

Step	Implementation
6. Recording	6. Have the client note praise, ignoring, reinforcers, and positive and negative responses on the recording form.
7. Monitoring and feedback	7. At least once a week review data and provide verbal praise for using the procedures. Offer additional training as needed.

SUMMARY

Human service professionals assisting older families can draw on a range of research and practice methods in addition to traditional casework and counseling methods. Practitioners can also consider methods being developed that promote family involvement. Community service linkages, or case-management methods, although continually recognized as vital in work with older clients, require additional development and backing to become a standard part of home support for the elderly. Finally, a rich practice and research base exists for training families to deal effectively with specific behavior problems. Both the parent-training methods previously tested with children and the behavioral gerontology literature show great promise of being applicable to older families in home settings. Preliminary research conducted by the ESP suggests a range of effective interventions to maximize family and community support of the impaired elderly.

CHAPTER 19

Working with Organizations
Serving Persons
with Disabilities

Harold E. Briggs

In this chapter, Briggs examines the combined contributions of the family-centered perspective, applied behavioral analysis, and program implementation methods to promoting the community adjustment of persons with developmental disabilities. The chapter examines the covariation between organizational behavior modification, therapeutic programming, and clinical outcomes for persons with developmental disabilities living in community-based environments. The reader of the chapter is provided an example of empirical practice at the agency level. The model development and design methods described earlier by William Reid and the evidence-based approaches highlighted by Bruce Thyer are integrated into this chapter, which includes a detailed case study of the role of knowledge development and empirically based approaches to enhance agency development and service outcomes. The chapter includes descriptive data to highlight the covariation between agency development, service, and clinical outcomes for persons with developmental disabilities. Briggs concludes with an agency practice model, which includes the intervention and consultation methodology and the resulting family-centered, empirically supported practice method that evolved as a result of combining empirical practice, family involvement, and evidence-based staff management approaches. The chapter includes a table of functions, tasks, and activities defined at each level of the agency infrastructure as a basis for replicating this nonprofit agency practice model of planning, implementing, ensuring quality control, and promoting service effectiveness.

Urban community organizations lack an empirically based multilevel planning, implementation, evaluation, and quality-assurance technology that is driven by the desirable outcomes and perspectives of families served by them. The purpose of this paper is to describe a research-based multilevel family-centered approach to community-based social service organizations. "Multilevel family-centered" refers to client-consumers including their families, staff, management, and the governing board of directors of an organization working in a coordinated way to pursue goals and objectives defined by families. Although this perspective incorporates many of the ideas in the empirically based intervention methods expressed by Pinkston, Levitt, Green, Linsk, and Rzepnicki (1982) and Bailey-Dempsey and Reid (1996) and the "client-centered" and "service effectiveness" perspectives expressed by Patti, Poertner, and Rapp (1987), it involves the family in all aspects of the organization, including policy development, planning, implementation, and evaluation.

The family-centered perspective in social work has been described theoretically in textbooks; in practice, staff, management, and policy makers of organizations each have their own definitions of what family centered means. Also, they each have their own personal and professional agendas that may conflict and interfere with the goal of designing supportive organizational cultures that promote goals defined by families. Although different organizations have different issues, one goal should nevertheless remain paramount: helping the client-consumer and his or her family move toward greater independence with an ability to function within the community. The central practice question for all organizational levels is, What can be done to assist the client-consumer, including his or her family, to achieve this goal?

In urban community organizations, the shift to a multilevel family-centered perspective can be completed if all levels of the organization's work are integrated. This will mean redefining environmental contingencies (Redmon & Wilks, 1991) and establishing new roles for the family and for management and staff (Friesen & Koroloff, 1990). Given the nature of urban community organizations, which generally involves work by both staff and volunteers to resolve a variety of client-consumer problems (including those of the physically disabled, the chronically mentally ill, the homeless, the elderly, the developmentally disabled, and many children and families with at-risk characteristics), the technology used to promote service effectiveness will need to be based in a generalist context (Reid, 1987).

PERSPECTIVES ON FAMILY-CENTERED PRACTICE

Practitioners and policy makers designing multilevel family-centered urban community organizations need to review a wide number of literature bases. Key areas to search include social work, children's mental health, and applied behavioral analysis.

Social Work

The family-centered perspective has been a major theory of practice in social work dating as far back as Hartman and Laird (1983). Germain (1979) defines family-centered practice as "a model of social work practice which locates the family in the center of the unit of attention or the field of action" (p. 4). Based in an ecological systems framework, family-centered practice in this context defines the role of the family primarily as a service beneficiary. The relationships between the family and other systems such as individuals, organizations, and community define the areas for social work assessment and intervention activities. Hartman and Laird (1983) conclude, "In short, the family can be in the center of attention whether one is working with individuals, groups, neighborhoods, or larger systems" (p. 5).

Adams and Nelson's (1995) definition of family-centered perspective extends the definition advanced by Hartman and Laird. It considers a number of added dimensions, such as culture and community, as relevant contextual variables for social work practice. At the core of their perspective is a different definition of family-centered practice. It embraces the key service delivery dimensions of family-centered systems of care including neighborhood-based care, collaboration, and partnership between private service providers and families. This particular approach to family-centered practice incorporates the key components of power and authority. Adams and Nelson's family-centered perspective also embraces the concepts of empowerment, informal networks, and service coordination within a culturally responsive and community context. Formally known as the Patch approach, it has been tested in Britain and the United States. Serving as a mechanism to redirect human services, its experience has been realized in systems of care in Iowa and Pennsylvania. Patch is another way for professionals, community workers, and family members to work in a coordinated fashion aimed at supporting, strengthening, and preserving families. The practice technology that makes up Patch incorporates many of the strategies used in children's mental health practice, which has been influenced by the family support movement.

Children's Mental Health

The family-support movement includes the critical concepts of interagency collaborations, service coordination, partnerships, case management, and cultural competence, with a strengths-based family-centered perspective. It differs from the family-centered practice discussed above. In children's mental health, the family-centered practice is accompanied by considerable practice innovations that add up to the "cultural revolution" that has taken place over the past decade, according to Friesen (1993). Friesen and Huff (1996) provide a positive account of the shift to a family-centered perspective in children's mental health. Hunter and Friesen (1996) provide a succinct definition of family-centered practice in children's mental health in terms of three key practice principles:

1. Services to children with emotional disorders and their families flow out of an expanded ecological view of the family within the context of the greater community.
2. Services for children with emotional disorders and their families are designed to meet the unique needs of all family members and employ a wide variety of both formal and informal support strategies.
3. Parents and other family members are involved in all aspects of service planning, delivery, and evaluation in partnership with formal service providers and policy makers.

The rise in popularity of the family-centered perspective in children mental health has been accompanied by a new practice strategy that contributes the added dimensions of family advocacy. Bryant-Compstock, Huff, and Vandenberg (1996) describe the evolution of family advocacy networks. These organizational arrangements emerged as a result of the need for parent input on ways to enhance the circumstances of families of children with serious emotional and behavioral disorders. These families are pursuing a better, flexible, seamless service delivery system based on the idea that the family is a key player in the planning, implementation, and quality-assurance activities that characterize emerging family-centered/culturally competent systems of care.

The initial development of statewide family networks was described by staff of the Portland Research and Training Center on Family Support and Children's Mental Health (Briggs, Koroloff, Richards, & Friesen, 1993; Briggs, Carrock, & Koroloff, 1994). These early program development and evaluation reports have provided guidelines for the development and further enhancement of family advocacy networks. In subsequent research, Friesen and her associates have written additional empirically based articles that portray and highlight the development of statewide family organizations using sponsoring organizations (Briggs & Koroloff, 1995), delineate the predictable stages of growth and development as these particular organizations pass through stages of their life cycle (Koroloff & Briggs, 1996), and describe the contributions these organizations have made to system change (Briggs, 1996b; Briggs, Smith, Leary, & Johnson, under review) in promoting culturally competent systems of care (Briggs, Carrock, Williams-Murphy, Leary, & Johnson, under review).

Between 1990 and 1993, fifteen statewide family networks received consultation, monitoring, and program evaluation capability building supports. Four of the fifteen received technical assistance and consultation on a multi-level approach (Briggs, 1996b). Results of their successful growth and development were reported by Briggs et al. (1993). An evaluation of the first year of funding revealed that these organizations have been able to secure additional funding, involve families from non-Anglo backgrounds in their activities, and affect systems change in a positive way (Briggs, 1996b; Briggs & Carrock, 2000).

Although the family-centered perspective advanced in children's mental health is not the only valid approach to including families in key, nontraditional roles, it encompasses other practice methods and approaches such as strategies based in an applied behavioral analysis framework.

Applied Behavioral Analysis

The multilevel practice model incorporated a number of relevant practice theories such as operant conditioning, social learning theory, and task-centered practice into a culturally responsive, strengths-based, performance-driven, family-centered perspective to promote system-wide behavior modification. The consultation model used with the four family networks previously mentioned was developed by Briggs, Pinkston, and the late Larry T. Byrd at an inner-city, African-American managed community organization in Chicago, Illinois. The aim is to enhance goals and objectives defined by families, staff, and management. The consultant's philosophy, style, and strategy of working as mentor, teacher, parent, and friend (as depicted in Table 19-1), aided management and staff in facilitating broad-scale behavior change. Teaching staff and management effective ways to develop proactive relationships to pursue desirable outcomes for African-American children and families is consistent with an Afrocentric perspective (see Everett, Chipungu, & Leashore, 1991).

Initially referred to as performance management in human services, its aim was to promote the achievements of client-consumers, including their families, staff, and management, by using a multilevel approach that considers the actions and activities of every player of the organization as a basis to achieve family and consumer outcomes. All activities of the organization were systematically planned, implemented, and evaluated in terms of enhanced functional capacity, advocacy and political empowerment, community and economic development. Family members and community residents were key players in the policy development and decisions that affect the organization and its beneficiaries. The organization is now positioned and governed by professionals and scholars who are inextricably linked to the founding community residents and families. Many of the families and community residents remain involved in policy, service delivery, and quality-assurance activities.

To achieve system-wide behavior modification, the intervention design and development process served as the framework to pilot test the development of the multilevel technology described below. The design and development technology was described by Reid early on as model development (1979) and later presented as design and development for organizational innovation by Thomas in Patti et al. (1987) and almost ten years later as intervention design and development (Bailey-Dempsey & Reid, 1996). It is a useful way to enhance and develop organizational environments and promote the service effectiveness and the performance of staff, management, and client-consumers and their families.

The intervention design and development paradigm incorporates elements of the traditional problem-solving process. Given the fact that some practitioners avoid using a problem focus because it engenders a cultural deficit view, they can begin the process by defining issues as discrepancies between where the client system is versus where it wants to go (see Mager & Pipe, 1984). The design and development approach allows the social worker to use a four-step process: 1) identification of discrepancies (problem identification), 2) design and development, 3) initial testing and preliminary evaluation, and 4) retesting and further evaluation.

TABLE 19-1   Intervention Design and Development Plan

	Information Analysis	Program Development	Staff Development	Organizational Development	Personal Support
STAFF	Staff perceptions Resource needs Supervisory support Case-management issues Skill-training needs	Social leisure activity program Assessment tools Tracking tasks Clinical consultation Case collaboration Family participant and service delivery	Case management Record keeping Community linkages Implementation tasks Brief treatment methods	Policies and procedures Methods to evaluate Focus on strengths and outcomes Administrative support	Advocate Advisor Feedback On-the-job training
GROUP HOME RESIDENTS AND FAMILIES	Behavior management issues Activity planning Positive and corrective feedback	Weekly meetings between residents and staff Administrative support Training Quarterly treatment staffings	Behavioral management Parent-training methods Collaboration with biological family and staff	Administrative support with case coordination unit Staff support Meeting with management Joint activity between staff, residents, faculty, and management	Advocate Training consultant
UPPER AND EXECUTIVE MANAGEMENT	Staff performance indicators (or lack of) Negative licensure evaluations Environmental contingencies	Annual training program Additional training supports Performance evaluations Administrative participation Recognition Organizational support	Professional development Supervision Planning, evaluation Quality assurance	Staff support Management consultation	Confidant Advisor Volunteer Trainer Feedback Advocate
BOARD OF DIRECTORS	Feedback Recommendations Supports	Review of progress at annual board, staff, and management retreats	Participation in training with staff and management at annual retreats	Advisors Consultants	Advocate

SOURCE: Briggs (1996b).

DESIGN AND DEVELOPMENT ISSUES: A CASE STUDY

The multilevel family-centered approach to urban community organizations was pilot tested at an African-American–governed community organization as part of an academic/community partnership with the University of Chicago School of Social Service Administration. A design and development process was used initially in one service division that later became two separate and distinct divisions: 1) child welfare and 2) residential services. As the technology proved useful, it was transferred to the remaining seven service divisions of the organizations. This case example delineates the application of the multilevel family-centered perspective to a program aimed at promoting the community adjustment of persons with developmental disabilities.

Problem Analysis and Project Planning

This system-wide behavior modification intervention grew out of several concerns involving a number of systems such as 1) zoning regulations, 2) funding sources, 3) community, 4) family, and 5) individual group home residents. Essentially, the unions representing the employees of large state institutions and the trade associations representing the interests of families of adults with developmental disabilities had concerns about community-based care. It was their express desire that the institutions remain the service provider and they were concerned that the community was not safe or equipped to address the unique needs of their relatives with disabilities. The funding source had concerns about the readiness of the organization to provide this service and expressed the need for operating and training manuals, staff, equipment, and all other necessary items needed to open and maintain a community residential service delivery system. In addition to the issues raised through zoning, family members had concerns about the staff being able to provide safe and individual care. The individual residents initially did not want to leave the institution. They were accustomed to routines, practices, and contingency systems that seemed familiar and comfortable.

Information-Gathering Process

Information was collected from staff, management, and funding sources concerning the structural and programmatic areas that need to be addressed before this particular community service system could remain open. In a series of meetings with staff of the local office of the Department of Mental Health and Developmental Disabilities, it was clear that a policy and procedure manual was needed. This manual would define how to operate a group home program through standard operating policies and procedures, ways and means to train staff on how to provide individualized habilitation programs and services, and procedures for training clients. A consultant was hired to complete this task. In addition to infrastructure-related issues, the executive director was working with other key staff and local service providers on trying to get the zoning requirements changed so that both locations could be in close proximity and be able to house residents with developmental disabilities.

After the program had been open for a period of sixty days, it was evaluated for compliance by the newly hired operations manager. This internal evaluation uncovered a number of major licensure violations. Major problems involved record keeping, lack of staff training, very little evidence of client-consumer training, and no contact with families except when there was a critical incident. Interviews with staff revealed the lack of staff supervision, quality assurance, and adequate resources to program the residents in the community. Interviews with executive management provided evidence that a self-corrective planning, implementation, and quality-assurance process was needed. As part of his discussions with key board members who were community residents and family members of children with developmental disabilities, the executive director shared the facts of the situation with them and they concurred with his decision. Each level of the organization shared the goal of promoting the community adjustment of persons with developmental disabilities.

Design and Development

The community adjustment of persons with developmental disabilities was considered a function of a supportive organizational environment. Four intervention strategies were developed: 1) change in program administration, 2) staff training, 3) family involvement in service delivery, and 4) support and advocacy for all levels of the program that are described by Briggs, Carrock, Mason, and Williams-Murphy (1996). In designing this plan of intervention it was clear that at the basis of our vision was the building of positive relationships for group home residents inside and outside the organization. Chief among the strategies used to facilitate this outcome was hiring a consultant to assist us in developing a self-perpetuating program infrastructure that focused on the strengths and positive aspects of the client-consumers, staff, and management of the program.

Early Development and Pilot Testing

The consultant worked with all levels of the organization to promote system-wide behavior modification as reflected in Table 19-1. In the group home system, the consultants taught staff and consumers how to ensure self-determination through meetings in which each gave input and made decisions regarding a structured social leisure activity program. They participated in the initial planning meeting with staff, consumers, and program supervisory staff so that they could assist in program development and provide a linkage to upper and executive management personnel. Meetings with upper and executive management during initial planning and implementation phases of the social leisure program intervention provided the consultant with the opportunity to share positive feedback about staff and consumers. They in turn used this information in supervising other service divisions of the organization and in progress reports to the board of directors.

Evaluation and Advanced Development

As staff and consumers met with the consultant weekly for social leisure activities there was a decrease in the number of critical incidents due to behavior management. Staff defined a range of self-care skills for clients to complete prior to social leisure activity participation. Results of their efforts were reviewed monthly by executive management through meetings with the consultant and program supervisor. As the data provided support for social leisure activity as a consequence for conducting self-care and behavior, the program supervisor, consultant, and executive management decided that a better way to track data and use it to make decisions concerning the consumers' community participation was needed. They also felt that staff who were committed to goals of community integration and client self-determination were needed. Young staff working primarily part time for additional money were the staff of this program until management engaged in a staff change intervention.

In addition to changing the culture of staff and consumer interactions, a staff change intervention provided management the opportunity to hire staff with a practical orientation to training consumers to link with family, friends and community settings. During this phase, three additional strategies were defined and implemented: 1) family intervention, 2) community service intervention, and 3) staff training intervention. Each of these established opportunities for clients to transfer to permanent residence and participation in the community. The family intervention was restructured in a way so as to provide families few opportunities to hear negative feedback. This was done to replace the old way of connecting with the family by giving them opportunities to assist in activity planning, arrange visits for their relatives, and share good news about their relatives' performance overall.

The family involvement in service delivery was also extended to a community service intervention. They were given opportunities to assist staff in teaching residents community survival skills such as grocery shopping, using public transportation, and using community facilities, i.e., movies, restaurants, and so on. The community service intervention provided staff, consumers, and family members the opportunity to transfer learning that was taking place in the group home residence to other natural settings such as family members' homes, restaurants, movies, and other public gathering places so that the generalization of self-care and social skills across environments could be established.

Dissemination and Adoption

As staff and consumers were able to keep a balanced schedule of in-home events and out-of-home activities, the need for a consultant was lessened. Thus, activities designed and tested by staff with assistance by the consultant were packaged, and procedures that describe how to implement them were established and used to conduct program development and implementation tasks.

As the staff, management, and consultant developed improved policies, procedures, and practices for planning, implementing, record keeping, and ensuring quality control, this technology was being adapted for agency-wide use and distribution. The annual agency retreats included staff from the group home system. Their participation allowed for the adaptation of staff, consumer, and quality-assurance training materials and activities to other programs and services throughout the agency. The retreats were held annually, with board members comprised of client-consumer family members, community residents, interested professionals, and civic-minded people. Quarterly staff and management retreats were held to design materials to be used throughout the agency and in preparation for the next annual meeting, which included the board of directors.

As depicted in Table 19-2, the multilevel family-centered approach to urban community organizations takes into account the diversity of the people served and the variability of organizations. It is driven by a vision and the nine interrelated components as described below.

Vision. The vision of any organization that is driven by the perspectives of families and other key stakeholders such as staff, management, and volunteers must be based on the dreams, aspirations, and hopes of all the people involved. The vision of an organization characterizes the place, the ways, and the actions of people involved in the organization after it has achieved its official purpose, its primary mission. For example, when scientists, professionals, families, and communities, having witnessed countless victims of polio, thought of a world without this devastating, crippling, fatal illness, their eyes were on the preservation of life combined with preserving the quality of life for youth, adults, and families, the kind of life that gives people hope and the commitment to do their personal best. This vision was part of the philosophy of proponents and leaders of the March of Dimes, whose mission was to develop a treatment to fight against the onset and spread of polio.

Martin Luther King's "I Have a Dream" speech is another example that can be used to distinguish a vision from a mission. Clearly the passage of the Civil Rights Act was not the final destination as he envisioned it; that destination was the dream for his daughter and others regardless of race, culture, gender, or any other at-risk characteristic persecuted in American society.

Mission. In multilevel family-centered urban community organizations, there are a few things to remember about mission statements. The mission is the official purpose of the organization. It is the reason why the entity exists. Mission statements that incorporate a family-centered perspective means that the perspective, input, and participation by families in all aspects of the organization's infrastructure is sanctioned and valued. The mission is empirically based.

As its reason for being, the mission of an organization is arrived at by establishing vehicles by which families, staff, management, boards of directors, community residents, and funding representatives can provide ideas and answers to five questions: 1) Who are we? 2) Why did we establish this organization? 3) Where is the organization going? 4) What is the nature of our organization? and 5) Who will receive our services? To keep in touch with both the vision and mission, the answer to only one question should be considered: Why do we provide these services?

Having a clear mission requires a consensus of the people throughout the organization about its official purpose. To facilitate a change in the mission of an organization to include a multilevel family-centered perspective, establishing a committee of representatives across all levels of the organization is the first step. The committee's composition should include board members, management, staff, and client-consumers including family members; in this way the committee will represent people who have a knowledge of the organization and of the community and who understand the need for their coexistence. Upon completion of a new or revised mission statement, this committee will need to go back to their constituencies or systems for review and feedback. Because each group will recommend a statement based on their particular agendas and priorities, the committee will need to devise a process or involve a party who can assist in designing a statement that supports the beneficiaries' and stakeholders' buy-in to the organization.

Final review of the new mission statement will need to be submitted to the governing board of directors for further refinement and subsequent adoptions. The new mission statement is discussed with staff, management, and key resources and supplemented by written feedback that provides steps to implementing the mission. These steps are necessary because organizations seeking buy in at all levels will want the implementation of the mission to be based on a team approach that includes people with varying roles and functions. These people need to help in the design and development of guidelines so that they can see themselves in the process as well as own the product of such change.

The organization bears some costs as a result of changing the mission, but these costs need not be exorbitant. Hiring a consultant to participate in the planning process can be helpful (Eubanks, O'Driscoll, Hayward, Daniels, & Connor, 1990). An alternative is to use senior management, former executives, or technical assistance from the United Way or another supportive liaison or trade association. Funding from foundations can also be sought as well

TABLE 19-2 Multilevel Family-Centered Perspective in Urban Community Organizations

	Definition of Mission	Conceptual Model of Service Delivery	Definition of Structure	Care Cycle	Definition of Outcomes	Plan of Intervention	Monitoring the Process	Evaluation of Outcomes	Enhancement and Development
BOARD OF DIRECTORS	Sanction family member participation on board. Facilitate modification of mission to reflect measurable objectives for family participation in planning, implementation, and evaluation. Adopt agency philosophy that sanctions family-centered participation in planning, implementation, and evaluation. Sanction family outcomes and mission statement.	Define scope of organizational policies and procedures to reflect philosophical orientation, with disability groups, practice theories, and anticipated outcomes at family and organizational levels. Develop clear policy on methods and theoretical orientation used to deliver family-centered services.	Create board committee with families, professionals, and community residents. Set policy and review operations of organization to ensure 1) family participation and evaluation, 2) that services are available to meet family needs, 3) that fund-raising plans are implemented to raise unrestricted service delivery, and 4) that time and resources are spent in accordance with family objectives.	Set policies on how families need to access services as well as the coordination of visible services and objectives of the organization.	Define measurable objective in mission statement. Define job description for board committees, terms of family objectives, and outcomes. Define measurable indicators for family, staff, and management performance.	Define plan of action to pursue short- and long-range family objectives. Assess/plan fund-raising needs. Assess/plan budget needs. Identify process for strategic planning with staff and family participation.	Assess the way services are provided via quality-assurance reports. Monitor financial practices.	Through program evaluation, track family responses to service delivery via satisfaction of service effectiveness. Track staff performance. Track board objectives.	Do needs assessment to determine relevance of current programs and service to address community needs. Review management recommendation for budget and plan in accordance with family needs and outcomes. Celebrate agency change and family/staff accomplishments.
MANAGEMENT	Educate/clarify mission within and outside of the organization. Expand participation of staff, family members, and board in defining mission. Meet with family members and staff in program to seek input about organizational focus.	Management task staff ways to understand theories of human behavior and practice technology that promote family participation and family achievement.	Define infrastructure on team of major objectives. Promote participating management philosophy practices. Use team management group to get task and activities completed. Use feedback from staff to facilitate service delivery.	Arrange case-management, therapy, and training process to facilitate enhanced independent functioning.	Identify client outcomes in job description, in agency program plans, and in program operating policies and procedures.	Define family objectives and input in program plans. Develop linkages with outside agencies educating them about focus on family outcomes.	Develop staff, family, and management quality-assurance review. Learn to ensure delivery of services in focus of the family use of supervision.	Evaluate service effectiveness in focus on family accomplishments and behavior change. Evaluate staff performance in accordance with family behavior change and community adjustment.	Plan activities to achieve objectives not previously met. Increase positive attention on how well staff and families are performing responsibilities. Assess staff for training or supervision in context of promoting family behavior change and participation to service delivery.

STAFF	Identify service outcomes with family member outcomes and mission statement. Adapt principles of family-centered practice.	Staff and family collaborate on service methods and treatment approaches to promote family achievement.	Participate in committees with families and management to plan board organization, staff training and activities and services.	Use policies and procedures to revise ways for families to enter and exit system.	Use time-management plan to identify service tasks and outcomes.	Use family service plans, treatment contracts, and joint family, staff, and management committees to lay out activities to pursue family outcomes.	Use time management to evaluate tasks, activities, objectives. Use quality-assurance procedures to assess progress.	Track trend and frequency of service outcomes (family reaction to treatment) by individual and caseload.	Focus on family treatment gains. Provide more support to family in areas in which they have demonstrated small behavior change.
FAMILY MEMBERS	Arrange meeting between family member groups and management to get family input on primary purpose of organization.	Family members inform staff of the services they are seeking to promote family achievement.	Participate in board committees, quality-assurance committee and activity planning meetings with staff and management.	Participate in defining service plan to address family statement of problem.	Resolve outcomes in observable and measurable actions and behaviors.	Plan activities and services with staff to correspond with self-identified objectives. Learn self-reinforcement skills. Identify reinforcement for task completion.	Involve family in tracking staff activities. Share feedback about staff and organization delivery treatment review.	Use family member satisfaction. Maintain log of family outcomes.	Use self-reinforcement skills. Increase contact with support system.

SOURCE: Briggs (1996b).

as developing arrangements with academic consultants. Compared with the cost associated with retaining a management consultant unfamiliar with the organization, other options may be more cost effective.

Structure. The form that an urban organization takes to achieve its primary purpose is reflected by the infrastructure and organization of the agency environment. The infrastructure defines the structural boundaries of the organization, which are usually reflected in the form of an organizational chart. The chart depicts the reporting relationships of the client-consumers, including families, staff, management, and board of directors. The chart may also reflect the mission of the organization through identifying the way the particular objectives are programmatically addressed through the division and departments of the organization.

The chain of command delineates how the organization is set up to accomplish the mission and who is responsible and accountable to whom at every level. In urban community organizations that use a multilevel family-centered perspective, the family members are involved in a number of roles and functions across levels of the organizationís infrastructure. This structure determines the way members of the organization relate to one another in accomplishing the mission, remembering of course that form (structure) follows function (goals and objectives).

How an organization is designed to accomplish the mission is as important as having a specific purpose. Placing emphasis on the desired inputs and perceptions of each level, especially those of the family, changes the way people interact. It certainly changes the parameters of accountability (Koroloff & Briggs, 1996). Rothman (1989) suggests a way to include clients in all aspects of the helping process. In his scheme, the practitioner retains responsibility for using competency-based skills, while the client-consumer provides input at any stage of the process. If clients disagree with the plan of action, they reserve the right to exercise their veto. However, person and environmental circumstances exist that challenge and, in some cases, limit the self-determination of clients in social services (for a review, see Rothman, 1989): client participation is possible but difficult to arrange. In this study, opportunities for client-consumer participation and input on all levels of the organization were highlighted.

Modifying the structure and environment of organizations by defining new roles and responsibilities for family (Kruzich & Friesen, 1984; Friesen & Koroloff, 1990) participation at all levels legitimizes their input in setting policies and decision making. Changing the way families participate in service delivery depends on the catalyst and process used to incorporate their perspective. According to Resnick (1978), change often occurs in organizations where there is a change catalyst (a person or group of people who have the commitment and resources to initiate change), an action system (a team or group motivated to work with the catalyst), and a change goal ("mechanism, process, or idea that would improve a particular policy, program procedure, or administrative arrangement for the purpose of improving services to clients," p. 30). In a multilevel family-centered urban community organization, the catalyst and process of change begins with a clearly stated vision, a measurable mission statement, and support for improved outcomes and services, all facilitated by interested and affected families, staff, management, community residents, and board members of an agency.

The design of an organizational culture that promotes goal attainment across multiple levels of an infrastructure within a family-centered perspective will need to consider the way in which the contingencies are defined and managed. Redmon and Wilks (1991) recommend changing the reinforcing consequences and contingencies as defined by the funding and regulatory agencies that provide the funds and licenses to urban community organizations. If adopted, changing the environmental contingencies of funding and accreditation of organizations may facilitate a host of behavior changes across multiple levels. Briggs et al. (1994, 1996) highlighted the changes in client-consumer, family, staff, and management behaviors after the implementation of multilevel strategy that involved changing the antecedents and consequences of behavior across levels of the organization's infrastructure.

Care cycle.   The care cycle defines the values, practice principles, and practice methods used to deliver goods and services. It defines the process by which client-consumers enter and exit the organization. It also defines the host of services provided. All in all, it is the vehicle used by management and staff to specifically define their roles and responsibilities to client-consumers.

In community organizations, the design of the care cycle is both community and market driven. This policy development process includes input from all levels of the organization's infrastructure. The executive director in collaboration with key committees of the board of directors needs to be responsible for overseeing this process. Although the design of the mix of programs and services should be directly tied to the needs and interests of community residents and families, the following must be taken into consideration: 1) availability of funding, 2) availability of additional community supports, and 3) technical assistance and support to secure additional resources (e.g., financial and in-kind supports).

Urban community organizations using multilevel family-centered perspectives include family members, staff, and management in defining the care cycle. At the board of directors' level, these particular stakeholders set policies on how families gain access to services and how services will be coordinated. The policies and procedures developed are the necessary structural parameters used to communicate to family members, staff, management, and board members acceptable and normative behaviors that are legally and administratively sanctioned.

While the board of directors proposes policies and procedures that govern the care cycle, the management and staff disposes of and executes them. Management, with the assistance of staff and client-consumers, designs or chooses the case-management, therapy, and client-training systems. The selection or design of each of these service types was based on how consistent they were with the practice model and philosophical orientation of the organization. In the organization in which this multilevel technology was initially tested, case management was based in a philosophy that considered the strengths and cultural and community context of the client-consumer and which was also performance driven as defined through a collaborative process involving the perspectives of clients, families, and staff.

The implementation of the care cycle by staff of multilevel family-centered urban organizations is primarily the role of staff and the client-consumer including the family. Staff of child and family services participates in weekly or biweekly interagency staff meetings, which include the affected youth, family, foster parents, staff, and program supervisor in order to review service plan progress, obstacles and barriers to service delivery, and plans of action that focus on defining the ways and means to achieve service effectiveness.

Family members participate in the care cycle so that their perspectives will assist in guiding the actions and activities of staff and program management. Staff interested in strengthening, preserving, and supporting families receiving community services receive early orientation and ongoing training. The focus of staff development at this juncture is to educate staff and management about the relevance of family and community participation in service delivery and the significance of their input as it relates to the organization's mission and overall vision.

Definition of outcomes. As the organization begins to direct the performance of each level, it must focus on the specific needs and the measurable objectives of a client-consumer (including the family) to enable them to become more independent within a supportive community environment. The outcomes of multilevel family-centered urban community organizations must bear a direct relationship to the mission statement, as in the studies by Christian (1983) and Briggs et al. (1994, 1996). If the organization can demonstrate to the funding source, the neighborhoods it serves, and its own staff and management that it can deliver, continued support is likely.

Behaviorally specific and measurable time-management, supervision, and quality-assurance tools are useful as a means to achieve a particular set of objectives (Christian, 1983; Maher, 1983). Staff develops each of these tools with input from each level of the infrastructure. To implement the policies and procedures, the staff needs to understand their goals and how they relate to the overall goals of the organization. They also need to know how to define their performance aims as they relate to family-centered goals and objectives.

At the board of directors' level, the definition of outcomes is relevant because all board committees must have descriptions that are performance driven and whose measures tie directly to the organization's mission. For example, in most urban community organizations the board has at least one executive committee and four standing committees: 1) membership, 2) finance, 3) programs and plans, and 4) development. The chairs of each of these committees make up the organization's executive committee. Take Agency X's mission as of November 1989:

The mission of Agency X is to enhance economic development, political empowerment, and ultimately community development by assisting less advantaged individuals to become more capable and self-reliant through the use of scientifically based methods along with sound management practices. As part of the membership committee's charge during this time it was well poised to recruit new board members that would enable the organization to enhance its economic base and the economic base of its stakeholders, including the staff, client-consumers, and community residents.

The same kind of logical connections can be made between the programs and plans of the committee of the board, which sanctioned a number of infrastructure development efforts at Agency X between 1984 and 1989 as a means for enhancing the management and direct practices of the staff and management. This focus results in a number of strategic actions and activities aimed at the design and implementation of an operating system that aided staff and management in assisting client-consumers and families enhance their functional capacities and "become more capable and self-reliant."

Plan of intervention.   The plan of intervention is coordinated by different individuals at different levels of the organization. In multilevel family-centered urban community organizations, the plan of intervention emphasizes the removal of conditions and practices that do not favor client-consumers including their families. One objective of the plan of intervention is to programmatically ensure the use of practice methods that incorporate family participation in activities across all levels of the organization. Administrative sanction of family-centered activities is critical to implementing a multilevel family-centered plan of intervention.

The plan of intervention at the board of directors' level includes 1) a plan of action to pursue short- and long-range family-centered objectives, 2) an assessment and plan to address fund-raising needs, and 3) the identification of a strategic planning process that includes staff, management, and family participation. The plan of intervention needs to include a vehicle by which standing committees of the board of directors may develop plans to facilitate the adoption or modification in policies and practices that promote a multilevel family-centered perspective. Such a process will facilitate accountability between the policy-making and management levels of the organization.

The plan of action at the management level includes 1) a description of the program plan that is based in a family-centered context, 2) service coordination plans that include the client-consumer and family as full partners,

3) supervisory processes that function as a means for establishing checks and balances with respect to family-centered goals and objectives, and 4) involving families as allies in the service delivery process.

Program plans are similar to treatment and services plans. The unit of attention for each differs. For individuals and families the plan is focused on treatment and services needed to assist consumers and families enhance functional capacity, and for organizations the focus is on the resources and supports needed to achieve family and client-centered objectives such as economic self-sufficiency and political and community empowerment. Similar to the program plan, the service coordination or community linkage plan needs to be written in such a manner that the perspectives and anticipated outcomes of all people involved with the organization are articulated with an emphasis on the perspectives of the client-consumer including the family.

The supervision process is fundamental to the implementation of the plan of intervention. The data collected from supervision is useful in making decisions on each level. Client-consumers and family members who do not perform at expected levels are provided opportunities to have their aims redefined into smaller, achievable, steps. Staff whose performance requires enhancement are provided opportunities similar to those provided to client-consumers to redefine their performance into smaller steps. If needed, they are provided training, periodic feedback, incentives, or a combination of enhancement strategies to improve their performance (Mager & Pipe, 1984; Ziarnik & Bernstein, 1982).

As allies to service delivery, family members are involved in planning and implementing a broad array of activities (Briggs et al. 1996). Friesen and Koroloff (1990) discussed the implications of using the family in planning and implementing services and recommended new roles for parents. They pinpointed the programmatic, fiscal, and administrative roles of families and the skills that clients, staff, and management need to foster a family-centered agenda. Porterfield, Evans, and Blunden (1985) effectively used families in the delivery and monitoring of community-based services. Their participation informed staff and management of those activities that had particular value and those that were less desirable. As natural helpers, family members must be involved in service delivery to increase opportunities for the client-consumer to have additional reinforcing experiences (Pinkston et al., 1982), as well as provide an important source of data to monitor the effectiveness of service delivery.

Monitoring the process. Monitoring the process is the quality-assurance component of the model. It provides the checks and balances system needed to ensure desirable performance and an enhanced organizational culture. This process involves an assessment of the way services are provided. This process is driven by the question, Are we doing what we set out to do? Throughout the organization, a number of quality-assurance activities are used to provide answers to that question. The process of feedback is a very useful tool for promoting accountability. The feedback at each level should bear a direct relationship to the organization's family-centered objectives. Much of what is discussed at most board of directors' meetings focuses on the fiscal health, development, and fund-raising needs of the organization. With assistance, even these inquiries can be connected to the goals and objectives of the organization as well as those stated in service plans for client-consumers including family development. At the board level, this could be monitored by looking at the number of jobs in a neighborhood that are the result of new programs and services. This same data could also be used to determine the number of jobs filled by client-consumers and family members as well as the change in the amount of family income for clients and community residents who were employed in these particular vacant positions.

Evaluation of outcomes.   Outcome evaluations inform funding sources, client-consumers, staff, and management about the benefits of the organization. In multilevel family-centered organizations, the objectives of each level are assessed through program evaluation. At the board of directors, level, the evaluation of outcomes can be assessed by looking at an evaluation that shows the progress of each program and service in relationship to the mission. The basis of such an evaluation is the extent to which the organization has been able to achieve service effectiveness along client-consumer, family member, staff, and management performance goals and objectives.

As illustrated in the study by Briggs et al. (1994), single-case study methods were used as a means for tracking consumer, staff, and program objectives. As agency practices were modified, there was an increase in the number of foster parent adoptions, a reduction in staff turnover, and an increase in the number of foster parents interested in providing care and support to nonwhite children.

Enhancement and development.   Techniques for maintaining treatment gains have been studied by Goldstein and Kanfer (1979) and Pinkston et al. (1982). An elaboration of this approach by Rzepnicki (1991) defines the major practice principles and steps for enhancing the durability of treatment gains. These practice principles include creating similarity between the intervention situation and the client-consumer's natural environment, increasing environmental support for improved client functioning, and providing opportunities for thorough learning of new behavior.

Pinkston and coworkers used these procedures to change and maintain positive behaviors of staff working with consumers in institutional settings. They applied this same technology to ensure the continuation of training and program implementation activities of staff, management and client-consumers at Agency X as reported by Briggs et al. (1994, 1996).

CONCLUSION

As multilevel technology is adapted and used in other organizational settings, a comprehensive evaluation of the usefulness of this approach will need to be completed. The multilevel family-centered approach has practical utility for client-consumers including their families, staff, and management of urban community organizations. The study of its effectiveness in other organizational setting and community environments needs further investigation, especially in fields of practice that place emphasis on family participation, such as child welfare.

One question that guides future studies is how does the multilevel approach enhance long-term, supportive relationships and positive alternatives for youth growing up in foster care? Although Briggs et al. (1994) provide a detailed account of how organizational environments can be shaped to produce desirable consequences for all organizational actors involved in permanency planning of foster parent adoptions, more is needed to understand how these new family arrangements have fared and what supports they used to remain intact.

In conclusion, a multilevel family-centered approach has practical utility for practitioners seeking to focus on broad-scale behavior change. More research is needed to test the usefulness of this approach in an interorganizational context. As youth with multiple service providers seek community-based service systems and supports, the usefulness of the multilevel approach will be important to professional and family members seeking effective service coordination technology. Affected families and professionals seeking flexible, seamless, wraparound services for youth with substance abuse, mental health, and juvenile justice issues may be able to develop intervention designs and development strategies that address the complex coordination of systems of care factors that threaten the service effectiveness for this emerging population. So far, the systems of care that address issues for youth are not linked in philosophy, theory, or practice. More research needs to be done in this area so that data may be used to design practice guidelines for professionals, service providers, and family members faced with the challenges of negotiating multiple service systems on behalf of children and youth with multiple needs and service requirements. A family-centered approach that incorporates empirically based and culturally responsive strategies may be useful to give these youth sufficient administrative supports and research and development resources.

CHAPTER 20

Clinical Practice with Involuntary Clients in Community Settings

Ronald H. Rooney

Anthony A. Bibus

In this chapter, Rooney and Bibus examine the issues involved with working with involuntary, or mandated, clients in social work practice. They examine ways in which practitioners can think about their work with mandated clients and the incongruence between the practice principles of self-determination and the perspectives of empowerment- and strengths-based methods and practice with involuntary clients. This chapter describes for students the way the profession looks at people who do not seek social work assistance. It provides the reader with an historical overview of social work's response to mandated clients and delineates the types of problems and settings involved in providing these social services. The chapter also provides for the reader the foundation knowledge and skills that practitioners need to know when working with involuntary clients. The reader learns the legal and ethical bases for practice with mandated clients and the best practice wisdom for goal setting. Practice guidelines are provided to the reader as professional tips or advice to follow when preparing to practice with mandated clients. The chapter also provides the student with a discussion about ways to ensure the effectiveness of social work practice with mandated clients and presents case examples and related evidence to support the usefulness of this type of social work practice. The chapter describes the challenges to the social worker practitioner when working at multiple levels of care, and students are given a few practice suggestions and factors to consider in this case. The chapter ends with practice guidelines for social workers and a discussion and caution to the reader about the critical issues to consider when working with involuntary clients.

Social work practice has been built on the model of providing service to those who desire it. Yet throughout our profession's history we have also provided service to those who, rather than seeking help, are required to have it or are seen by others as needing it. Other chapters in this book address practice with troubled youth (LeCroy, chapter 11), persons with drug or alcohol problems (Fischer, chapter 12), persons with phobias (Thyer, chapter 9), and persons experiencing marital discord (Cobb & Jordan, chapter 10). Sometimes such persons acknowledge these problems, admitting "I am addicted and need help," "I am getting in difficulty with the law," "I have a mental illness," or "Our marriage needs help." In such cases, persons have difficulties seen by others and they own responsibility for those concerns. In other instances, persons in such situations do not acknowledge the problems attributed to them by others (Reid, 1978). That is, they do not see themselves as having problems beyond the pressures brought by others.

Productive work with such clients is thus complicated by who owns the problem, who has the right to determine the problem, and the direction in which work will proceed (Cingolani, 1984). What happens then to a potential client whose problems are recognized by others rather than self-acknowledged? The answer depends on the nature of the problem, whether a violation of the law has occurred, and whether pressure or persuasion can be brought to bear on the intervention.

In addition, such work with clients who do not acknowledge problems creates ethical difficulties for social workers influenced by the values of client self-determination, empowerment, and pursuit of strengths (Freeberg, 1989; Gutierrez, 1990; Saleeby, 1997). Must we forgo these values to work with persons who have not requested our service?

In addressing this question, this chapter is about social work practice with persons who have not sought our assistance. They come under many names: hard to reach, reluctant, resistant, involuntary, and high risk. No matter how involuntary clients are labeled, it is important to recognize that practice with them is critical, even inevitable, and can be consistent with social work values. This chapter will describe the dynamics of involuntary status, offer principles for practice with involuntary clients that are legal, ethical, and effective, and provide practice guidelines for such work at multiple systems levels.

WHO ARE INVOLUNTARY CLIENTS? WITH WHAT KINDS OF PROBLEMS AND IN WHAT TYPES OF SETTINGS DO INVOLUNTARY TRANSACTIONS OCCUR?

Involuntary clients are persons who receive social and psychological services from human service agencies but do not actively seek them (Ivanoff, Blythe, & Tripodi, 1994; Rooney, 1992). Involuntary clients can be further divided into two groups based on the presence or absence of legally mandated contact. Hence, legally mandated clients are those who experience the threat or actuality of court orders (Hutchison, 1987). For example, social workers in probation and parole and other correctional settings routinely serve court-ordered clients (Harris & Watkins, 1987). Others have legally mandated contact with families regarding allegations of child abuse and neglect (Diorio, 1992; Weakland, Jordan, & Dimmock, 1992). Furthermore, persons with serious and persistent mental illness are also often under legal mandates to receive services (Scheid-Cook, 1993). In addition, social workers often work with perpetrators of partner or spouse abuse (Williams, 1992).

In addition to legally mandated clients, other clients experience formal and informal pressures to accept services. These clients are called nonmandated or nonvoluntary (Ivanoff et al., 1994, p. 6; Rooney, 1992). They are found in settings in which others have the power to attribute problems and influence their acceptance or at least minimal compliance with such services. For example, school children are frequently referred for services from a helping professional that they have not voluntarily sought (Franklin & Streeter, 1995). In addition, clients with substance abuse problems often experience pressure to seek and accept help (Burke & Clapp, 1997). Persons with disabilities may feel compelled to work with case managers in order to obtain benefits otherwise unavailable to them, such as housing (Mackelprang & Salsgiver, 1996). In instances of marital or family discord, frequently one party sees a problem and brings another reluctant party for assistance (McCown & Johnson, 1993). Finally, workfare programs pressure persons on welfare to seek work or face limits on their ability to draw on welfare funds (Mills, 1996; Hasenfeld & Weaver, 1996).

Involuntary transactions also frequently include encounters between clients and practitioners who are different from one another in many characteristics such as race, culture, ethnicity, power, socioeconomic status, and education. Further, members of historically oppressed groups are overrepresented in involuntary situations (Longres, 1991; Horejsi, Craig, & Pablo, 1992; Rooney & Bibus, 1996).

What Are the Goals for Involuntary Contact?

In practice with voluntary clients, the goal typically is to achieve outcomes mutually agreed upon with the client. When clients are mandated to receive services, some goals are required, whether or not the client agrees to them. For example, if a client is on probation or parole, then parts of the treatment plan will be mandated by court order or according to the plan of the probation officer. On the other hand, even in mandated situations, it is often helpful for there to be some fit in motivation and goals between practitioner, agency, and client such that the mandated client perceives personal benefit from the outcome in addition to carrying out the mandate (Videka-Sherman, 1988). Similarly, when nonvoluntary clients experience strong nonlegal pressures to participate in services, finding a fit in goals also increases the chances that the nonvoluntary client experiences more than a superficial involvement with services. When this motivational congruence is present, research findings from a variety of fields of clinical practice suggest that clients are more likely to avoid premature termination and to experience successful completion of their goals (Rooney, 1992; Bibus, 1992; Videka-Sherman, 1988).

How Are We Guided Legally?

Increasingly, laws, along with the policies, rules, and procedures they dictate, govern social work practice. This is particularly true for work with involuntary clients. Legal regulations often mandate contact between practitioners and clients, and they necessitate that social workers consider the interests and safety of other members of the community besides clients. They also provide some protection from unwarranted intrusion into involuntary clients' freedom or privacy. For example, parents facing charges of neglecting their children because of suspected alcohol abuse may be required by the court to meet with the child protective services social worker to assess whether or not they need treatment. These parents have rights to due process, informed consent, and confidentiality during the assessment so that only those aspects of their lives directly related to the care of their children should come under scrutiny and so that they have some choices over courses of action or treatment to follow as long as the children's needs are met.

Similarly, people with mental illness, physical impairments, or alcohol or drug addictions are sometimes found to be legally incompetent and placed under compulsory care. Yet social workers serving these committed patients, in addition to supervising their care, should also advocate for their legal rights. Under due process, those rights include adequate notice of legal proceedings and allegations, open hearings before impartial examiners, legal counsel, opportunities to cross-examine and present witnesses on their own behalf, written decisions based on fact, and the right to appeal (Saltzman & Proch, 1990). Other procedural standards and safeguards also are in place to curb inappropriate imposition of mandated treatments and arbitrary exercise of professional or agency discretion and to guarantee fundamental fairness. These include the laws protecting data privacy, confidentiality, and privileged communications, although all are subject to limitations and the rights of others, such as protection from harm or threats to life, can override them. In addition, clients have rights related to imposed treatment, including freedom from unnecessary treatment and access to needed treatment. To justify involuntary commitments, service settings must be the least restrictive or intrusive to meet the mandated needs. Clients must be found to be not competent to manage their own affairs or to be at immediate risk for harming themselves or others (Murdach, 1996).

Most importantly in work with involuntary clients, the legal and ethical requirements to ensure that clients are fully informed are of the highest priority (Senna, 1974). Informed consent must be upheld in the spirit of individualized, respectful, open collaboration between practitioners and clients and not just in the standardized forms often presented for routine signature (Regehr & Antle, 1997). The *Code of Ethics* provides the following guidance: "In instances when clients are receiving services involuntarily social workers should provide information about the nature and extent of services and the extent of clients' rights to refuse services" (NASW, 1996, p. 8). Asserting that, "Social workers often work in situations in which they have a responsibility for the interests not only of the client, but also of significant others in the community," Regehr and Antle (1997, p. 301) outline a number of obstacles to informed consent with mandated clients. Assessments and other interviews are often unstandardized, unstructured, and open ended. "As a result it is impossible to consider and inform the person of all the possible risks and benefits of consent" (Regehr & Antle, 1997, p. 303). Regehr and Antle continue that "for court-mandated clients to be fully informed, they would need to know in advance of participation that there is no guarantee of confidentiality and that others outside the court process may become aware of the social worker's findings, that the findings may not be in the client's favor, that there is no way to predict in advance what information will be received in the assessment process, and that there is no way to predict how the information collected will influence the conclusions reached in the social worker's report" (p. 303). They observe that in the presence of potentially coercive dynamics, it is difficult for clients to assess their vulnerability and the meaning of their relationship with the practitioner and indeed whether they are the primary clients. Hence, "social workers must similarly identify for all parties at the onset of the contract both the limitations of their role and the extent of their obligation to the safety of others" (pp. 303-304). Moreover, the therapeutic alliance is powerful such that relationship skills can inadvertently serve the purpose of social control (with a smiling face). "The client, assuming that the social worker will provide an assessment that is in his or her best interest despite the nature of the referral, may be completely honest with the worker, who is then obligated to use the information from the assessment to address the needs, interest and safety of others and not those of the client" (p. 301).

Inevitably, the shadow of professional liability also overcasts practice with involuntary clients, but this chapter may provide some reassurance that the best management of our heightened liability when clients face restrictions on their freedom is good practice. Good practice includes careful collaborative negotiation of service plans with clients, identification and usually compliance with the laws that apply, scrupulous record keeping, and regular supervision, using ethics committees or consultation groups if available. Since involuntary clients are disproportionately members of oppressed groups, such as women, children, and people of color, good practice also frequently requires focused competence in cross-cultural communication and services as well as acute sensitivity to the vulnerable position of people from oppressed groups. Social workers involved with involuntary clients must advocate for socially just laws and policies as part of their practice.

Accompanying this trend toward a legalistic context for practice is a tendency for social workers and agencies to refrain from intervening in clients' lives unless specific laws require their involvement, and then to do so coercively. Practitioners must transcend the false dichotomy of having only the options of inaction when there are no obvious legal grounds or, when there is a mandate, full-scale use of court orders and restrictive intrusive services. This chapter provides some guidance for a middle road wherein practitioners can attempt to influence clients' decisions and actions. In the following two sections we will review legal and ethical guidelines for when practitioners should try to influence involuntary clients and when they should refrain from influence attempts. These guidelines lead to an integrative framework for ethical practice with involuntary clients.

When first meeting with involuntary clients, families, groups, or organizations, practitioners should follow these steps:

1. State the reason for the contact clearly and nonjudgmentally, including the legal mandates.
2. Describe what is required of both the practitioner and client, not as conditions or threats, but in a matter-of-fact, business-like tone.
3. Identify fully the client's legal rights.
4. Explain the objectives and goals of the service intervention, especially the rationale for those goals that the client may not share.

Thus, a critical first step in working with involuntary clients is to identify what the client and practitioner alike are required to do by law. What laws apply to the contact between practitioner and clients? What policies, rules, and procedures pertain? What specifically must the practitioner and clients do to meet the mandates?

To identify the mandates in a given situation, social workers must not only know the immediate legal status of clients and the particular laws that govern their contact, but also the wider context of laws, regulations, and rights related to the clients' situations and the services being offered or planned. For example, a social worker assigned to supervise a youth on probation must become familiar with general rules covering probationers and court jurisdiction as well as the particular court order or sentence imposed on this youth. A social worker serving people in an overnight shelter must distinguish between guests' behavior that might be legal but in violation of the shelter's rules, such as drinking alcohol, and behaviors that are illegal, such as selling drugs. A case manager whose client is suffering from mental illness, is under supervised care in a hospital pending a commitment hearing, and is threatening others faces specific legal obligations such as the duty to warn potential victims as well as assessment reports required by the court overseeing the commitment. Likewise, a social worker supervising visiting arrangements for parents engaged in a custody dispute must inform all parties of the social worker's obligations as a mandated reporter of child abuse and neglect as well as make the required assessment regarding custody of the children.

This explicit and pervasive presence of legal requirements can create a climate of suspicion and fear even for seasoned practitioners and certainly for

most clients. Instead of the helping relationship growing in a nurturing interpersonal exchange marked by honesty and presumption of good will, contacts
between practitioners and clients can begin as adversarial and become hostile.
Hence, in addition to being knowledgeable about the particular and general
legal context of the client's situation, social workers involved in involuntary
transactions must be aware of the social control function of the profession. At
the same time, they must maintain a daily, active dedication to the professional ethical principles, especially the dignity and worth of each person and
the importance of partnership in human relationships (NASW, 1996).

HOW WE ARE GUIDED ETHICALLY

We are often the legally mandated agents for restitution, correctional sen-
tences, compulsory treatment, changes in behavior, incarceration, and other
restrictions of freedom imposed by the law on clients. However, the profession
in its commitment to human dignity recognizes that social workers will also
strive to act in accordance with universal human rights and ethical standards
that may supersede local, state, and national laws. In England, for example,
social workers are taking the lead in bringing the jurisdiction of the United
Nations Declaration of the Rights of the Child to bear on local child welfare
proceedings as well as national law, asserting children's rights over parents'
rights in some cases (Thomas & O'Kane, 1998). In addition, although social
workers' legal obligations are dictated and the range of potential decisions as
well as clients' choices are likely to be constrained by mandates, there is also
likely to be room for some professional discretion. Ethical dilemmas frequently
arise, especially when deciding to use or avoid influence attempts when
clients' actions threaten the safety of themselves or others. Should we intervene to protect the community or vulnerable persons from harm threatened
by clients? Or should we protect the client from undue interference in their
lives and their right to self-determination? The latest version of the NASW
Code of Ethics (1996) added the phrase "socially responsible" to self-determination for the first time, stating that, "Social workers promote clients' socially
responsible self-determination" (p. 5).

The NASW *Code of Ethics* goes on to say, "Social workers respect and promote the right of clients to self-determination and assist clients in their efforts
to identify and clarify their goals. Social workers may limit clients' right to self-
determination when, in the social worker's professional judgment, clients'
actions or potential actions, pose a serious, foreseeable, and imminent risk to
themselves or others" (p. 7).

Thus, social workers must sometimes engage in ethical paternalism, that
is, intervene beneficently in the client's own interest whether the client wants
it or not (Rooney, 1992; Reamer, 1995a). Murdach (1996) defines paternalistic beneficence "as protective interventions (at times despite the client's objections) intended to enhance the client's quality of life" (p. 27). Since exercising

such beneficence is prone to abuse, we must justify its necessity; the ethical burden of proof is on practitioners; clients do not have to prove that such interventions are unnecessary. The concept of beneficence can be useful for social workers today who are "increasingly required to intervene protectively in the lives of clients, many of whom are unable to fend for themselves" (p. 26). Murdach suggests a model for selecting the extent of intervention into clients' lives dependent on both the clients' level of impairment in their capacity to make decisions in their own interests and the risks they face. Limited beneficence may be appropriate for those situations in which a client with low impairment in decision-making capacity faces low risks to personal safety or harm of others. "For example, a psychiatric hospital social worker may recommend that a patient's visits with family members be limited despite the patient's objections if such contacts are perceived as detrimental to the patient's welfare. Although this intervention places some restrictions on the patient's right to have visitors, it does not abrogate the right entirely and hence constitutes a limited exercise in beneficence" (p. 28). A more extensive intervention into certain clients' rights and freedom for their own protection or that of others may be appropriate when the client's decision-making capacity is subject to a moderate or temporary level of impairment and when the risk faced is moderate to severe; Murdach calls this level selective beneficence: "For example, physically ill patients deemed incompetent may be deprived of the right to refuse medical treatment" (p. 29). The most extensive level of beneficence may be appropriate when the client's impairment in decision-making capacity is substantial and the risk to his or her own life or to the lives of others is pervasive. "Patients suffering from major psychoses, developmental disabilities, brain trauma, or stroke are examples of individuals who may require extensive paternalistic interventions [beneficence] to function satisfactorily" (p. 30). Since extensive beneficence represents the extreme end of this model both in terms of the restrictiveness of interventions and the risks faced by clients if the social worker does not intervene, Murdach urges caution in its judicious application. "Obviously, care needs to be taken that the patients' desires are not needlessly or heedlessly overridden. The need for careful assessment, therefore, is paramount" (p. 31).

Another model to assist practitioners in deciding whether to exercise ethical paternalism in work with involuntary clients is the empirically based framework developed by Rothman and colleagues (Rothman, 1989; Rothman, Smith, Nashima, Paterson, & Mustin, 1996). This framework presents a continuum of practitioner responses to clients' situations from less to more directive. There are four degrees of directiveness on this continuum, beginning with less directive, reflective responses, in which the social worker reflects with clients on their goals. Next is the suggestive response, during which the social worker explores options with clients and expresses a tentative preference for a particular direction in which the clients may choose to proceed. More directive is a prescriptive response, whereby the social worker clearly indicates a specific course of action. And most directive is a determinative response as the social worker takes independent action. Rothman and colleagues found that the degree of directiveness of intervention chosen as appropriate by practitioners depends on certain factors in the particular client situation. Constraints on self-determination can arise in clients' capacity, external restrictions, and the need to override self-determination based on other professional considerations or primary values. Practitioners may be less directive if the client has the mental acuity and skill to carry out reasonable decisions, if there are many helping resources, if the client has reason to distrust helpers and will react negatively to direction from the practitioner, or if the social worker knows of no research showing that one direction is more helpful than another. Practitioners may be more directive if there is serious danger to health or well-being, if extreme disability interferes with informed or rational choice, or if the client overtly disregards others' needs or threatens their safety.

The following guidelines provide a framework for legal and ethical practice with involuntary clients and offers guidance for when and how to exercise professional discretion:

1. Assure informed consent and due process as discussed above.
2. Utilize beneficence and paternalism within appropriate limits as discussed above.
3. Promote empowerment; within legal limits affirm worth, dignity, uniqueness, strengths, and ability to resolve problems.
4. Provide notice of requirements, negotiable items, and possible choices.
5. Make a commitment to honest communication. Since clients cannot leave help without consequences, avoid using deceptive methods, which are prohibited by the *Code of Ethics* (NASW, 4.04: "Social workers should not participate in, condone, or be associated with dishonesty, fraud, or deception," including withholding information, having hidden plans, inappropriate professional distance, etc.).
6. Advocate for social justice and fair treatment, challenging demeaning, unfair discriminatory practices and institutional restraints.

In deciding on a level of intervention that is legally and ethically supported, practitioners must consider the potential effectiveness of their helping efforts.

What Do We Know about Effectiveness?

Conventional wisdom about involuntary services has been that they are unlikely to be successful. In fact, studies reviewed in the social work literature suggest that those persons who are under court order do as well as others who are not court ordered (Videka-Sherman, 1988). A similar conclusion is drawn in a review of the psychology literature by Brehm and Smith: "Though many therapists and counselors are firmly convinced that successful therapeutic outcomes are substantially more difficult to achieve with nonvoluntary client populations, the results of applied (and therefore, necessarily correlational) research on this issue have not provided support for this belief" (Brehm & Smith, 1986, p. 88).

Perceived choice to remain in treatment may be a more powerful variable than initial referral status. That is, voluntarism can be enhanced by extending choices and a perceived sense of personal control (Brehm & Smith, 1986; Videka-Sherman, 1988). When a client perceives that he or she has a choice, even a constrained one, that client is more likely to be successful than the person who perceives no choice. Similarly, results are more promising when there is motivational congruence or an overlap or fit between the goals of the practitioner and those of the client (Videka-Sherman, 1988). Further, involuntary clients appear to benefit from role socialization or preparation through explaining expectations for client and practitioners roles (Garfield & Bergin, 1986). In addition, contracts that are more behaviorally specific have been more successful than less specific contracts (Kravetz & Rose, 1973; Mayer & Timms, 1970). Finally, clients are more likely to complete tasks in which they have participated in selecting (Meichenbaum & Turk, 1987).

In a recent survey of clients receiving outpatient services in a mental health center, motivations for treatment were compared between those who were court ordered to receive help and those who were not. Court-ordered clients were expected to express less concern about their problems and to be less ready for change than voluntary clients. While court-ordered clients expressed fewer concerns than voluntary clients, it does not follow that they were unwilling or unable to change; one-fourth of them expressed that they were thinking about changing, doing something about making a change, or attempting to maintain a change (O'Hare, 1996). O'Hare suggests, similar to the above recommendations, that the first goal is to accustom court-ordered clients to clienthood by accepting their initial reluctance, avoiding premature confrontation, clarifying dual roles, and providing some sense of control and choice in selecting methods and goals. Hence, we avoid a "muddled enterprise where clinicians pretend to treat and clients pretend to comply" (p. 421).

How Do We Approach Intake and Assessment?

Preparation for intake and assessment may begin in the office as the practitioner reviews available case information. The practitioner must be clear about legal mandates and policies that guide what he or she and the client must do. In addition, however, the practitioner should be equally clear about client rights, remaining freedoms, and choices, even though they may be constrained ones. That is, while participation in a chemical dependency assessment may be legally mandated, the practitioner may be able to offer constrained alternatives within the provider of the assessment. In addition, the practitioner may prepare to avoid prejudgment by focusing more on the facts leading to the contact and less on the interpretation of those facts or labels attached to them in the file. For example, it is important to distinguish observed facts in a police report of domestic violence from speculation about the perpetrator's motivation.

The actual assessment needs to begin with a clarification of roles and a specification of both what is required and nonnegotiable and what may be negotiable. This explanation should be conducted in a respectful fashion that avoids judgment and labeling. Even when conducted in such a fashion, many involuntary clients express anger and resentment in having such contact. Rather than label negative responses as evidence of resistance or pathology, it is more useful to consider negative responses to be the expected responses to perceived threats to valued freedoms (Brehm, 1976). Hence, if the practitioner expects the negative response and considers it normal, it is possible to act to reduce that negative response. For example, by avoiding labeling, providing choices, and emphasizing remaining freedoms, negative responses can be reduced (Brehm, 1976; Rooney, 1992).

In addition, if the client anticipates that the practitioner's opinion and report will be significant in determining the client's future regarding key goals, the practitioner may anticipate efforts by the involuntary client to influence the impression the practitioner has of him or her. Specifically, client efforts may include attempts to ingratiate the practitioner (you are better than the last worker I had), to intimidate him or her, to selectively confess to a part but not the whole of the allegations, or in general to present oneself in the best possible light (Jones & Pittman, 1982). Rather than label such efforts as manipulative, it is more useful for the practitioner to anticipate them as normal efforts to influence the practitioner's impression. The practitioner can then be clear about what kinds of data will influence his or her report, and such efforts at making an impression may become less necessary.

Finally, since efforts to engage the client in motivational congruence will require some linkage with client goals and values, the practitioner should pay attention to those values expressed by the client. For example, if a parent who is alleged to have abused or neglected his or her child expresses love and concern for the child's safety, that value can be drawn on in attempting to contract with the client in ways that preserve the child's safety.

What Are the Principles of Intervention?

Building on the above process of engagement, socialization, and assessment, the practitioner should attempt to develop a contract that includes some measure of motivational congruence. That is, in addition to including nonnegotiable, legally mandated items, the practitioner should seek to include client goals and motivations. Four types of agreement that seek to enhance motivational congruence are described below (Rooney, 1992).

Agreeable mandate. In some instances, the practitioner may be able to find a goal or problem that the involuntary client perceives as overlapping with the problem or goal that he or she is mandated to address. For example, people with children in out of home care may perceive the problem as "my child is in foster care" and have the goal of regaining custody. In order to reach this goal, the client will have to acknowledge the conditions that led to the removal of the child. In other instances, persons with serious and persistent mental illness rarely see their problem as "not taking psychotropic medication." Rather, the goal as they perceive it is likely to be "live independently" or "avoid hospitalization." In order to meet this goal, taking medication may be selected as a means to an end.

Quid pro quo or "let's make a deal." Some clients do not perceive any inherent value in working on a mandated goal or problem. On the other hand, they may be willing to barter or work on a mandated problem in exchange for an incentive or a problem of their own concern. It should be noted that mandated clients do not have the option of refusing to work on mandated problems. Their participation may, however, be enhanced by provision of incentives.

Get rid of the pressure or mandate. Many involuntary clients do not perceive a reason for working on the mandated problem and incentives are not readily visible. However, "getting other people out of my business" may be a goal that they would find attractive. Some might think that such motivation is insufficient since the client may not acknowledge the problem attributed to him or her. This "get rid of the pressure" strategy is based on the premise that motivation may be enhanced over time and that failure to capitalize on current motivation may handicap efforts by not including areas of congruence.

Informed consent. If the involuntary client does not choose to voluntarily participate on any of the levels suggested above, the social work practitioner should clarify his or her intention to proceed to carry out the legal requirements and to solicit client input on them.

The above contracting strategies encourage the exploration for fit or congruence in motivation between the practitioner and client. Lack of fit often leads to ineffective work in which involuntary clients evade meaningful involvement in the work and practitioners experience frustration. Should the practitioner successfully negotiate a contract, additional principles can be used to facilitate ongoing work.

Completion of disagreeable tasks. Even when involuntary clients agree with all or parts of contracts, they often find themselves faced with disagreeable tasks. Such tasks are not inherently reinforcing but rather necessities toward a larger goal (Rooney, 1992). For example, completing random urinalyses may be a disagreeable task for some. There are several ways to facilitate the completion of disagreeable tasks. First, practitioners can solicit client input in selecting the order of tasks. If all cannot be addressed simultaneously, then the client can participate in selecting those that will be explored first. In some instances this might be done in a shared fashion: the client suggests the first task and the practitioner suggests the second task. Second, the client might have some influence on when, where, and how the task might be completed. For example, a client might be able to pick from several alternative locations where urinalyses could be completed. Third, the client can be reminded that he or she is completing this task for his or her own reasons. For example, a client ordered to complete parenting education may remind him- or herself that the task is being done to regain custody of their child.

Contract around specific agreed-upon outcomes.   The contracting process is designed to share power in an otherwise largely unbalanced power situation in which the agency and practitioner may have more power to influence the contents of the contract than the client. Involuntary clients can experience their involvement as open ended such that the prospects of living outside involuntary scrutiny become ever more remote. For example, if the practitioner or agency continues to add new demands beyond those specified in the original contract, the involuntary client can experience the demoralization of a continually moving marker. Circumstances in which new expectations might need to be added should be specified in the original contract. That is, new law violations or serious threats to health and safety might constitute grounds for unilateral changes to contracts. Should the agency or practitioner reserve the right to add other indicators of success before termination of the contract will be considered, the power of the involuntary client to influence the contract and his or her motivation to complete it can be reduced.

How Do We Practice at Multiple Systems Levels?

Dynamics of interaction between practitioners and individual involuntary clients are complicated and subject to change as both parties become more or less willing to work with each other or share each other's goals for the work. Of course, if the practitioner is working with larger systems such as families, groups, organizations, and communities, the complexity of interactions among system members multiplies. Fortunately, so do the opportunities for mutual influence and change. The principles for intervention reviewed above still apply and promise to increase the likelihood that practice with these larger systems will be effective and ethical. Indeed, a practice focus that is community based as opposed to one based in psychotherapy is seen by some social workers as the defining characteristic that distinguishes social work from other helping professions (Adams & Nelson, 1995; Specht & Courtney, 1994; Haynes, 1998). In addition, members of larger systems are likely to experience the full range of normal reactions to being threatened with the loss of valued freedoms, so social workers should be prepared for premature drop outs, technical compliance with the letter of the law, going through the motions while seeking loopholes to escape perceived unfair restrictions or prerequisites, and outright hostility toward the practitioners themselves (Chovanec & Kuechler, 1999). These reactions should be carefully assessed and understood rather than labeled as indications that members of the systems involved are uncooperative or resistant simply for reacting to their involuntary status. The principles of practice outlined here in addition to other sound practice strategies including contracting can be useful in responding to initial reactions, preventing a dangerously adversarial encounter, and focusing energy on concerns shared by most of the members of the systems and by the practitioner.

While most models for working with families, groups, organizations, and communities presume that at least one member of the client system has acknowledged a problem or need for help from the practitioner, few social workers are wholeheartedly invited by members of a family, group, organization, or community to work with them. And even when an invitation is extended, the system or members within the system often have different views of the problem than outsiders and different goals from those set forth in the laws mandating social work intervention or from those shared by the practitioner. For example, a social worker might arrive at a community focus-group meeting called to engage community members in providing wraparound supports for families whose children are returning to their care from institutional settings and discover that instead of the expected embrace of a troubled family by the community, participants in the focus group want the social service agency to move "those" families out of the neighborhood. Similarly, a school social worker may be called on to persuade a family whose children have lice to submit to home visits by school nursing and county public health officials and find that the family refuses all contact and plans to pull the children out of the public schools. Hospital social workers routinely are involved in helping families negotiate supervised living arrangements for loved ones when there are deep and agonizing differences among family members and perhaps with the patients themselves regarding where they should be allowed to live. These sensitive negotiations often take place under pressures of mandates to free up a bed or shortages in ideal resources for dignified living arrangements and treatment. Family-based practitioners may provide family counseling for families facing placement of an adolescent into foster care, and the parent may be going through the motions of the program figuring that it will fail and that the preferred outcome of placement of the adolescent will finally be authorized. A social worker providing rehabilitative job counseling may be assigned to give the mandatory orientation to the work requirements, time limits, and sanctions built into new welfare reform legislation to a group of parents more interested in day-care subsidies, health care, housing, transportation assistance, or grants to support them in caring for infant children in their home than they are in seeking minimum wage employment. On occasion, a practitioner might be asked by the upper management of a social service agency to provide training for staff in an important area such as cultural competence and discover at the first meeting with the quite hostile agency staff that the goal of training is understood to be "Discovering the Racist Within." Much of group work is frequently in settings where some or all of the group members are required or under outside pressure to attend, such as in correctional institutions or drug and alcohol treatment programs.

Thus, as indicated above, a critical first step when working with larger systems is to identify what the practitioner is required to do, what members of the system are required to do, what is negotiable, and where there are opportunities for free choices not governed by legal mandates or subject to formal and informal pressures. Then, practitioners should clearly identify how they and their agencies define the problems faced by the members of the family, group, organization, or community and what the primary outcome of their interventions is intended to be. This definition of the problem and of the goals should then be compared with each member of the system's own definition of the problem and their own goals. This step could lead to discovering some potential for motivational congruence. For example, the parent who is willing to participate in family counseling only as a means for her daughter to be placed out of the home and the daughter who is frustrated by what she views to be unreasonable rules and demands on her time may both be willing to use the mandated family sessions to negotiate and test out a new set of expectations that might make their household more peaceful and safe from the violent fights they had experienced before. If such an agreeable mandate is not feasible, the mother in this case-example might agree to participate in a certain number of sessions in exchange for the practitioner's help in referral to a "tough love" support group and the daughter's agreement to meet with a school social worker individually. Or both mother and daughter might agree to be present at the minimum four in-home family counseling sessions as required by the placement policies and at the end of those sessions be done with the family-based services option whether successful or not. And if none of these attempts to reach some motivational congruence work, then the practitioner should review with the family the legal consequences, including placement of the daughter, but probably at the mother's expense. All of the rights of the parents and the children in these situations should be explained thoroughly. In the experience of the authors, social workers are sometimes reluctant to fully disclose options available to parents, such as seeking police holds to bypass agency procedures for authorizing placements, fearing that clients might actually exercise their rights to these options. But keeping these legal options secret may backfire and certainly could lead to fostering long-standing distrust of the helping system. Contracting provides a useful mechanism for forming the basis of motivational congruence and for providing fully informed consent.

Social work educators and group workers Chovanec and Kuechler have been studying work with involuntary groups and how groups faced with mandated purposes and goals differ from voluntary task groups (Chovanec & Kuechler, 1999). They have found that "social work literature appears to be limited in providing both theoretical and practice knowledge applicable to working specifically with this client population" (p. 2). Nevertheless, after a thorough review of the existing research and practice models applicable to work with groups whose members are legally required or under external pressure to participate, they suggest guidelines for the beginning, middle, and ending phases. In the beginning phase, leaders of involuntary groups need to tune in to expressed concerns of involuntary clients in order to reach for motivational congruence. They also need to clarify the nonnegotiable norms and purpose of the group as well as seek group input into the negotiable norms and purpose. They suggest that anger is expected during the middle phase and the leaders are responsible for channeling it productively. Finally, the termination phase is more focused on completion of requirements than on a sense of loss as the group comes to an end.

Supervision, consultation, and teaming when working with larger systems are critical. The dynamics of being a practitioner with involuntary clients, maintaining hope, replenishing our professional energies, and sustaining ethical and effective practice strategies in organizational climates that are stagnating or sterile require us to secure a support network of like-minded practitioners within and without our own clinical settings (Rooney, 1992; Sherman & Wenocor, 1983). Again, we must be part of healthy systems to intervene helpfully with other systems.

SUMMARY

This chapter has suggested that work with involuntary clients is common in social work practice and that such practice can often be conducted congruently with the social work principles of maximizing self-determination, utilizing strengths, pursuing empowerment, and facilitating motivational congruence. On the other hand, social work actions to protect individuals from self-harm and the community from danger are sanctioned by the profession. Social workers now practice in an environment in which many clients experience multiple pressures from simultaneous time lines. For example, drug-dependent parents participating in concurrent planning face one-year time limits to demonstrate that they can successfully parent. Similarly, clients in workfare programs experience time limits to secure employment. Such requirements increase pressures on involuntary clients to succeed and to do so within time limits. It falls to social workers and other helping professionals to assist them in efforts to succeed. Such assistance includes not only counseling and encouragement, but also access to needed resources and skills to complete their tasks.

References

Abbot, P., Weller, S., Delaney, H., & Moore, B. (1998). Community reinforcement approach in the treatment of opiate addicts. *American Journal of Drug and Alcohol Abuse, 24,* 17–30.

Abramson, M. (1985). The autonomy-paternalism dilemma in social work practice. *Social Casework, 66*(7), 387–393.

Achatz, M., & MacAllum, C. (1994). *Young unwed fathers: Report from the field.* Philadelphia, PA: Public/Private Ventures.

Adams, P., & Nelson, K. (Eds.). (1995). *Reinventing human services: Community- and family-centered practice.* New York: Aldine de Gruyter.

Adler, G. (1985). *Borderline psychopathology and its treatment.* New York: Jason Aronson.

Advocate Internet. (1998, September 18). New AIDS drug.

Airaksinen, T. (1998). Professional ethics. In R. Chadwick (Ed.), *Encyclopedia of applied ethics* (Vol. 3, pp. 671–682). San Diego: Academic Press.

Albanese, H., & Gardner, K. (1977). Biofeedback treatment of tardive dyskinesia: Two case reports. *American Journal of Psychiatry, 134,* 1149–1150.

Allen-Meares, P. (1984). Adolescent pregnancy and parenting: The forgotten adolescent father and his parents. *Journal of Social Work and Human Sexuality, 3*(1), 27–38.

Allgood-Merten, B., Lewinsohn, P., & Hops, H. (1990). Sex differences and adolescent depression. *Journal of Abnormal Psychology, 99*(1), 55–63.

American Medical Association (1995). Ethical issues in managed care. *Journal of the American Medical Association, 273,* 330–335.

American Psychiatric Association (1980). *Diagnostic and statistical manual of mental disorders.* (3rd ed.). Washington, DC: APA.

American Psychiatric Association (1987). *Diagnostic and statistical manual of mental disorders.* (3rd., revised ed.). Washington, DC: American Psychiatric Press.

American Psychiatric Association (1994). *Diagnostic and statistical manual of mental disorders* (4th ed.). Washington, DC: APA.

American Psychiatric Association (1995). Practice guidelines for the treatment of patients with substance use disorders: Alcohol, cocaine, opioids. *American Journal of Psychiatry, 152,* 3–50.

Ammerman, R. T., Last, C. G., & Hersen, M. (Eds.). (1993). *Handbook of prescriptive treatments for children and adolescents.* Boston, MA: Allyn & Bacon.

Ammerman, R. T., & Van Hasselt, V. B. (1988). The Callner-Ross Assertion Questionnaire. In M. Hersen & A. S. Bellack (Eds.), *Dictionary of behavioral assessment techniques.* New York: Pergamon.

Anderson, C. M. (1989). Goal-setting in social work practice. In B. R. Compton & B. Galaway (Eds.), *Social work processes.* Belmont, CA: Wadsworth.

Anderson, C. M., Reiss, D. J., & Hogarty, G. E. (1986). *Schizoprenia and the family.* New York: The Guilford Press.

Anderson, E. (1989). Sex codes and family life among poor inner-city youths. *Annals of the American Academy of Political and Social Science,* 59–78.

407

Anderson-Smith, L. (1988). Black adolescent fathers: Issues of service provision. *Social Work, 33*(3), 269–271.

Andolfi, M. (1980). Prescribing the families' own dysfunctional rules as a therapeutic strategy. *The Journal of Marital and Family Therapy, 6,* 29–36.

Aneshensel, C., & Stone, J. (1982). Stress and depression: A test of the buffering model of social support. *Archives of General Psychiatry, 39,* 1392–1396.

Annis, H. M. (1986). A relapse prevention model for treatment of alcoholics. In W. R. Miller & N. Heather (Eds.), *Treating addictive behaviors: Processes of change.* New York: Plenum.

Arkava, M., & Lane, T. (1983). *Beginning social work research.* Boston, MA: Allyn & Bacon.

Armelius, B., Kullgrean, G., & Renberg, E. (1985). Borderline diagnosis from hospital records. *Journal of Nervous and Mental Disease, 173,* 32–34.

Arnold, S. (1970). Confidential communication and the social worker. *Social Work, 15,* 61–67.

Astor, A. R., Behre, J. W., Wallace, J. M., & Fravil, K. A. (1998). School social workers and school violence: Personal safety, training, and violence programs. *Social Work, 43,* 223–232.

Atherton, C. R. (1993). Empiricists versus social constructionists: Time for a cease-fire. *Families in Society: The Journal of Contemporary Human Services, 74*(10), 617–624.

Au, C. (1996). Rethinking organizational effectiveness: Theoretical and methodological issues in the study of organizational effectiveness for social welfare organizations. *Administration in Social Work, 20*(4), 1–21.

Auslander, G. K. (1996). Outcome evaluation in host organizations: A research agenda. *Administration in Social Work, 20*(2), 15–27.

Austin, D. M. (1997). The profession of social work in the second century. In M. Reisch & E. Gambrill (Eds.), *Social work in the 21st century* (pp. 396–407). Thousand Oaks, CA: Pine Forge Press.

Austin, K. M., Moline, M. E., & Williams, G. T. (1990). *Confronting malpractice: Legal and ethical dilemmas in psychotherapy.* Newbury Park, CA: Sage Publications.

Austin, M. J., Kopp, J., & Smith, P. L. (1986). *Delivering human services.* New York: Longman.

Axelrod, R. (1984). *The evolution of cooperation.* New York: Basic Books.

Azrin, N. (1976). Improvements in the community reinforcement approach to alcoholism. *Behaviour Research and Therapy, 14,* 339–348.

Azrin, N., Flores, T., & Kaplan, S. (1975). Job-finding club: A group assisted program for obtaining employment. *Behaviour Research and Therapy, 13,* 17–22.

Azrin, N. H., Naster, J., and Jones, R. 1973. Reciprocity counseling: A rapid learning-based procedure for marital counseling. *Behaviour Research and Therapy, 11,* 365–382.

Azrin, N., Sisson, W., Meyers, R., & Godley, M. (1982). Alcoholism treatment by disulfiram and community reinforcement therapy. *Journal of Behavior Therapy and Experimental Psychiatry, 11,* 365–382.

Baer, D. M., & Wolf, M. M. (1970). The entry into natural communities of reinforcement. In R. Ulrich, T. Staachnki, & J. Maabry (Eds.), *Control of Human Behavior* (Vol. 2, pp. 319–324). Glenview, IL: Scott Foresman.

Baer, D. M., Wolf, M. M., & Risley, T. R. (1968). Some current dimensions of applied behavior analysis. *Journal of Applied Behavior Analysis, 1,* 91–97.

Baer, D. M., Wolf, M. M., & Risley, T. R. (1987). Some still-current dimensions of applied behavior analysis. *Journal of Applied Behavior Analysis, 20,* 313–327.

Bailey-Dempsey, C., & Reid, W. J. (1996). Intervention design and development: A case study. *Research on Social Work Practice, 6*(2), 208–228.

Baines, D. (1997). Feminist social work in the inner-city: The challenges of race, class and gender. *Affilia, 12*(3), 297–317.

Baker, B. L., Cohen, D. C., & Saunders, J. T. (1973). Self-directed desensitization for acrophobia. *Behavior Research and Therapy, 11,* 79–89.

Baker, T. B., & Cannon, D. S. (Eds.). (1988). *Assessment and treatment of addictive disorders.* New York: Praeger.

Baltes, M. M., & Barton, E. M. (1977). New approaches toward aging: A case for the operant model. *Educational Gerontology, 2,* 383–405.

Baltes, M. M., & Zerbe, M. B. (1976). Independent training in nursing home residents. *The Gerontologist, 16,* 428–432.

Bandler, R., & Grinder, J. (1975). *Patterns of the hypnotic techniques of Milton H. Erickson, M.D.* (Vol. 1). Cupertino, CA: Meta Publications.

Bandler, R., & Grinder, J. (1982). *Reframing.* Moab, UT: Real People Press.

Bandura, A. (1977a). Self-efficacy: Toward a theory of behavior change. *Psychological Review, 84,* 191–215.

Bandura, A. (1977b). *Social learning theory.* Englewood Cliffs, NJ: Prentice-Hall.

Bandura, A. (1986). *Social foundations of thought and action.* Englewood Cliffs, NJ: Prentice-Hall.

Barber, J. G., & Gilbertson, R. (1996). An experimental investigation of a brief unilateral intervention for the partners of heavy drinkers. *Research on Social Work Practice, 6,* 325–336.

Barber, J. G., & Gilbertson, R. (1997). Unilateral interventions for women living with heavy drinking. *Social Work, 42,* 69-78.

Barker, R. (1984). *Treating couples in crises.* New York: Free Press.

Barker, R. L., & Branson, D. M. (1993). *Forensic social work.* New York: Haworth Press.

Barker, R. (Ed.). (1995). *The social work dictionary* (2nd ed.). Washington, DC: NASW Press.

Barlow, D. (1988). *Anxiety and its disorders.* New York: Guilford.

Barlow, D. H., Hayes, S. C., & Nelson, R. O. (1984). *The scientist practitioner: Research and accountability in clinical and educational settings.* New York: Pergamon Press.

Barry, V. (1986). *Moral issues in business.* (3rd ed.). Belmont, CA: Wadsworth.

Barry, W. A. (1968). Conflict in marriage: A study of the interactions of newlywed couples (Doctoral Dissertation). University of Michigan: University Microfilms, 68–13, 273.

Barth, R. P. (1996). *Reducing the risk: Building skills to prevent pregnancy, STD and HIV.* (3rd ed.). Santa Cruz, CA: ETR Associates.

Bartlett, H. M. (1970). *The common base of social work practice.* Silver Spring, MD: NASW Press.

Bartolome, F. (1983). The work alibi: When it's harder to go home. *Harvard Business Review, 61*(2), 76–74.

Bartolome, F., & Evans, L. P. A. (1980). Must success cost so much? *Harvard Business Review, 58*(2), 137–148.

Bass, E., & Davis, L. (1988). *The courage to heal: A guide for women survivors of child sexual abuse.* New York: Harper and Row.

Bates, L. W., McGlynn, F. D., Montgomery, R. W., & Mattke, T. (1966). Effects of eye–movement desensitization versus no treatment on repeated measures of fear of spiders. *Journal of Anxiety Disorders, 10,* 555–569.

Baucom, D. H. (1982). The relative utility of behavioral contracting and problem solving/communications training in behavioral marital therapy: A controlled outcome study. *Behavior Therapy, 13,* 162–174.

Baucom, D. H., & Hoffman, J. A. (1986). The effectiveness of marital therapy: Current status and application to the clinical setting. In N. S. Jacobson & A. S. Gurman (Eds.), *Clinical handbook of marital therapy* (pp. 597–620). New York: Guilford Press.

Bay-Hinitz, A. K., Peterson, R. F., & Quilitch, H. R. (1994). Cooperative games: A way to modify aggressive and cooperative behaviors in young children. *Journal of Applied Behavior Analysis, 27,* 435–446.

Beck, D. F. (1976). Research findings on the outcomes of marital counseling. In H. L. Olsen (Ed.), *Treating relationships.* Lake Mills, IA: Graphic.

Beck, T. T. (1976). *Cognitive therapy and the emotional disorders.* New York: International Universities Press.

Beck, T. T. (1988). *Love is never enough.* New York: Harper and Row.

Beidel, D. C., Turner, S. M., & Morris, T. L. (1995). A new inventory to assess childhood social anxiety and phobia: The Social Phobia and Anxiety Inventory for Children. *Psychological Assessment, 7,* 73–79.

Bellah, R. N., Madsen, R., Sullivan, W. M., Swidler, A., & Tipton, S. M. (1985). *Habits of the heart: Individualism and commitment in American life.* New York: Harper and Row.

Belle, D. (1982). Lives in stress: *Women and depression.* Beverly Hills, CA: Sage Publications.

Benbenishty, R. (1996). Integrating research and practice: Time for a new agenda. *Research on Social Work Practice, 6*(1), 77–82.

Benbenishty, R. (1997). Outcomes in the context of empirical practice. In E. J. Mullen & J. L. Magnabosco (Eds.), *Outcomes measurement in the human services.* Washington, DC: NASW Press.

Berliner, A. K. (1989). Misconduct in social work practice. *Social Work, 34,* 69–72.

Bernstein, B. (1981). Malpractice: Future shock of the 1980's. *Social Casework, 62*(3), 175–181.

Bernstein, E. M., & Putman, F. W. (1986). Development, reliability, and validity of a dissociation scale. *Journal of Nervous and Mental Disease, 174,* 727–735.

Bernstein, S. (1960). Self–determination: King or citizen in the realm of values. *Social Work, 5*(1), 3–8.

Berube, M. S. (Ed.). (1991). *American heritage dictionary of the English language* (3rd ed.). Boston: Houghton Mifflin.

Besa, D. (1994). Evaluating narrative family therapy using single-system research designs. *Research on Social Work Practice, 4*(3), 309–325.

Besharov, D. J. (1985). *The vulnerable social worker: Liability for serving children and families.* Silver Spring, MD: National Association of Social Workers.

Besharov, D. J., & Besharov, S. H. (1987). Teaching about liability. *Social Work, 32*(6), 517–522.

Bibus, A. A. (1992). *The influence of supervisors on social workers' practice with involuntary clients: An exploratory study of a child welfare training project.* Unpublished doctoral dissertation.

Bierman, K. L., & Greenberg, M. T. (1996). Social skills training in the fasttrack. In R. D. Peters & R. J. McMahon (Eds.), *Preventing childhood disorders, substance abuse, and delinquency.* Thousand Oaks, CA: Sage.

Biestek, F. P. (1957). *The casework relationship.* Chicago: Loyola University Press.

Biestek, F. P., & Gehrig, C. C. (1978). *Client self-determination in social work: A fifty-year history.* Chicago: Loyola University Press.

Biglan, A. (1995). *Changing cultural practices: A contextualist framework for intervention research.* Reno, NV: Context Press.

Biglan, A. (1996). Sexual coercion. In M. A. Mattaini & B. A. Thyer (Eds.), *Finding solutions to social problems: Behavioral strategies for change* (pp. 289–316). Washington, DC: APA Books.

Biglan, A., Glasgow, R., & Singer, G. (1990). The need for a science of larger social units: A contextual approach. *Behavior Therapy, 21,* 195–215.

Biglan, A., Sverson, H., Ary, D., & Faller, C. (1987). Do smoking prevention programs really work? Attrition and the internal and external validity of an evaluation of a refusal skills training program. *Journal of Behavioral Medicine, 10,* 159–171.

Billups, J. O. (1992). The moral basis for a radical reconstruction of social work. In P. N. Reid & P. R. Popple (Eds.), *The moral purposes of social work* (pp. 100–119). Chicago: Nelson–Hall.

Bissell, L., Fewell, L., & Jones, R. (1980). The alcoholic social worker: A survey. *Social Work in Health Care, 5*(421–432).

Bissell, L., & Haberman, P. W. (1984). *Alcoholism in the professions.* New York: Oxford University Press.

Black, P. N., Hartley, E. K., Whelley, J., & Kirk-Sharp, C. (1989). Ethics curricula: A national survey of graduate schools of social work. *Social Thought, 15*(3/4), 141–148.

Blackman, D. K., Gehle, C., & Pinkston, E. M. (1979). Modifying eating habits of the institutionalized elderly. *Social Work Research and Abstracts, 15,* 18–24.

Blackman, D. K., Howe, M., & Pinkston, E. M. (1976). Increasing participation in social interaction of the institutionalized elderly. *The Gerontologist, 16,* 69–76.

Blackman, D. (1981, May). *Applied behavioral analysis in institutions for the elderly.* Paper presented at the 7th Annual Convention of the Association for Behavior Analysts, Milwaukee, WI.

Blades, J. (1984). Mediation: An old art revisited. *Mediation Quarterly, 3,* 59–95.

Bloom, M. (1975). *The paradox of helping: Introduction to the philosophy of scientific practice.* New York: Wiley.

Bloom, M. (Ed.). (1985). *Life span development.* New York: Macmillan.

Bloom, M., & Fischer, J. (1982). *Evaluating practice: Guidelines for the accountable professional.* Englewood Cliffs, NJ: Prentice-Hall.

Bloom, M., Fischer, J., & Orme, J. G. (1995). *Evaluating practice: Guidelines for the accountable professional.* (2nd ed.). Boston: Allyn and Bacon.

Bloom, M., Fischer, J., & Orme, J. G. (1999). *Evaluating practice: Guidelines for the accountable professional.* (3rd ed.). Boston: Allyn and Bacon.

Blythe, B. J. (1995). Single-system design. In R. L. Edwards (Ed.), *Encyclopedia of social work* (19th ed., pp. 2164–2168). Washington, DC: NASW Press.

Blythe, B. J., & Rodgers, A.Y. (1993). Evaluating our own practice: Past, present, and future trends. *Journal of Social Service Research, 18,* 101–119.

Blythe, B. J., & Tripodi, T. T. (1989). *Measurement for direct social work practice.* Newbury Park, CA: Sage Publications.

Bodenmann, G. (1997). Can divorce be prevented by enhancing the coping skills of couples? *Journal of Divorce and Remarriage, 27*(3/4), 177–194.

Borduin, C., Mann, B., Cone, L., & Henggeler, S. (1995). Multisystemic treatment of serious juvenile offenders: Long term prevention of criminality and violence. *Journal of Consulting and Clinical Psychology, 63,* 569–578.

Botvin, G. J. (1996). Substance abuse prevention through life skills training. In R. D. Peters & R. J. McMahon (Eds.), *Preventing childhood disorders, substance abuse, and delinquency.* Thousand Oaks, CA: Sage.

Bouchard, T. (1972). Training, motivation, and personality as determinants of the effectiveness of brainstorming groups and individuals. *Journal of Applied Psychology, 56,* 324–331.

Boudin, H. M., et al. (1977). Contingency contracting with drug abusers in the natural environment. *International Journal of the Addictions, 12,* 1–16.

Bourgeois, M. S. (1990). Enhancing conversation skills in patients with Alzheimer's disease using a prosthetic memory aid. *Journal of Applied Behavior Analysis, 23,* 29–42.

Bourgeois, M. S. (1994). Teaching caregivers to use memory aids with patients with dementia. *Seminars in Research and Language, 15,* 291–305.

Bourgeois, M. S., Burgio, L. D., Schulz, R., Beach, S., & Palmer, B. (1997). Modifying repetitive verbalizations of community-dwelling patients. *The Gerontologist, 371,* 30–39.

Bourgeois, M., Schulz, R., & Burgio, L. (1996). Interventions for caregivers of patients with Alzheimer's disease: A review and analysis of content, process, and outcomes. *The International Journal of Aging and Human Development, 43,* 35–92.

Bowman, P. (1989). Research perspectives on Black men: Role strain and adaptation across the adult life cycle. In R. Jones (Ed.), *Black adult development and aging* (pp. 117–150). Berkeley, CA: Cobbs and Henry.

Boyd-Franklin, N. (1989). *Black families in therapy: A multi-systems approach.* New York: Guilford Press.

Boyd-Franklin, N., Steiner, G., & Boland, M. (1994). *Children, families and HIV/AIDS.* New York: Guilford Press.

Bratter, T. E., & Forrest, G. G. (Eds.). (1985). *Alcoholism and substance abuse: Strategies for clinical intervention.* New York: Free Press.

Breckenridge, J., Zeiss, A., Thompson, L., & Munoz, R. (1987). *The life satisfaction course: An intervention for the elderly.* In R. Munoz (Ed.), Depression prevention: Research directions (pp. 185–196). Washington, DC: Hemisphere.

Brehm, S. S. (1976). *The application of social psychology to clinical practice.* New York: John Wiley.

Brehm, S. S., & Smith, T. W. (1986). Social psychological approaches to psychotherapy and behavior change. In S. L. Garfield & A. E. Bergin (Eds.), *Handbook of pyschotherapy and behavior change* (pp. 69–115). New York: John Wiley.

Brekke, J. S. (1986). Scientific imperatives in social work research: Pluralism is not skepticism. *Social Services Review, 50,* 538–555.

Briar, S. (1973). Effective social work intervention in direct practice: Implications for education. In S. Briar, et al. (Eds.), *Facing the challenge.* New York: Council on Social Work Education.

Briar, S. (1977). Incorporating research into education for clincial practice in social work: Toward a clinical science in social work. *Sourcebook on research utilization* (pp. 132–140). Washington, DC: Council on Social Work Education.

Bricker-Jenkins, M., & Hooyman, N. (1984). Feminist practice project: Summary of pretest findings, *Unpublished paper sponsored by NCOWI under auspices of NASW*. Silver Spring, MD: NASW.

Bricker-Jenkins, M., & Hooyman, N. (1986). *Not for women only*. Silver Spring, MD: NASW Press.

Brieland, D. (1995). Social work practice: History and evolution. In R. L. Edwards (Ed.), *Encyclopedia of social work* (19th ed., Vol. 3, pp. 2247–2258). Washington, DC: NASW Press.

Briggs, H. E. (1996a). Creating independent choices: The emergence of statewide family advocacy networks. *Journal of Mental Health Administration, 23*(4), 447–457.

Briggs, H. E. (1996b). Enhancing community adjustment of persons with developmental disabilities: Transferring multilevel behavioral technology to an inner city community organization. *Journal of Applied Social Sciences, 20*(2), 177-190.

Briggs, H. E., & Carrock, S. (2000). *Working outside the boxes: Final Report of the national evaluation of statewide family networks*. Portland, OR: Portland State University, Research and Training Center of Family Support and Children's Mental Health.

Briggs, H. E., Carrock, S., Williams-Murphy, T., Leary, J., and Johnson, W. (under review). Promoting culturally competent systems of care through statewide family advocacy networks. *Journal of Community Practice*, 1–23.

Briggs, H. E., Carrock, S., & Koroloff, N. M. (1994). *The driving force: The influence of statewide family networks on family support and systems of care*. Portland, OR: Portland State University, Research and Training Center on Family Support and Children's Mental Health.

Briggs, H. E., Carrock, S., Mason, J., & Williams-Murphy, T. (1996). Promoting culturally competent systems of care through statewide family advocacy networks. *Journal of Community Practice*, 1–23.

Briggs, H. E., & Koroloff, N. M. (1995). Enhancing statewide family advocacy networks: An analysis of the roles of sponsoring organizations. *Community Mental Health Journal, 31*(4), 317–333.

Briggs, H. E., Koroloff, N. M., Richards, K., & Friesen, B. J. (1993). *Family advocacy organizations: Advances in support and system reform*. Portland, OR: Portland State University, Research and Training Center on Family Support and Children's Mental Health.

Briggs, H. E., Smith, S., Carrock, S., Leary, J., & Johnson, W. (Under review). Talking the talk and walking the walk: Family participation in systems change. *Journal of Mental Health Administration*.

Bright, P. B., & Robin, A. L. (1981). Ameliorating parent-adolescent conflict with problem-solving communication training. *Journal of Behavior Therapy and Experimental Psychiatry, 12*, 275–280.

Brigham, T. A., Meier, S., & Goodner, V. (1995). Increasing designated driving with a program of prompts and incentives. *Journal of Applied Behavior Analysis, 28*, 83–84.

Brindis, et al. (1995). A case management program for chemically dependent clients with multiple needs. *Journal of Case Management, 4*, 22–28.

Brittan, A. (1973). *Meanings and situations*. London: Routledge and Kegan Paul.

Bromberger, J., & Matthews, K. (1994). Employment status and depressive symptoms in middle-aged women: A longitudinal investigation. *American Journal of Public Health, 84*(2), 202–206.

Bronson, D. E. (1994). Is a scientist-practitioner model appropriate for direct social work practice? No. In W. W. Hudson & P. S. Nurius (Eds.), *Controversial issues in social work research*. Boston: Allyn and Bacon.

Brown, G., & Harris, T. (1978). *The social origins of depression: A study of psychiatric disorders in women*. London: Tavistock Publications.

Brown, J. A., & Brown, C. S. (1977). *Systematic counseling: A guide for the practioner.* Champaign, IL: Research Press.

Brown, L. (1995). Cultural diversity in feminist therapy: Theory and practice. In H. Landrine (Ed.), *Bringing cultural diversity to feminist psychology: Theory, research and practice.* Washington, DC: APA Press.

Brownell, K. D. (1984). The addictive disorders. In C. M. Franks (Ed.), *Annual Review of behavior therapy* (Vol. 10,). New York: Guilford Press.

Broxmeyer, N. (1978). Practioner-research in treating a borderline child. *Social Work Research and Abstracts, 14,* 5–10.

Bryant-Compstock, S., Huff, B., & Vandenberg, J. (1996). The evolution of the family advocacy movement. In B. A. Stroul (Ed.), *Children's mental health: Creating systems of care in a changing society.* Baltimore: Paul H. Brookes Co.

Buchanan, A. (1978). Medical paternalism. *Philosophy and Public Affairs, 7,* 370–390.

Buie, D., & Adler, G. (1982). The definitive treatment of the borderline patient. *International Journal of Psychoanalytic Psychotherapy, 9,* 51–87.

Bullis, R. K. (1995). *Clinical social worker misconduct.* Chicago: Nelson-Hall.

Bunck, T., & Iwata, B. (1978). Increasing senior citizen participation in a community-based nutritious meal program. *Journal of Applied Behavior Analysis, 11,* 75–86.

Bunge, M. (1993). Realism and antirealism in social science. *Theory and Decision, 35,* 207–235.

Bureau of Justice Statistics. (1986). *Children in custody* (NCJ–102457, p. 2): Bureau of Justice Statistics, Department of Justice.

Burgio, L. D., & Burgio, K. L. (1986). Behavioral gerontology: Applications of behavioral methods to the problem of older adults. *Journal of Applied Behavior Analysis, 19,* 321–328.

Burke, A. C., & Clapp, J. D. (1997). Ideology and social work practice in substance abuse settings. *Social Work, 42*(6), 552–561.

Burns, D. (1980). *Feeling good: The new mood therapy.* New York: Signet Books.

Caccioppo, J., & Petty, R. (1981). Social psychological procedures for cognitive response assessment: The thought listing technique. In T. V. Merluzzi, C. R. Glass, & M. Genest (Eds.), *Cognitive assessment.* New York: Guilford Press.

Caldarola, T., & Helquist, M. (1989). Counseling mixed antibody status couples. *Focus: A Guide to AIDS Research and Counseling, 4*(9), 1–2.

Callahan, D., & Bok, S. (Eds.). (1980). *Ethics teaching in higher education.* New York: Plenum Press.

Capra, F. (1996). *The web of life.* New York: Anchor Books.

Carkhuff, R. R. (1971). Training as a preferred mode of treatment. *Journal of Counseling Psychology, 18,* 123–131.

Carroll, J. F. X. (1984). Substance abuse problem checklist: A new clinical aid for drug and/or alcohol dependency. *Journal of Substance Abuse Treatment, 1,* 31–36.

Carroll, L. (1960). *The annotated Alice: Alice's adventures in Wonderland.* Cleveland: Forum Books, World Publishing Company.

Carstensen, L. L. (1988). The emerging field of behavioral gerontology. *Behavior Therapy, 19,* 259–281.

Carter, R. (1977). Justifying paternalism. *Canadian Journal of Philosophy, 7,* 133–145.

Carter, R. D., & Thomas, E. J. (1975). Modification of problematic marital communication. In A. S. Gurman & D. G. Rice (Eds.), *Couples in conflict.* New York: Jason Aronson.

Cautela, J. R. (1967). Covert sensitization. *Psychological Record, 20,* 459–468.

Caughey, A., & Sabin, J. (1995). Managed care. In D. Calkins, R. J. Fernandopulle, & B. S. Marino (Eds.), *Health care policy* (pp. 88–101). Cambridge, MA: Blackwell Science.

Cazenave, N. (1979). Middle-income Black fathers: An analysis of the provider role. *Family Coordinator, 28*(4), 645–653.

Centers for Disease Control (1997). *HIV surveillance report* (Year-end edition, Vol. 9, no. 2): CDC: Centers for Disease Control and Prevention, US Department of Health and Human Services, Public Health Service.

Centers for Disease Control. 2000. Surveillance report (Vol. 11, no. 2): CDC: Centers for Disease Control and Prevention, U.S. Department of Health and Human Services, Public Health Service.

Cervera, N. (1991). Unwed teenage pregnancy: Family relationships with the father of the baby. *Families in Society: The Journal of Contemporary Human Services, 72*(1), 29–37.

Chambless, D. L., & Holon, S. D. (1998). Defining empirically supported theories. *Journal of Consulting and Clinical Psychology, 66*(1), 7–18.

Chambless, D., Sanderson, W., Shoham, V., Johnson, S., Pope, K., Crits-Cristoph, P., Baker, M., Johnson, B., Woody, S., Sue, S., Beutler, L., Williams, D., & McCurry, S. (1995). An update on empirically validated therapies. *The Clinical Psychologist, 49*(2), 5–18.

Chambless, D., Sanderson, W., Shoham, V., Johnson, S., Pope, K., Crits-Cristoph, P., Baker, M., Johnson, B., Woody, S., Sue, S., Beutler, L., Williams, D., & McCurry, S. (1998). Update on empirically validated theories II. *The Clinical Psychologist, 51,* 3–16.

Chandler, S. M. (1994). Is there an ethical responsibility to use practice methods with the best empirical evidence of effectiveness? No. In W. W. Hudson & P. S. Nurius (Eds.), *Controversial issues in social work research* (pp. 105–111). Boston: Allyn and Bacon.

Charlesworth, E. A., Williams, B. J., & Baer, P. E. (1984). Stress management at the worksite for hypertension: Compliance, cost-benefit, health care, and hypertension-related variables. *Psychosomatic Medicine, 46*(5), 387–397.

Cheatham, J. (1987). The empirical evaluation of clinical practice: A survey of four groups of practioners. *Journal of Social Services Research, 10,* 163–177.

Cherin, D., & Meezan, W. (1998). Evaluation as a means of organizational learning. *Administration in Social Work, 22*(2), 1–21.

Chetkow-Yanoov, B. (1997). *Social work approaches to conflict resolution: Making fighting obsolete.* New York: The Haworth Press.

Chovanec, M., & Kuechler, C. (1999). *Group skills with involuntary clients: Integrating theory and practice into the graduate curriculum.* Paper presented at the Council on Social Work Education Annual Program Meeting, March, San Francisco.

Christenson, R. M., & Wilson, W. P. (1985). Assessing pathology in the separation-individuation process by an inventory: A preliminary report. *Journal of Nervous and Mental Disease, 173*(561–565).

Christian, W. (1983). A case study in programming and maintenance of institutional change. *Journal of Organizational Behavior Management, 5*(3/4), 99–153.

Christmon, K. (1990a). Parental responsibility of African American unwed adolescent fathers. *Adolescence, 25,* 645–653.

Christmon, K. (1990b). Parental responsibility and self-image of African-American fathers. *Families in Society: The Journal of Contemporary Human Services, 71*(3), 563–567.

Chun, K. T., Cobb, S., & French, J. (1975). *Measures for psychological assessment.* Ann Arbor, MI: Institute for Social Research.

Ciminero, A. R., Calhoun, K. S., & Adams, H. E. (1986). Self-monitoring procedures. In A. R. Ciminero, K. S. Calhoun, & H. E. Adams (Eds.), *Handbook of behavioral assessment.* New York: Wiley.

Cingolani, J. (1984). Social conflict perspective on work with involuntary clients. *Social Work, 29,* 442–446.

Clark, D. C., & Fawcett, J. (1992). Review of empirical risk factors for evaluation of the suicidal patient. In B. Bongar (Ed.), *Suicide: Guidelines for assessment, management, and treatment.* New York: Oxford University Press.

Clum, G. A. (1989). Psychological interventions vs. drugs in the treatment of panic. *Behavior Therapy, 20,* 429–457.

Cochran, D. (1997). African American fathers: A decade review of the literature. *Families in Society: The Journal of Contemporary Human Services, 78*(4), 340–350.

Cochran, S., & Mays, V. (1994). Depressive distress among homosexually active African American men and women. *American Journal of Psychiatry, 151*(4), 524–529.

Cohen, C. B. (1988). Ethics committees. *Hastings Center Report, 18,* 11.

Cohen, M. B. (1998). Perceptions of power in client/worker relationships. *Families in Society, 79,* 433–442.

Cohen, R. E. (1970). *Preventive mental health programs for ethnic minority populations: A case in point.* Paper presented at the Congresso Internacional de Americanistas, Lima, Peru.

Cohen, R. J., & Mariano, W. E. (1982). *Legal guidebook in mental health.* New York: Free Press.

Colletti, G., & Brownell, K. D. (1982). The physical and emotional benefits of social support: Application to obesity, smoking and alcoholism. In M. Hersen (Ed.), *Progress in behavior modification* (Vol. 13, pp. 109–178). New York: Academic Press.

Comas-Diaz, L. (1988). *Feminist therapy with Hispanic/Latina women: Myth or reality?* Paper presented at the Paper delivered for the Trans-Cultural Mental Health Institute, Washington, DC.

Comery, A. L., et al. (1973). *A source book for mental health measures.* Los Angeles, CA: Human Interaction Research Institute.

Committee on National Needs for Biomedical and Behavioral Research Personnel (1994). *Meeting the nation's needs for biomedical and behavioral scientists.* Washington, DC: National Academy Press.

Compton, B. R., & Galaway, B. (Eds.). (1989). *Social work processes.* Belmont, CA: Wadsworth.

Conrad, A. P. (1989). Developing an ethics review process in a social service agency. *Social Thought, 15*(3/4), 102–115.

Consortium on the school-based promotion of social competence. (1996). The school-based promotion of social competence: Theory, research, practice, and policy. In R. J. Haggerty, L. R. Sherrod, N. Garmezy, & M. Rutter (Eds.), *Stress, risk, and resilience in children and adolescents.* Cambridge, MA: Cambridge University Press.

Conte, H. R., Plutchik, R., Karasu, T. B., & Jerrett, I. (1980). A self-report borderline scale: Discriminative validity and preliminary norms. *Journal of Nervous and Mental Disease, 174*, 727–735.

Coontz, S. (1992). *The way we never were: American families and the nostalgia trap.* New York: Basic Books.

Coontz, S. (1997). *The way we really are: Coming to terms with America's changing families.* New York: Basic Books.

Cooper, N. A., & Clum, G. A. (1989). Imaginal flooding as a supplementary treatment for PTSD in combat veterans: A controlled study. *Behavior Therapy, 20*, 381–391.

Corcoran, K. J. (1982). Behavioral and non-behavioral methods of developing two types of empathy: A comparative study. *Journal of Education for Social Work, 18*, 85–93.

Corcoran, K. (1985). Clinical practice with non-behavioral methods: Strategies for evaluation. *Clinical Social Work Journal, 13*(3), 78–86.

Corcoran, K. (1993). Practice evaluation: Problems and promises of single-system designs in clinical practice. *Journal of Social Service Research, 18*, 147–159.

Corcoran, K. (1997). The use of rapid assessment instruments as outcomes measures. In E. Mullin & J. L. Magnabosco (Eds.), *Outcomes measurements in the human services* (pp. 137–143). Washington, DC: NASW Press.

Corcoran, K., & Fischer, J. (2000a). *Measures for clinical practice: A sourcebook.* (3rd ed.). (Vol. 1, Couples, families and children). New York: Free Press.

Corcoran, K., & Fischer, J. (2000b). *Measures for clinical practice: A sourcebook.* (3rd ed.). (Vol. 2, Adults). New York: Free Press.

Corcoran, K., & Gingerich, W. (1994). Practice evaluation in the context of managed care: Case recording methods for quality assurance review. *Research on Social Work Practice, 4*, 326–337.

Corcoran, K., & Vandiver, V. L. (1996). *Maneuvering the maze of managed care: Skills for mental health practitioners.* New York: Free Press.

Corcoran, K., & Winslade, W. J. (1994). Eavesdropping in the 50-minute hour: Managed mental health care and confidentiality. *Behavioral Sciences and the Law, 12*, 331–365.

Cordon, J., & Preston-Shoot, M. (1987). *Contracts in social work.* Hants, England: Gower.

Cormier, W. H., & Cormier, L. S. (1985). *Interviewing strategies for helpers.* (2nd ed.). Belmont, CA: Brooks/Cole.

Corrigan, P., Reedy, P., Thadani, D., & Ganet, M. (1995). Correlates of participation and completion in a job club for clients with psychiatry disability. *Rehabilitation Counseling Bulletin, 39*, 42–53.

Costello, E. J. (1990). Child psychiatric epidemiology: Implications for clinical research and practice. In B. B. Lahey & A. E. Kazdin (Eds.), *Advances in clinical child psychology* (Vol. 13, pp. 53–90). New York: Plenum.

Costin, L. B. (1964). Values in social work education: A study. *Social Service Review, 38*, 271–280.

Coulton, C. J., & Solomon, P. L. (1977). Measuring outcomes intervention. *Social Work Research and Abstracts, 13*, 3–9.

Council on Social Work Education. (1988). *Handbook of accreditation standards and procedures.* Washington, DC: Council on Social Work Education.

Council on Social Work Education. (1994). *Curriculum policy statement for Master's degree programs in social work education.* Alexandria, VA: Author.

Cox, W. J., & Kenardy, J. (1993). Performance anxiety, social phobia, and setting effects in instrumental music students. *Journal of Anxiety Disorders, 7,* 49–60.

Cox, W. M. (Ed.). (1987). *Treatment and prevention of alcohol problems: A resource manual.* New York: Academic Press.

Cranford, R. E., & Doudera, E. (Eds.). (1984). *Institutional ethics committees and health care decision making.* Ann Arbor, MI: Health Administration Press.

Crow Dog, L., & Erdoes, R. (1995). *Crow Dog: Four generations of Sioux medicine men.* New York: HarperCollins.

Cuellar, I., Arnold, B., & Maldonado, R. (1995). Acculturation Rating Scale for Mexican Americans-II: A revision of the original ARSMA Scale. *Hispanic Journal of Behavioral Sciences, 17,* 275–304.

Curran, J. P., & Monti, P. M. (1982). *Social skills training: A practical handbook for assessment and treatment.* New York: Guilford.

Curtis, J. D., & Detert, R. A. (1981). *How to relax: A holistic approach to stress management.* Palo Alto, CA: Mayfield.

Curtis, L. C., & Hodge, M. (1995). Boundaries and HIV-related case management. *Focus: A Guide to AIDS Research and Counseling, 10*(2), 5–6.

Daley, D. C. (1986). *Relapse prevention workbook.* Holmes Beach, FL: Learning Publications, Inc.

Daniels, A. C. (1994). *Bringing out the best in people.* New York: McGraw-Hill.

Danziger, S., & Radin, N. (1990). Absent does not equal uninvolved: Predictors of fathering in teen mother families. *Journal of Marriage and the Family, 52,* 636–642.

Davidson, A. (1994). *Endangered peoples.* San Francisco, CA: Sierra Club Books.

Davidson, J. (1978). *Effective time management: A practical workbook.* New York: Hinnan Science Press.

Davidson, J., Miner, C. M., DeVeaugh-Geiss, J., & Tupler, L. (1997). The Brief Social Phobia Scale: A psychometric evaluation. *Psychological Medicine, 27,* 161–166.

Deloria, V., Jr. (1995). *Red earth, white lies.* New York: Scribner.

Denicola, J., & Sandler, J. (1980). Training abusive parents in cognitive-behavioral techniques. *Behavior Therapy, 11,* 263–270.

DeRoos, Y. S., & Pinkston, E. M. (1997). Training adult day-care staff. In D. M. Baer & E. M. Pinkston (Eds.), *Environment and behavior* (pp. 249–257). Boulder, CO: Westview Press.

DeRubeis, R. J., & Crits-Christoph, P. (1998). Empirically supported individual and group psychological treatments for adult mental disorders. *Journal of Consulting and Clinical Psychology, 66,* 37–52.

DeRubeis, R. J., & Feeley, M. (1990). Determinants of change in cognitive therapy for depression. *Cognitive Therapy and Research, 14*(5), 469–482.

deSchmidt, A., & Gorey, K. M. (1997). Unpublished social work research: Systemic replication of a recent meta-analysis of published intervention effectiveness research. *Social Work Research, 21*(1), 58–62.

Deschner, J. (1984). *The hitting habit.* New York: The Free Press.

Deutsch, C. (1985). A survey of therapists' personal problems and treatment. *Professional Psychology: Research and Practice, 16,* 305–315.

Dew, M., Bromet, E., & Penkower, L. (1992). Mental health effects of job loss in women. *Psychological Medicine, 22*(3), 751–764.

Dewey, J. (1938). *Logic: The theory of inquiry.* New York: Holt, Rinehart & Winston.

Dickson, D. T. (1998). *Confidentiality and privacy in social work.* New York: Free Press.

DiNardo, P. A., Mora, K., Barlow, D. H., & Rapee, R. M. (1993). Reliability of the DSM-III-R anxiety disorder categories: Using the Anxiety Disorders Interview Schedule–Revised (ADIS–R). *Archives of General Psychiatry, 50,* 251–256.

Diorio, W. D. (1992). Parental perceptions of the authority of public child welfare workers. *Families in Society, 73*(4), 222–35.

Donahue, B. C., Van Hasselt, V., & Hersen, M. (1994). Behavioral assessment and treatment of social phobia: An evaluative review. *Behavior Modification, 18,* 262–288.

Donovan, B. M., & Marlatt, G. A. (1988). Assessment of addictive behaviors: Implications of an emerging biopsychosocial model. In B. M. Donovan & G. A. Marlatt (Eds.), *Assessment of addictive behaviors: Behavioral, cognitive, and physiological procedures.* New York: Guilford Press.

Dryfoos, J. G. (1990). *Adolescents at risk: Prevalence and prevention.* New York: Oxford University Press.

Duehn, W. (1985). The problem-solving process. In R. M. Grinnell (Ed.), *Social work research and evaluation* (2nd ed.). Itasca, IL: Peacock.

Dunn, G., Dunn, K., & Price, G. (1975). *Learning Style Inventory.* Lawrence, KS: Price Systems Inc.

Dunnette, M., Campbell, J., & Joasted, K. (1963). The effect of group participation on brainstorming effectiveness for two industrial samples. *Journal of Applied Psychology, 47,* 30–37.

Dworkin, G. (1971). Paternalism. In R. Wasserstrom (Ed.), *Morality and the law* (pp. 107–126). Belmont, CA: Wadsworth.

East, J. (1998). In-dependence: A feminist postmodern deconstruction. *Affilia, 13*(3), 273–288.

Eckblad, M., & Chapman, L. J. (1983). Magical ideation as an indicator of schizotypy. *Journal of Consulting and Clinical Psychology, 51,* 215–225.

Eckrich, S. (1985). Identification and treatment of borderline personality disorder. *Social Work, 30,* 166–171.

Ehlers, A., Hofman, S. G., Herda, C. A., & Roth, W. T. (1994). Clinical characteristics of driving phobia. *Journal of Anxiety Disorders, 8,* 323–339.

Ehrenreich, B. (1983). *The hearts of men: American dreams and the flight from commitment.* Garden City, NY: Anchor/Doubleday Press.

Einstein, A. (1979). *The world as I see it.* New York: Citadel Press.

Elder, J. P., Edelstein, B. A., & Narick, M. M. (1979). Modifying aggressive behavior with social skill training. *Behavior Modification, 3,* 161–178.

Elias, M. J., & Clabby, J. R. (1992). *Building social problem-solving skills.* San Francisco, CA: Jossey-Bass Publishers.

Elliott, L. J. (1931). *Social work ethics.* New York: American Association of Social Workers.

Emmet, D. (1962). Ethics and the social worker. *British Journal of Psychiatric Social Work, 6,* 165–172.

Epstein, L. H., & Wing, R. R. (1984). Behavioral contracting: Health behaviors. In C. M. Franks (Ed.), *New developments in behavior therapy.* New York: Haworth Press.

Erickson, B. (1992). Feminist fundamentalism: Reactions to Avis, Kaufman, and Bograd. *Journal of Marital and Family Therapy, 18*(3), 263–267.

Erwin, E. (1993). Current philosophical issues in the scientific evaluation of behavior therapy and outcome. *Behavior Therapy 23,* 151–171.

Eubanks, J. L., O'Driscoll, M. P., Hayward, G. B., Daniels, J. A., & Connor, S. H. (1990). Behavioral competency requirements for organizational development consultants. *Journal of Organizational Behavior Management, 11*(1), 77–97.

Evarts, W., Greenstone, J., Kirkpatrick, G., & Leviton, S. (1983). *Winning through accomodation: The mediator's handbook.* Dubuque, IA: Kendall/Hunt.

Everett, J. E., Chipungu, S. S., & Leashore, B. (1991). *Child welfare: An Africentric perspective.* New Brunswick, NJ: Rutgers University Press.

Ewalt, P. (1979). *Toward a definition of clinical social work: National Conference Proceedings,* Washington, DC.

Ewart, C. K., Taylor, C. B., Kraemer, H. C., & Agras, W. S. (1984). Reducing blood pressure reactivity during interpersonal conflict: Effects on marital communication training. *Behavior Therapy, 15*(5), 473–484.

Farella, J. R. (1984). *The main stalk: A synthesis of Navaho philosophy.* Tucson, AZ: University of Arizona Press.

Farrington, D. P. (1995). The challenge of teenage antisocial behavior. In M. Rutter (Ed.), *Psychosocial disturbances in young people.* Cambridge, MA: Cambridge University Press.

Feindler, E. L., & Gutterman, J. (1994). Cognitive–behavioral anger control training. In C. W. LeCroy (Ed.), *Handbook of child and adolescent treament manuals* (pp. 170–199). New York: Lexington Books.

Ferner, J. (1980). *Successful time management.* New York: Wiley.

Ferner, J. (1995). *Successful time management: A self-teaching guide.* New York: Wiley.

Feske, U., & Chambless, D. L. (1995). Cognitive behavioral versus exposure only treatment for social phobia: A meta-analysis. *Behavior Therapy, 26,* 695–720.

Filsinger, E. E., & Thoma, S. J. (1988). Behavioral antecedents of relationship stability and adjustment: A five-year longitudinal study. *Journal of Marriage and the Family, 50,* 785–795.

Fingarett, H. (1988). Alcoholism: The mythical disease. *Utne Reader, 30,* 64–68.

First, M. B., Gibbon, M., Williams, J. B. W., & Spitzer, R. L. (1995). *Structured Clinical Interview for the DSM-IV.* Washington, DC: American Psychiatric Press.

Fischer, J. (1973). Is casework effective: A review. *Social Work, 18,* 5–20.

Fischer, J. (Ed.). (1976). *The effectiveness of social casework.* Springfield, IL: Charles Thomas Press.

Fischer, J. (1978). *Effective casework practice: An eclectic approach.* New York: McGraw-Hill.

Fischer, J., & Corcoran, K. (1994). *Measures for clinical practice: A sourcebook.* (2nd ed.). New York: The Free Press.

Fletcher, J. C. (1986). The goals of ethics consultation. *Biolaw, 2,* 36–47.

Fletcher, J. C., Quist, N., & Jonsen, A. R. (1989). *Ethics consultation in health care.* Ann Arbor, MI: Health Administration Press.

Florsheim, P., Moore, D., & Suth, A. (1997). *He says, she says: Factors related to the quality of partnerships between expectant adolescent mothers and fathers.* Unpublished paper presented at the National Council on Family Relations Annual Conference in Arlington, VA.

Fogg, R. (1985). Dealing with conflict: A repertoire of creative, peaceful approaches. *Journal of Conflict Resolution, 29,* 330–358.

Foreyt, J. P. (1987). The addictive disorders. In G. T. Wilson (Ed.), *Review of Behavior Therapy* (Vol. 10). New York: Guilford Press.

Fortune, A. E., & Reid, W. J. (1999). *Research in social work*. (3rd ed.). New York: Columbia University Press.

Foy, D. W., Cline, K. A., & Laasi, N. (1987). Assessment of alcohol and drug abuse. In T. D. Nirenberg & S. A. Maisto (Eds.), *Developments in the assessment and treatment of addictive behaviors*. Norwood, NJ: Ablex.

Frailberg, S. (1977). *Insights from the blind*. New York: Basic Books, Inc.

Frankel, C. (1959). Social philosophy and the professional education of social workers. *Social Service Review, 33*, 345–359.

Frankena, W. K. (1973). *Ethics*. (2nd ed.). Englewood Cliffs, NJ: Prentice-Hall.

Franklin, C. (1995). Expanding the vision of the social constructionist debates: Creating relevance for practioners. *Families in Society: The Journal of Contemporary Human Services, 76*, 395–407.

Franklin, C., & Streeter, C. L. (1995). School reform: Linking public schools with human services. *Social Work, 40*, 773–782.

Fraser, M., & Kohlert, N. (1988). Substance abuse and public policy. *Social Service Review, 62*, 103–126.

Fredman, N., & Sherman, R. (1987). *Handbook of measurements for marriage and family therapy*. New York: Brunner/Mazel.

Freeberg, S. (1989). Self-determination: Historical perspectives and effects on current practice. *Social Work, 34*, 33–38.

Freed, A. O. (1980). The borderline personality. *Social Casework, 61*, 548–558.

Freedman, B. J., Rosenthal, C., Donahoe, C. P., Schlundt, D. G., & McFall, R. M. (1978). A social-behavioral analysis of skill deficits in delinquent and nondelinquent adolescent boys. *Journal of Consulting and Clinical Psychology, 48*, 1448–1462.

Freeman, E. (1994). African-American women and the concept of cultural competence. *Journal of Multicultural Social Work, 3*(4), 61–75.

Friere, P. (1994). *Pedagogy of the oppressed*. (Rev. ed.), New York: Continuum.

Friedman, R., & Dermit, S. (1988). Popular stress management: A selected review. *Behavioral Medicine, 14*(4), 186–189.

Friesen, B. J. (1993). *Advances in child mental health in the 1990's: Curricula for the graduate and undergraduate professional education*. (pp. 12–19). Rockville, MD: US Department of Health and Human Services.

Friesen, B. J., & Huff, B. (1996). Family perspectives on systems of care. In B. A. Stroul (Ed.), *Children's mental health: Creating systems of care in a changing society* (pp. 41–67). Baltimore: Paul H. Brookes Co.

Friesen, B. J., & Koroloff, N. M. (1990). Family centered services: Implications for mental health administration and research. *Journal of Mental Health Administration, 17*(1), 13–25.

Friman, P. (in press). Behavioral, family-style residential care for troubled out-of-home adolescents: Recent findings. In J. E. Carr & J. Austin (Eds.), *Handbook of applied behavior analysis*. Reno, NV: Context Press.

Friman, P., Osgood, D., Smith, G., Shanahan, D., Thompson, R., Larzelere, R., & Daly, D. (1996). A longitudinal evaluation of prevalent negative beliefs about residential placement for troubled adolescents. *Journal of Abnormal Child Psychology, 24*, 299–324.

Galatner, M. (1983). *Recent developments in alcoholism*. (Vols. I and II). New York: Plenum.

Gambrill, E. (1997). *Social work practice: A critical thinker's guide*. New York: Oxford.

Gambrill, E., & Richey, C. (1985). *Taking charge of your social life*. Belmont, CA: Behavioral Options.

Gant, L. (1996). HIV/AIDS care givers in African-American communities: Contemporary issues. In V. Lynch (Ed.), *Caring for the HIV care giver*. Westport, CT: Auburn House.

Garfield, S. L., & Bergin, A. E. (Eds.) (1986). *Handbook of psychotherapy and behavior change*. New York: John Wiley.

Garrison, R., & Eaton, W. (1992). *Women and Health, 18*(4), 53–76.

Gechtman, L., & Bouhoutsos, J. (1985). *Sexual intimacy between social workers and clients*. Paper presented at the annual meeting of the Society for Clinical Social Workers, University City, CA.

Gendlin, E. T. (1973). Experiential psychotherapy. In R. Corsini (Ed.), *Current psychotherapies*. Itasca, IL: Peacock.

Gendlin, E. (1978). *Focusing*. New York: Bantam.

Gerber, R. (1988). *Vibrational medicine: New choices for healing ourselves*. Sante Fe, NM: Bear and Company.

Germain, C. B. (1968). Social study: Past and future. *Social Casework, 49*(403–409).

Germain, C. B. (Ed.). (1979). *Social work practice: People and environments: An ecological perspective*. New York: Columbia University Press.

Germain, C. B., & Gitterman, A. (1980). *The life model of social work practice*. New York: Columbia University Press.

Germain, C. B., & Gitterman, A. (1996). *The life model of social work practice: Advances in theory and practice*. (2nd ed.). New York: Columbia University Press.

Gerson, M. J. (1984). Splitting: The development of a measure. *Journal of Consulting and Clinical Psychology, 40*(157–162).

Ghosh, A., & Marks, I. M. (1987). Self–treatment of agoraphobia by exposure. *Behavior Therapy, 18*, 3–16.

Gifis, S. H. (1991). *Law dictionary*. (3rd ed.). Hauppauge, NY: Barron's.

Gil, D. G. (1998). *Confronting injustice and oppression: Concepts and strategies for social workers*. New York: Columbia University Press.

Giles, T. R. (Ed.). (1993). *Handbook of effective psychotherapy*. New York: Plenum.

Gillman, R. (1996). Women care givers in HIV, A strengths perspective. In V. Lynch (Ed.), *Caring for the HIV care giver*. Westport, CT: Auburn House.

Gingerich, W. J. (1983). Significance testing in single-case research. In A. Rosenblatt & D. Waldfogel (Eds.), *Handbook of clinical social work*. San Francisco, CA: Jossey-Bass.

Gingerich, W. J. (1984). Generalizing single-case evaluation from classroom to practice. *Journal of Education for Social Work, 20*, 74–82.

Gingerich, W. J. (1990). Rethinking single-case evaluation. In L. Videka-Sherman & W. J. Reid (Eds.), *Advances in clinical social work*. Silver Spring, MD: National Association of Social Workers.

Girdano, D., & Everly, G. S. (1986). *Controlling stress and tension: A holistic approach*. Englewood Cliffs: Prentice-Hall.

Girodo, M. (1974). Yoga meditation and flooding in the treatment of anxiety neurosis. *Journal of Behavior Therapy and Experimental Psychiatry, 5*, 157–160.

Gitterman, A. (1989). Testing professional authority and boundaries. *Social Casework, 70*, 165–171.

Glenn, S. S. (1991). Contingencies and metacontingencies: Relations among behavioral, cultural, and biological evolution. In P. A. Lamal (Ed.), *Behavioral analysis of societies and cultural practices* (pp. 39–73). New York: Hemisphere.

Gochros, H. L., Gochros, J. S., & Fischer, J. (1986). *Helping the sexually oppressed.* Englewood Cliffs, NJ: Prentice-Hall.

Gochros, H. (1988). Risks of abstinence. *Social Work, 33*(3), 254–256.

Gochros, H. (1992). The sexuality of gay men with HIV infection. *Social Work, 37*(2), 105–111.

Gochros, H. (1996). The stresses of volunteer and professional care givers. In V. Lynch (Ed.), *Caring for the HIV care giver.* Westport, CT: Auburn House.

Golan, N. (1979). Crisis theory. In F. J. Turner (Ed.), *Social work treatment.* New York: Free Press.

Golding, J. (1990). Division of household labor, strain, and depressive symptoms among Mexican-Americans and non-Hispanic Whites. *Psychology of Women Quarterly, 14*(1), 103–117.

Goldman, B., & Sanders, J. (1974). *Directory of unpublished experimental mental measures.* (Vol. 1). New York: Behavioral Publications.

Goldman, B., & Busch, J. (1978). *Directory of unpublished experimental mental measures.* (Vol. 2). New York: Human Sciences Press.

Goldman, B., & Busch, J. (1982). *Directory of unpublished experimental mental measures.* (Vol. 3). New York: Human Sciences Press.

Goldstein, A. P., & Glick, B. (1987). *Aggression replacement training.* Champaign, IL: Research Press.

Goldstein, A. P., & Kanfer, F. H. (1979). *Maximizing treatment gains: Transfer enhancement in psychotherapy.* New York: Academic Press.

Goldstein, E. G. (1995). *Ego psychology and social work practice.* (2nd ed.). New York: Free Press.

Goldstein, H. (1998). Education for ethical dilemmas in social work practice. *Family in Society, 79*(3), 241–253.

Goldstein, W. M. (1988). Beginning psychotherapy with the borderline patient. *American Journal of Psychotherapy, 42,* 561–573.

Goodman, S., Cooley, E., Sewell, D., & Leavitt, N. (1994). Loss of control and self-esteem in depressed, low-income African-American women. *Community Mental Health Journal, 30*(3), 259–269.

Gordon, T. (1970). *P. E. T. Parent effectiveness training: The tested new way to raise responsible children.* New York: Widen.

Gordon, W. E. (1962). A critique of the working definition. *Social Work, 7*(6).

Gordon, W. E. (1965). Knowledge and value: Their distinction and relationship in clarifying social work practice. *Social Work, 10*(3), 32–39.

Gorey, K. M. (1996). Effectiveness of social work intervention research: Internal versus external evaluations. *Social Work Reseach, 20*(2), 119–128.

Gorovitz, S. (Ed.). (1971). *Mill: Utilitarianism.* Indianapolis, IN: Bobbs-Merrill.

Gottman, J. M. (1979). *Marital interaction: Experimental investigations.* New York: Academic Press.

Gottman, J. M. (1983). How children become friends. *Monographs of the Society for Research in Child Development, 48,* 410–423.

Gottman, J. M. (1993). A theory of marital dissolution and stability. *Journal of Family Psychology, 7,* 57–75.

Gottman, J. M. (1994). *Why marriages succeed or fail.* New York: Simon & Schuster.

Gottman, J. M., & Leiblum, S. R. (1974). *How to do psychotherapy and how to evaluate it.* New York: Holt, Rinehart and Winston.

Gottman, J. M., Notarius, C., Gonso, J., & Markman, H. (1976). *A couples guide to communication.* Champaign, IL: Research Press.

Granvold, D. (1988). Treating marital couples in conflict and transition. In J. McNeil & S. Weinstein (Eds.), *Innovations in health care practice: Papers from the health/mental health conference.* New Orleans, LA: National Association of Social Workers.

Greene, B. F. (1994). Diversity and difference: Race and feminist psychotherapy. In M. Mirkin (Ed.), *Women in context: Toward a feminist reconstruction of psychotherapy* (pp. 333–351). New York: The Guilford Press.

Greene, B. F., Norman, K. R., Searle, M. S., Daniels, M., & Lubeck, R. C. (1995). Child abuse and neglect by parents with disabilities: A tale of two families. *Journal of Applied Behavior Analysis, 28,* 417–434.

Greene, B. F., Winett, R., Houten, R., Geller, E., & Iwata, B. (1987). *Behavior analysis in the community.* Lawrence, KS: Society for the Experimental Analysis of Behavior.

Green, G. R., Linsk, N. L., & Pinkston, E. M. (1986). Modification of verbal behavior of mentally impaired elderly by their spouses. *Journal of Applied Behavior Analysis, 4,* 329–336.

Greenhaus, J. H., & Beutell, N. J. (1985). Sources of conflict between work and family roles. *Academy of Management Review, 10,* 76–88.

Greenwood, C. R., Todd, N. M., Hops, H., & Walker, H. M. (1979). Behavior change targets in the assessment and behavior modification of socially withdrawn preschool children. *Behavioral Assessment, 4,* 273–297.

Griffith, J. D., Joe, G. W., Chatham, L. R., & Simpson, D. D. (1998). The development and validation of a Simpatia Scale for Hispanics Entering Drug Treatment. *Hispanic Journal of Behavioral Sciences, 20,* 468–482.

Grinnell, R. (Ed.). (1993). Social work research and evaluation (4th ed.). Itasca, IL: F. E. Peacock.

Grinnell, R. M., & Williams, M. (1990). *Research in social work: A primer.* Itasca, IL: Peacock.

Gross, E. (1998a). Reevaluation feminist thought for social work practice. *Affilia, 13*(1), 5–8.

Gross, E. (1998b). Deconstructing the liberal consensus on what is feminist. *Affilia, 13*(2), 143–146.

Guay. (1989, April). *Psychotherapy and HIV disease.* Paper presented at the Seventh National AIDS Forum, San Francisco, CA.

Gunderson, J. G., Franks, A. F., Runningstam, E. F., Wachter, S., Lynch, V. J., & Wolf, P. J. (1989). Early discontinuance of borderline patients from psychotherapy. *The Journal of Nervous and Mental Disease, 177,* 38–42.

Gunderson, J. G., & Kolb, K. (1978). Discriminating features of borderline patients. *American Journal of Psychiatry, 135,* 792–796.

Gunderson, J. G., Kolb, J. E., & Austin, V. (1981). Discriminating features of borderline patients. *American Journal of Psychiatry, 138,* 896–903.

Gutierrez, L. M. (1990). Working with women of color: An empowerment perspective. *Social Work, 35,* 149–153.

Haggerty, R. J., Sherrod, L. R., Garmezy, N., & Rutter, M. (1996). *Stress, risk, and resilience in children and adolescents.* Cambridge, MA: Cambridge University Press.

Haley, J. (1973). *Uncommon therapy.* New York: W. W. Norton.

Hall, L. K. (1952). Group workers and professional ethics. *The Group, 15*(1), 3–8.

Hamilton, G. (1940). *Theory and practice of social casework.* New York: Columbia University Press.

Hamilton, G. (1951). *Social casework.* (2nd ed.). New York: Columbia University Press.

Hancock, R. N. (1974). *Twentieth-century ethics.* New York: Columbia University Press.

Hanson, N. (1958). *Patterns of discovery.* Cambridge: Cambridge University Press.

Hardman, D. G. (1975). Not with my daughter you don't! *Social Work, 20*(4), 278–285.

Harris, G. A., & Watkins, D. (1987). *Counseling the involuntary and resistant client.* College Park, MD: American Correctional Association.

Hartman, A. (1990). Many ways of knowing. *Social Work, 35,* 3–4.

Hartman, A. (1995/1978). Diagrammatic assessment of family relationships. *Families in Society, 76,* 111–122.

Hartman, A., & Laird, J. (1983). *Family centered social work practice.* New York: The Free Press.

Hasenfeld, Y. (1987). Power in social work practice. *Social Service Review, 61,* 469–483.

Hasenfeld, Y., & Weaver, D. (1996). Enforcement, compliance, and disputes in welfare-to-work programs. *Social Service Review, 70,* 235–256.

Hauenstein, E., & Boyd, M. (1994). Depressive symptoms in young women of the Piedmont: Prevalence in rural women. *Women and Health, 21*(2/3), 105–123.

Haussmann, M., & Halseth, J. (1983). Re-examining women's roles: A feminist group approach to decreasing depression in women. *Social Work with Groups, 6*(3/4).

Hayes, S. C., Nelson, R. O., & Jarrett, R. B. (1987). The treatment utility of assessment. *American Psychologist, 42,* 63–71.

Haynes, K. S. (1998). The 100-year debate: Social reform versus individual treatment. *Social Work, 43*(6), 501–509.

Heineman, M. B. (1981). The obsolete imperative in social work research. *Social Service Review, 55,* 371–397.

Heineman, M. P. (1994). Science, not scientisim: The robustness of naturalistic clinical research. In E. Sherman & W. J. Reid (Eds.), *Qualitative research in social work* (pp. 71–88). New York: Columbia University Press.

Helzer, J. E. (1987). Epidemiology of alcoholism. *Journal of Consulting and Clinical Psychology, 55,* 248–292.

Hendricks, L., Howard, C., & Caesar, P. (1981). Black unwed adolescent fathers: A comparative study of their problems and help-seeking behavior. *Journal of the National Medical Association, 73*(9), 863–868.

Hendricks, L., & Montgomery, T. (1983). A limited population of unmarried adolescent fathers: A preliminary report of their views on fatherhood and the relationship with the mothers of their children. *Adolescence, 18,* 201–210.

Henggeler, S. W., Schoenwald, S. K., Borduin, C. M., Rowland, M. D., & Cunningham, P. B. (1998). *Multisystemic treatment of antisocial behavior in children and adolescents.* New York: Guilford.

Hepworth, D., & Larsen, J. (1986). *Direct social work practice; Theory and skills.* Chicago: Dorsey Press.

Hepworth, D., Rooney, R. H., & Larsen, J. (1997). *Direct social work practice.* Pacific Grove, CA: Brooks/Cole.

Herbert, E. M., et al. (1973). Adverse effects of differential parental attention. *Journal of Applied Behavior Analysis, 6,* 15–30.

Herman, E. (1988). The twelve-step program: Cure or cover. *Utne Reader, 30,* 52–63.

Hersen, M., & Barlow, D. H. (1986). *Single case experimental designs*. New York: Pergamon.

Hersen, M., & Bellack, A. S. (Eds.). (1988). *Dictionary of behavioral assessment techniques*. New York: Pergamon.

Herzberg, A. (1941). Short term treatment of neuroses by graduated tasks. *British Journal of Medical Psychology, 19*, 22–36.

Hesse, M. (1980). *Revolutions and reconstructions in the philosophy of science*. Bloomington, IN: Indiana University Press.

Hester, R. K., & Miller, W. R. (1989). *Handbook of alcoholism treatment approaches*. New York: Pergamon.

Hibbs, E. D., & Jensen, P. S. (Eds.). (1996). *Psychosocial treatments for child and adolescent disorders: Empirically based strategies for clinical practice*. Washington, DC: American Psychological Association Press.

Higgins, S. T., Budney, A. J., Bickel, W. K., Hughes, J. R., Foerg, F., & Badger, G. (1993). Achieving cocaine abstinence with a behavioral approach. *American Journal of Psychiatry, 150*, 763–769.

Hilton, M. R., & Lokane, V. G. (1978). The evaluation of a questionnaire measuring severity of alcohol dependence. *British Journal of Psychiatry, 132*, 42–48.

Himle, J., & Thyer, B. A. (1989). Clinical social work and obsessive compulsive disorder: A single-subject investigation. *Behavior Modification, 13*, 459–470.

Hofferth, S. L., Kahn, J. R., & Baldwin, W. (1987). Premarital sexual activity among US teenage women over the past three decades. *Family Planning Perspectives, 19*, 46–53.

Hoffman, A. (1987). *Steal this urine test*. New York: Penguin.

Hofstadter, R. (1944). *Social Darwinism in American thought*. Boston, MA: Beacon.

Hogan, D. B. (1979). *The regulation of psychotherapists: A study in the philosophy and practice of professional regulation*. (Vol. I). Cambridge, MA: Ballinger.

Hogarty, G. E. (1993). Prevention of relapse in chronic schizophreneic patients. *Clinical Psychiatry, 54*(3).

Hogarty, G. E., Anderson, C., Reiss, D., Kornblith, S., Greenwald, D., Ulrich, R., & Carter, M. (1991). Family psychoeducation, social skills training, and maintenance chemotherapy in the aftercare treatment of schizophrenia, II: Two year effects of a controlled trial on relapse and adjustment. *Archives of General Psychiatry, 48*, 340–347.

Hohman, M., & Buchik, G. (1994). Adolescent relapse prevention. In C. LeCroy (Ed.), *Handbook of child and adolescent treatment manuals*. New York: Lexington Books.

Hollis, F. (1939). *Social casework in practice: Six case studies*. New York: Family Welfare Association of America.

Hollis, F. (1963). Contemporary issues for case–workers. In H. J. Parad & R. R. Miller (Eds.), *Ego-oriented casework* (pp. 83–98). New York: Family Service Association of America.

Honolulu Advertiser (1989, April 4). *Honolulu Advertiser,* p. D–2.

Honolulu Advertiser (1989, September 6). *Honolulu Advertiser,* p. A–4.

hooks, b. (1989). *Talking back: Thinking feminist, thinking black*. Boston, MA: South End Press.

Hops, H., Walker, H. M., & Greenwood, C. R. (1979). PEERS: A program for remediating social withdrawal in school. In L. A. Hamerlynch (Ed.), *Behavior systems for the developmentally disabled: I. School and family environments*. New York: Brunner/Mazel.

Horejsi, C., Craig, B. H. R., & Pablo, J. (1992). Reactions by Native American parents to child protection agencies: Cultural and community factors. *Child Welfare, 71,* 329–342.

Houston-Vega, M. K., Nuehring, E. M., & Daguio, E. R. (1997). *Prudent practice: A guide for managing malpractice risk.* Washington, DC: NASW Press.

Howard, G. S. (1980). Response-shift bias: A problem in evaluating interventions with pre/post self-report. *Evaluation Review, 4,* 93–106.

Howard, W. A., Shane, M. M., & Clark, J. C. (1983). The nature and treatment of fear of flying. *Behavior Therapy, 27,* 79–91.

Howe, G. S. (1974). Casework self-evaluation: A single subject approach. Social Service Review, 48, 1–24.

Howing, P. T., Wodarski, J. S., Gaudin, J. M., Jr., & Kurtz, P. D. (1989). Effective interventions to ameliorate the incidence of child maltreatment: The empirical base. *Social Work, 34,* 330–338.

Hoyer, W. J. (1973). Application of operant techniques for the modification of elderly behavior. *The Gerontologist, 13,* 18–22.

Hoyer, W. J., Kafer, R. A., Simpson, S. S., & Hoyer, F. W. (1974). A reinstatement of verbal behavior in elderly patients using operant procedures. *The Gerontologist, 14,* 149–152.

Hudson, W. (1982). *The clinical measurement package: A field manual.* Chicago: Dorsey Press.

Hudson, W. W. (1987). Future directions in clinical evaluation. In N. Gottliev, H. A. Ishisaka, J. Kropp, C. A. Richey, & E. R. Tolson (Eds.), *Perspectives on direct practice evaluation, [Monograph #5].* Seattle, WA: School of Social Work, University of Washington.

Hudson, W. W. (1990). *Computer assisted social services.* Tempe, AZ: Walmyr Publishing Company.

Hudson, W., & Thyer, B. A. (1987). Research measures and indices in direct practice. In A. Minahan (Ed.), *Encyclopedia of social work* (pp. 487–498). Washington, DC: National Association of Social Workers.

Hunt, S. W., Hyles, S. E., Frances, A., Clarkin, J. F., & Brent, R. (1984). Assessing borderline personality disorder with self-report, clinical interview, or semi-structural interview. *American Journal of Psychiatry, 141,* 1228–1231.

Hunter, R. W., & Friesen, B. J. (1996). Family-centered servcies for children with emotional, behavioral, and mental health disorders. In C. A. Heflinger & C. T. Nixon (Eds.), *Families and the mental health system for children and adolescents: Policy, services, and research.* Thousand Oaks, CA: Sage Publications.

Huston, T. L., & Vangelisti, A. L. (1991). Socioemotional behavior and satisfaction in marital relationships: A longitudinal study. *Journal of Personality and Social Psychology, 61,* 721–733.

Hutchison, E. D. (1987). Use of authority in direct practice with mandated clients. *Social Service Review, 61,* 581–598.

Ingram, J. A., & Salzberg, H. C. (1988). Cognitive-behavioral approaches to the treatment of alcoholic behavior. In M. Hersen (Ed.), *Progress in behavior modification.* New York: Academic Press.

Institute for Juvenile Research (1972). *Juvenile delinquency in Illinois, highlights of the 1972 adolescent survey.* Chicago: Institute for Juvenile Research.

Ito, J. K., & Donovan, D. (1986). Aftercare in alcoholism treatment: A review. In W. R. Miller & N. Heather (Eds.), *Treating addictive behaviors.* New York: Plenum.

Ivanoff, A., Blythe, B. J., & Briar, S. (1997). What's the story, morning glory? *Social Work Research, 21*(3), 194–196.

Ivanoff, A., Blythe, B. J., & Tripodi, T. (1994). *Involuntary clients in social work practice: A research-based approach.* New York: Aldine de Gruyter.

Ivanoff, A., & Reidel, M. (1995). Suicide. In R. I. Edwards (Ed.), *Encyclopedia of social work* (19th ed., pp. 2358–2372). Washington, DC: NASW Press.

Jackson, A. W., & Hornbeck, D. W. (1989). Educating young adolescents: Why we must structure middle grade schools. *American Psychologist, 44*, 837–840.

Jackson, G. M. (1980). *The behavior treatment of facial tardive dyskinesia.* Paper presented at the first Conference on Behavior Gerontology, Nova University.

Jackson, N., & Mathews, R. (1995). Using public feedback to increase contributions to a multipurpose senior center. *Journal of Applied Behavior Analysis, 28*, 449–455.

Jacobs, R. (1991). Iroquois great law of peace and the United States Constitution: How the founding fathers ignored the clan mothers. *American Indian Law Review, 16*, 496–531.

Jacobson, N. S. (1977). Problem solving and contingency contracting in the treatment of marital discord. *Journal of Consulting and Clinical Psychology, 45*, 92–100.

Jacobson, N. S. (1978). A stimulus control model of change in behavioral couples' therapy: Implications for contingency contracting. *The Journal of Marriage and Family Counseling, 4*, 29–35.

Jacobson, N. S. (1984). The modification of cognitive processes in behavioral marital therapy: Integrating cognitive and behavioral intervention strategies. In K. Hahlweg & N. S. Jacobson (Eds.), *Marital interaction.* New York: Guilford.

Jacobson, N. S., & Christensen, A. (1996). *Integrative couple therapy: Promoting acceptance and change.* New York: Norton.

Jacobson, N. S., & Dallas, M. (1981). Helping married couples improve their relationships. In W. E. Craighead, A. E. Kazdin, & M. J. Mahoney (Eds.), *Behavior modification.* Boston, MA: Houghton Mifflin.

Jacobson, N. S., & Gurman, A. S. (Eds.). (1986). *Clinical handbook of marital therapy.* New York: Guilford.

Jacobson, N. S., & Holtzworth-Munroe, A. (1986). Marital therapy: A social learning cognitive perspective. In N. S. Jacobson & A. S. Gurman (Eds.), *Clinical handbook of marital therapy.* New York: Guilford.

Jacobson, N. S., & Margolin, G. (1979). *Marital therapy.* New York: Brunner/Mazel.

Jacobson, N. S., & Martin, B. (1976). Behavioral marriage therapy: Current status. *Psychological Bulletin, 83*, 540–556.

Jacobson, N. S., & Moore, D. (1981). Behavior exchange theory of marriage: Reconnaissance and reconsideration. In J. P. Vincent (Ed.), *Advances in family intervention assessment and theory* (Vol. II,). Greenwich, Ct: JAI.

Jacobson, N. S., Waldron, H., & Moore, D. (1980). Toward a behavioral profile of marital distress. *Journal of Consulting and Clinical Psychology, 48*, 696–703.

Janis, I. L., & Mann, L. (1977). *Decision-making.* New York: Free Press.

Janzen, C., & Harris, O. (1997). *Family treatment in social work practice.* (3rd ed.). Itasca, IL: Peacock.

Jayaratne, S. (1978). Analytic procedures for single-subject designs. *Social Work Research and Abstracts, 14*(4), 30–40.

Jayaratne, S., Croxton, T., & Mattison, D. (1997). Social work professional standards: An exploratory study. *Social Work, 42*, 187–198.

Jayaratne, S., & Levy, L. (1979). *Empirical clinical practice*. New York: Columbia University Press.

Jensen, C. (1994). Psychosocial treatment of depression in women: Nine single-subject evaluations. *Research on Social Work Practice, 4*(3), 267–282.

Jensen, J. P., Bergin, A. E., & Greaves, D. W. (1990). *The meaning of eclecticism: New survey and analysis of components. Professional Psychology: Research and Practice, 21*(2), 124–130.

Jessor, R. (1982). Problem behavior and developmental transition in adolescence. *The Journal of School Health, 53*, 295–300.

Jimenez, A., Alegria, M., Pena, M., & Vera, M. (1997). Mental health utilization in women with symptoms of depression. *Women and Health, 25*(2), 1–21.

Jimenez, M. (1997). Gender and psychiatry: Psychiatric conceptions of mental disorders in women, 1960–1994. *Affilia, 12*(2), 154–175.

Johnson, A. (1955). Educating professional social workers for ethical practice. *Social Science Review, 29*(2), 125–136.

Johnson, E., Levine, A., & Doolittle, F. (1999). *Fathers' fair share: Helping poor men manage child support and fatherhood*. New York: Russell Sage.

Johnson, V. W. (1973). *I'll quit tomorrow*. New York: Harper & Row.

Johnson, W. (1993). *Perceptions and patterns of paternal role functioning among urban, lower socioeconomic status adolescent and young adult African American males: A social choice/social norms perspective*. Unpublished Doctoral Dissertation, University of Chicago.

Johnson, W. (1995). Paternal identity among urban, adolescent males. *African American Research Perspectives, 2*(1), 82–86.

Johnson, W. (1998). Paternal involvement in fragile, African American families: Implications for clinical social work practice. *Smith College Studies in Social Work, 68*(2), 215–232.

Johnson, W. (1999, August). *The determinants of paternal involvement among unwed fathers*. Paper presented at the Fragile Families and Welfare Reform Workshop, Institute for Research on Poverty, University of Wisconsin, Madison.

Johnson, W. (2000). Work preparation and labor market experiences among urban, poor, nonresident fathers. In S. Danziger & A. Lin (Eds.), *Coping with poverty: The social contexts of neighborhood, work, and family in the African-American community*. Ann Arbor, MI: University of Michigan Press.

Johnston, L. D., Bachman, J. G., & O'Malley, P. M. (1995). *Drug use rises among American teenagers* (News release). Ann Arbor, MI: Institute for Social Research, University of Michigan.

Johnston, L. D., O'Malley, P. M., & Bachman, J. G. (1986). *Drug use among American high school students, college students, and other young adults*. Rockville, MD: National Institute on Drug Abuse.

Jones, E. E., & Pittman, T. S. (1982). Toward a general theory of strategic self-presentation. In J. Sals (Ed.), *Psychological perspectives on the self*. Hillsdale, NJ: Erlbaum.

Jordan, C., Cobb, N., & McCully, R. (1989). Clinical issues of the dual-career couple. *Social Work, 34*(1), 29–32.

Jordan, C., & Franklin, C. (1995). *Clinical assessment for social workers: Quantitative and qualitative methods*. Chicago: Lyceum Books.

Jordan, C., Franklin, C., & Corcoran, K. (1997). Measuring instruments. In J. R. M.

Grinnell (Ed.), *Social work research and evaluation: Qualitative and quantitative.* Itasca, IL: Peacock Press.

Joseph, M. V. (1985). A model for ethical decision making in clinical practice. In C. B. Germain (Ed.), *Advances in clinical practice* (pp. 207–217). Silver Spring, MD: National Association of Social Workers.

Joseph, M. V. (1989). Social work ethics: Historical and comtemporary perspectives. *Social Thought, 15*(3/4), 4–17.

Kagle, J. D., & Giebelhausen, P. N. (1994). Dual relationships and professional boundaries. *Social Work, 39*(2), 213–220.

Kahn, R. S. (1965). *Comments, Proceedings of the York House Institute on mentally impaired aged.* Philadelphia, PA: Philadelphia Geriatric Center.

Kahn, R. S., Goldfarb, A. I., Pollock, M., & Peck, R. (1960). Brief objective measures for the determination of mental status in the aged. *American Journal of Psychiatry, 117,* 326–328.

Kanfer, F. H. (1986). Implications of a self-regulation model of therapy for treatment of addictive behaviors. In W. R. Miller & N. Heather (Eds.), *Treating addictive behavior.* New York: Plenum.

Kantor, S., & Zimring, F. M. (1976). The effects of focusing on a problem. *Psychotherapy: Theory, Research and Practice, 13*(3), 255–258.

Karoly, P., & Steffen, J. J. (Eds.). (1980). *Improving the long-term effects of psychotherapy.* New York: Gardner.

Kazdin, A. E. (1979). Unobtrusive measures in behavioral assessment. *Journal of Applied Behavior Analysis, 12,* 713–724.

Kazdin, A. E., & Weisz, J. R. (1998). Identifying and developing empirically supported child and adolescent treatments. *Journal of Consulting and Clinical Psychology, 66,* 19–36.

Keith, W., & Schafer, R. B. (1998). Marital types and quality of life: A re-examination of a typology. *Marriage and Family Review, 17,* 19–35.

Keith-Lucas, A. (1963). A critique of the principle of client self-determination. *Social Work, 8*(3), 66–71.

Keith-Lucas, A. (1977). Ethics in social work. In J. B. Turner (Ed.), *Encyclopedia of social work* (17th ed., Vol. I, pp. 350–355). Silver Spring, MD: National Association of Social Workers.

Kemp, A. (1994). *Women's work: Degraded and devalued.* Englewood Cliffs, NJ: Prentice Hall.

Kemp, S. P., Whittaker, J. K., & Tracy, E. M. (1997). *Person-environment practice.* New York: Aldine de Gruyter.

Kendler, K., Kessler, R., Neale, M., Heath, A., & Eaves, L. (1993a). The prediction of major depression in women: Toward an integrated etiologic model. *American Journal of Psychiatry, 150*(8), 1139–1148.

Kendler, K., Kessler, R., Neale, M., Heath, A., & Eaves, L. (1993b). Alcoholism and major depression in women: A twin study of the causes of comorbidity. *Archives of General Psychiatry, 50*(9), 690–698.

Kendler, K., Kessler, R., Neale, M., Heath, A., & Eaves, L. (1993c). A longitudinal twin study of personality and major depression in women. *Archives of General Psychiatry, 50*(11), 853–862.

Kendler, K., Neale, M., Kessler, R., Heath, A., & Eaves, L. (1992). Childhood parental loss and adult psychopathology in women: A twin study perspective. *Archives of General Psychiatry, 49*(2), 109–116.

Kendler, K., et al. (1995). Stressful life events, genetic liability, and onset of an episode of major depression in women. *American Journal of Psychiatry, 152*(6), 833–842.

Kenmore, T. (1987). Negotiating with clients: A study of clinical practice experience. *Social Services Review, 61,* 132–144.

Kernberg, O. F. (1975). *Borderline conditions and pathological narcissism.* New York: Jason Aronson.

Kernberg, O. F. (1976). *Object-relations theory and clinical psychoanalysis.* New York: Jason Aronson.

Kernberg, O. F., Burstein, E. E., Coyne, L., Applebaum, A., Horwitz, L., & Voth, H. (1972). Psychotherapy and psychoanalysis: Final report of the Menninger Foundation's psychotherapy research project. *Bulletin of the Menninger Clinic, 36,* 1–277.

Kernberg, O. F., Goldstein, E. G., Carr, A. C., Hunt, H. F., Bauer, S. F., & Blumenthal, R. (1981). Diagnosing borderline personality: A pilot study using multiple diagnosis methods. *Journal of Nervous and Mental Disease, 169,* 225–231.

Kessler, R., McGonagle, K., Zhao, S., Nelson, C., Hughes, M., Eshleman, S., Wittchen, H., & Kendler, K. (1994). Lifetime and 12–month prevalence of DSM-III-R psychiatric disorders in the United States. *Archives of General Psychiatry, 51,* 8–19.

Kilgore, D. K. (1995). *Task-centered group treatment of sex offenders: A developmental study.* Unpublished doctoral dissertation, State University of New York, Albany, NY.

King, J. J. (1980). The therapeutic utility of abbreviated progressive relaxation: A critical review with implications for clinical practice. In M. Hersen, R. Eisler, & P. Miller (Eds.), *Progress in behavior modification* (Vol. 10,). New York: Academic Press.

Kiresak, T. J., & Sherman, R. (1968). Goal attainment scaling: A general method for evaluating comprehensive mental health programs. *Community Mental Health Journal, 4,* 443–453.

Kiresak, T. S., Smith, A., & Cardillo, J. E. (Eds.). (1994). *Goal attainment scaling: Applications, theory, and measurement.* Hillsdale, NJ: Erlbaum.

Kirk, S. A. (1990). Research utilization: The substructure of belief. In L. Videka-Sherman & W. J. Reid (Eds.), *Advances in clinical social work research* (pp. 233–250). Washington, DC: NASW Press.

Kirk, S. A., & Kutchins, H. (1988). Deliberate misdiagnosis in mental health practice. *Social Service Review, 62,* 225–237.

Kirk, S. A., & Penka, C. E. (1992). Research utilization and MSW education: A decade of progress? In A. J. Grasso & I. Epstein (Eds.), *Research utilization in the social services* (pp. 407–419). New York: Haworth Press.

Kitcher, P. (1993). *The advancement of science.* New York: Oxford University Press.

Klein, W. C., & Bloom, M. (1995). Practice wisdom. *Social Work, 40*(2), 799–807.

Klinman, D., Sander, J., Rosen, J., & Longo, K. (1986). The teen father collaboration: A demonstration and research model. In M. Lamb & A. Elster (Eds.), *Adolescent fatherhood.* Hillsdale, NJ: Lawrence Erlbaum.

Kohut, H., & Wolff, E. S. (1978). The disorders of the self and their treatment: An outline. *International Journal of Psychoanalysis, 59,* 413.

Kolb, D. (1983). *The mediators.* Cambridge, MA: MIT Press.

Kolb, J. E., & Gunderson, J. G. (1980). Diagnosing borderline patients with a semi-structural interview. *Archives of General Psychiatry, 37,* 37–41.

Koroloff, N. M., & Briggs, H. E. (1996). The life cycle of family advocacy organizations. *Administration in Social Work, 20*(4), 23–42.

Kravetz, D., & Rose, S. (1973). *Contracts in groups: A workbook.* Dubuque, IA: Kendall-Hunt Publishing Company.

Krieger, I. (1988). An approach to coping with anxiety about AIDS. *Social Work, 33*(3), 263–264.

Kroll, J., Pyle, R., Zander, J., Martin, K., Lari, S., & Sines, L. (1981). Borderline personality disorder: Reliability of the Gunderson diagnostic interview for borderliners (DIB). *Schizophrenia Bulletin, 7,* 269–272.

Kruk, E. (Ed.). (1997). *Mediation and conflict resolution in social work and the human services.* Chicago: Nelson-Hall Publishers.

Kruzich, J. M., & Friesen, B. J. (1984). Blending administrative and community organization practice: The case of community residential facilites. *Administration in Social Work, 8*(4), 55–66.

Kubler-Ross, E. (1987). *AIDS: The ultimate challenge.* New York: Macmillan.

Kuhn, T. S. (1970). *The structure of scientific revolutions.* (2nd ed.). Chicago: University of Chicago Press.

Kurzman, P. A. (1995). Professional liability and malpractice. In R. L. Edwards (Ed.), *Encyclopedia of social work* (19th ed., Vol. 3, pp. 1921–1927). Washington, DC: NASW Press.

Kutchins, H., & Kirk, S. A. (1997). *Making us crazy, DSM: The psychiatric bible and the creation of mental disorders.* New York: Free Press.

LaGreca, A., & Stone, W. (1993). Social Anxiety Scale for children—Revised: Factor structure and concurrent validity. *Journal of Clinical Child Psychology, 22,* 17–27.

Laird, J. (1995a). Family-centered practice in the postmodern era. *Families in Society: The Journal of Contemporary Human Services, March,* 150–160.

Laird, J. (1995b, March). *Ideas for a postmodern/feminist approach to practice.* Paper presented at the Council on Social Work Education APM, San Diego, CA.

Lakatos, I. (1972). Falsification and methodology of scientific research programs. In I. Lakatos & A. Musgrave (Eds.), *Criticisms and the growth of knowledge.* Cambridge, MA: Cambridge University Press.

Lakein, A. (1973). *How to get control of your time and your life.* New York: New American Library.

Lamal, P. A. (Ed.). (1991). *Behavioral analysis of societies and cultural practices.* New York: Hemisphere.

Lamal, P. A. (Ed.). (1997). *Cultural contingencies: Behavior analysis of societies and cultural practices.* Westport, CT: Praeger.

Lamb, D. H., Presser, N. R., Pfost, K. S., Baum, M. C., Jackson, V. R., & Jarvis, P. A. (1987). Confronting professional impairment during the internship: Identification, due process, and remediation. *Professional Psychology: Research and Practice, 18,* 597–603.

Lamb, M. (1997). Fathers and child development: An introductory overview and guide. In M. Lamb (Ed.), *The role of the father in child development* (pp. 1–18). New York: Wiley.

Lamb, M., & Elster, A. (1986). *Adolescent fatherhood.* Hillsdale, NJ: Erlbaum.

Lamb, M., & Oppenheim, D. (1989). Fatherhood and father-child relations: Five years of research. In S. Cath, A. Gurwitt, & L. Gunsberg (Eds.), *Fathers and their families* (pp. 11–26). Hillsdale, NJ: Analytic Press.

Lankston, S., & Lankston, C. (1983). *The answer within.* New York: Brunner/Mazel.

La Puma, J., & Schiedermayer, D. L. (1991). Ethics consultation: Skills, roles, and training. *Annals of Internal Medicine, 114,* 155–169.

Lavelle, J., Hovell, M., West, M., & Wahlgren, D. (1992). Promoting law enforcement for child protection: A community analysis. *Journal of Applied Behavior Analysis,* *25*(885–892).

Leary, M. R., & Kowalski, R. M. (1993). The Interaction Anxiousness Scale. *Journal of Personality Assessment, 61,* 136–146.

LeCroy, C. W. (1983). Social skills training with adolescents: A review. In C. LeCroy (Ed.), *Social skills training for children and youth* (pp. 91–116). New York: Haworth Press.

LeCroy, C. W. (1994). A social skills group for children. In C. W. LeCroy (Ed.), *Handbook of child and adolescent treatment manual* (pp. 126–169). New York: Lexington.

Lee, P. R. (1930). Cause and function, National Conference on Social Work, *Proceedings: 1929* (pp. 3–20). Chicago: University of Chicago Press.

Leff, J. (1989). Family factors in schizophrenia. *Psychiatric Annals, 19,* 542–547.

Leff, J., & Vaughn, C. (1985). *Expressed emotion in families: Its significance for mental illness.* New York: Guilford Press.

Leiby, J. (1978). *A history of social work and social welfare in the United States.* New York: Columbia University Press.

Lennon, M. (1994). Women, work and well-being: The importance of work conditions. *Journal of Health and Social Behavior, 35*(3), 235–247.

Leon, A., Klerman, G., & Wickramaratne, P. (1993). Continuing female predominance in depressive illness. *American Journal of Public Health, 83*(5), 754–757.

Levendusky, P. G. 1978. Effects of Social Incentives On Task Performance in the Elderly. *Journal of Gerontology, 33,* 562–564.

Levi, A., & Benjamin, A. (1977). Focus and flexibility in a model of conflict resolution. *Journal of Conflict Resolution, 21,* 405–425.

Levine, C. (1991). AIDS and the ethics of human subjects research. In F. G. Reamer (Ed.), *AIDS and ethics* (pp. 77–104). New York: Columbia University Press.

Leviton, S., & Greenstone, J. (1997). *Elements of mediation.* New York: Brooks/Cole.

Levitt, J. L., & Reid, W. J. (1981). Rapid-assessment instrument for practice. *Social Work Research and Abstract, 17,* 13–20.

Levy, C. S. (1972). The context of social work ethics. *Social Work, 17,* 95–101.

Levy, C. S. (1973). The value base of social work. *Journal of Education for Social Work, 9,* 34–42.

Levy, C. S. (1976). *Social work ethics.* New York: Human Sciences Press.

Levy, R. L. (1981). On the nature of the clinical research gap: The problems with some solutions. *Behavioral Assessment, 3,* 235–242.

Lewis, E., & Kissman, K. (1989). Factors linking ethnic-sensitive and feminist social work practice with African-American women. *Arete, 14*(2), 23–31.

Lewis, H. (1972). Morality and the politics of practice. *Social Casework, 53,* 404–417.

Lewis, J. A., Dana, R. O., & Blevins, G. A. (1988). *Substance abuse counseling: An individualized approach.* Pacific Grove, CA: Brooks/Cole.

Lindsley, O. R. (1964). Geriatric behavioral prosthetics. In R. Kastenbaum (Ed.), *New thoughts on old age.* New York: Springer.

Linehan, M. M. (1993a). *Cognitive-behavioral treatment of borderline personality disorders.* New York: Guilford Press.

Linehan, M. M. (1993b). *Skills training manual for treating borderline personality disorder.* New York: Guilford Press.

Linehan, M. M., & Kehrer, C. A. (1993). Borderline personality disorder. In D. H. Barlow (Ed.), *Clinical handbook of psychological disorders* (pp. 396–441). New York: Guilford Press.

Linsk, J. L., Howe, M. W., & Pinkston, E. M. (1975). Behavioral group work in a home for the aged. *Social Work, 20,* 454–463.

Linsk, N. L., Pinkston, E. M., & Green, G. R. (1982). Home-based behavioral social work with the impaired elderly. In E. M. Pinkston, J. L. Levitt, G. R. Green, N. L. Linsk, & T. L. Rzepnicki (Eds.), *Effective social work practice: Advanced techniques for behavioral intervention with individuals, families, and institutional staff* (pp. 220–232). San Francisco, CA: Jossey-Bass Publishers.

Litman, G. K. (1986). Alcoholism survival: The prevention of relapse. In W. R. Miller & N. Heather (Eds.), *Treating addictive behaviors.* New York: Plenum.

Loch, C. S. (1899). Christian charity and political economy. *Charity Organization Review, 6,* 10–20.

Locke, E. A., Sarri, L. M., Shaw, K. N., & Latham, G. P. (1981). *Psychological Bulletin, 90,* 125–152.

Loewenberg, F., & Dolgoff, R. (1996). *Ethical decision for social work practice.* Itasca, IL: F. E. Peacock.

Longress, J. F. (1991). Toward a status model of ethnic sensitive practice. *Journal of Multicultural Social Work, 1*(1), 41–56.

Lowery, C. T. (1998). Social justice and international human rights. In M. A. Mattaini, C. T. Lowery, & C. H. Meyer (Eds.), *The foundations of social work practice: A graduate text* (2nd ed., pp. 20–42). Washington, DC: NASW Press.

Lowery, C. T. (1999). The sharing of power: Empowerment with Native American women. In L. Gutierrez & E. Lewis (Eds.), *Empowerment with women of color.* New York: Columbia University Press.

Lowery, C. T., & Mattaini, M. A. (in press). The co-construction of empowerment cultures in child welfare. In W. Shera & L. Wells (Eds.), *International perspectives on empowerment practice.* New York: Columbia University Press.

Lubove, R. (1965). *The professional altruist: The emergence of social work as a career.* Cambridge, MA: Harvard University Press.

Lum, D. (1986). *Social work practice and people of color.* Pacific Grove, CA: Brooks/Cole.

Lundy, M. (1993). Explicitness: The unspoken mandate of feminist social work. *Affilia, 8*(2), 184–199.

Lynch, V. (Ed.). (1996). *Caring for the HIV care giver.* Westport, CT: Auburn House.

MacDonald, G., Sheldon, B., & Gillespie, J. (1992). Contemporary studies of the effectiveness of social work. *British Journal of Social Work, 22*(6), 625–643.

Mackelprang, G. W., & Salsgiver, R. O. (1996). People with disabilities and social work: Historical and contemporary issues. *Social Work, 41*(1), 7–14.

Mackenzie, A., & Waldo, K. C. (1981). *About time! A woman's guide to time management.* New York: McGraw-Hill.

Madden, R. G. (1998). *Legal issues in social work, counseling, and mental health.* Thousand Oaks, CA: Sage Publications.

Mager, R. F. (1972). *Goal analysis.* Belmont, CA: Fearon.

Mager, R. F., & Pipe, P. (1984). *Analyzing performance problems: Or you really oughta wanna.* Belmont, CA: Lake Publishing Company.

Maher, C. (1983). Description and evaluation of an approach to implementing programs in organizational settings. *Journal of Organizational Behavior Management, 34*(5), 69–98.

Mahler, M. S., Pine, F., & Bergman, A. (1975). *The psychological birth of the human infant.* New York: Basic Books.

Maisto, S. A., & Carey, K. B. (1987). Treatment of alcohol abuse. In T. D. Nirenberg & S. A. Maisto (Eds.), *Developments in the assessment and treatment of addictive behaviors.* Norwood, NJ: Ablex.

Malgady, R. G., Rogler, L. H., & Cortes, D. E. (1996). Cultural expressions of psychiatric symptoms: Idioms of anger among Puerto Ricans. *Psychological Assessment, 81,* 265–268.

Mallams, J., Godley, M., Hall, G., & Meyers, R. (1982). A social-systems approach to resocializing alcoholics in the community. *Journal of Studies on Alcohol, 43,* 1115–1123.

Malloy, P., & Levis, D. (1988). A laboratory demonstration of persistent human avoidance. *Behavior Therapy, 19,* 229–241.

Maluccio, A., & Marlow, W. (1974). The case for the contract. *Social Work, 19,* 28–36.

Mannuzza, S., Scheier, F. R., Chapman, T. F., & Leibowitz, M. R. (1995). Generalized social phobia: Reliability and validity. *Archives of General Psychiatry, 52,* 230–237.

Mantell, M. R. (1988). *Don't sweat the small stuff: P. S., it's all small stuff.* San Luis Obispo, CA: Impact.

Marin, G., Sabogal, F., Van Oss Marin, G., Otero-Sabogal, F., & Perez-Stable, E. J. (1987). Development of a short acculturation scale for Hispanics. *Hispanic Journal of Behavioral Sciences, 9,* 183–205.

Marino, R., Green, G. R., & Young, E. (1998). Beyond the scientist-practitioners model's failure to thrive: Social workers' participation in agency-based research activities. *Social Work Research, 22,* 188–191.

Markman, H. J. (1979). Application of a behavioral model of marriage in predicting relationship satisfaction of couples planning marriage. *Journal of Consulting and Clinical Psychology, 47,* 743–749.

Markman, H. J., Renick, M. J., Floyd, F. J., Stanley, S. M., & Clements, M. Preventing Marital Distress through Communication and Conflict Management Training: A Four and Five Year Follow Up. *Journal of Consulting and Clinicial Psychology, 61,* 70–77.

Marks, I. M. (1978). *Living with fear.* New York: McGraw-Hill.

Marks, I. M. (1987). *Fears, phobias, and rituals.* New York: Oxford University Press.

Marks, I. M., & Mathews, A. M. (1979). Brief standard self-rating for phobic patients. *Behavioral Research and Therapy, 17,* 263–267.

Marlatt, G. A. (1976). The drinking profile: A questionnaire for the behavioral assessment of alcoholism. In E. J. Mash & L. G. Terdal (Eds.), *Behavioral therapy assessment: Diagnosis, design, and evaluation.* New York: Springer.

Marlatt, G. A. (1979). Alcohol use and problem drinking: A cognitive-behavioral analysis. In P. C. Kendall & S. D. Hollon (Eds.), *Cognitive-behavioral interventions* New York: Academic Press.

Marlatt, G. A., & Gordon, J. R. (1985). Determinants of relapse: Implications of the maintenance of behavior change. In P. O. Davidson & S. M. Davidson (Eds.), *Behavioral medicine: Changing health lifestyles.* New York: Brunner/Mazel.

Marlatt, G. A., & Marques, J. K. (1977). Mediation, self-control and alcohol use. In R. B. Stuart (Ed.), *Behavioral self-management: Strategies, techniques and outcomes.* New York: Brunner/Mazel.

Marsiglio, W. (1988). Commitment to social fatherhood: Predicting adolescent males' intentions to live with their child and partner. *Journal of Marriage and the Family, 50,* 427–441.

Marsiglio, W. (1989). Adolescent males' pregnancy resolution preferences and family formation intentions: Does family background make a difference for Blacks and Whites? *Journal of Adolescent Research, 3,* 214–237.

Martin, L. I., & Kettner, P. M. (1997). Performance measurement: The new accountability. *Administration in Social Work, 21*(1), 17–29.

Masterson, J. F. (1972). *Treatment of the borderline adolescent: A developmental approach.* New York: Wiley.

Masterson, J. F. (1976). *Psychotherapy of the borderline adult: A developmental approach.* New York: Brunner/Mazel.

Matson, J. L. (1981). A controlled outcome study of phobias in mentally retarded adults. *Behavior Research and Therapy, 19,* 101–107.

Mattaini, M. A. (1993a). Behavior analysis and community practice: A review. *Research on Social Work Practice, 3,* 420–447.

Mattaini, M. A. (1993b). *More than a thousand words: Graphics for clinical practice.* Washington, DC: NASW Press.

Mattaini, M. A. (1996). Envisioning cultural practices. *The Behavior Analyst, 19,* 257–272.

Mattaini, M. A. (1998a). Knowledge for practice. In M. A. Mattaini, C. T. Lowery, & C. H. Meyers (Eds.), *The foundations of social work practice: A graduate text* (2nd ed., pp. 86–116). Washington, DC: NASW Press.

Mattaini, M. A. (1998b). Practice with individuals. In M. A. Mattaini, C. T. Lowery, & C. H. Meyer (Eds.), *The foundation of social work practice: A graduate text* (2nd ed., pp. 135–164). Washington, DC: NASW Press.

Mattaini, M. A. (1999a). *Clinical intervention with families.* Washington, DC: NASW Press.

Mattaini, M. A. (1999b). *Clinical practice with individuals.* (2nd ed.). Washington, DC: NASW Press.

Mattaini, M. A. (in press). Constructing cultures of non-violence: The PEACE POWER! strategy. *Education and Treatment of Children.*

Mattaini, M. A., & Lowery, C. T. (under review). *The science of sharing power: Native American thought and behavior analysis.*

Mattaini, M. A., Lowery, C. T., Herrara, K.,& DiNoia, J. (in press). *PEACE POWER! Developmental research for constructing alternatives to youth violence.*

Mattaini, M. A., Lowery, C. T., & Meyer, C. H. (Eds.). (1998). *The foundations of social work practice: A graduate text* (2nd ed.). Washington, DC: NASW Press.

Mattaini, M. A., McGowan, B. G., & Williams, G. (1996). Child maltreatment. In M. A. Mattaini & B. A. Thyer (Eds.), *Finding solutions to social problems: Behavioral strategies for change* (pp. 223–266). Washington, DC: APA Books.

Mattaini, M. A., & Thyer, B. A. (Eds.). (1996). *Finding solutions to social problems: Behavioral strategies for change.* Washington, DC: American Psychological Association Books.

Matuscha, P. R. (1985). The psychopharmacology of addiction. In T. E. Bratter & G. G. Forrest (Eds.), *Alcoholism and substance abuse.* New York: Free Press.

Mawson, D., Marks, I. M., Ramm, L., & Stern, R. S. (1981). Guided mourning for morbid grief: A controlled study. *British Journal of Psychiatry, 138,* 185–193.

Maxman, J. S. (1986). *Essential psychopathology.* New York: W. W. Norton.

Mayer, J. E., & Timms, N. (1970). *The client speaks: Working class impressions of casework.* London: Routledge & K. Paul.

McCann, C. W., & Cutler, J. P. (1979). Ethics and alleged unethical. *Social Work, 24,* 5–8.

McClannahan, L. E., & Risley, T. R. (1974). Designs of living environments for nursing home residents: Recruiting attendance in activities. *The Gerontologist, 14,* 236–240.

McClellan, A. T., et al. (1980). An improved evaluation instrument for substance abuse patients: The addiction severity index. *Journal of Nervous and Mental Disorders, 168,* 26–33.

McCleod, D., & Meyer, H. (1968). A study of values of social workers. In E. Thomas (Ed.), *Behavioral science for social workers* (pp. 401–416). New York: The Free Press.

McCown, W. F., & Johnson, J. (1993). *Therapy with treatment resistant families: A consultation-crisis intervention model.* New York: Haworth Press.

McCrady, B. S., & Sher, K. (1985). Treatment variables. In B. S. McCrady, N. E. Noel, & T. D. Nirenberg (Eds.), *Future directions in alcohol abuse treatment research.* Washington, DC: US Department of Health and Human Services.

McCready, D. J., Pierce, S., Rahn, S. L., & Were, K. (1996). Third generation information systems: Integrating costs and outcomes, tools for professional development and program evaluation. *Administration in Social Work, 20*(1), 1–15.

McDermott, F. E. (1975). Against the persuasive definition of "self-determination". In F. E. McDermott (Ed.), *Self-determination in social work* (pp. 118–137). London: Routledge & Kegan Paul.

McFall, R. M. (1982). A review and reformulation of the concept of social skills. *Behavioral Assessment, 4,* 1–33.

McFarlane, W. R. (1991). Family psychoeducational treatment. In A. S. Gurman & D. P. Kniskern (Eds.), *Handbook of family therapy* (Vol. II, pp. 363–395).

McGadney, B. F., Goldberg-Glen, R., & Pinkston, E. M. (1987). Clinical issues for assessment and intervention with the black elderly. In L. L. Carstensen & B.A. Edelstein (Eds.), *Handbook of clinical gerontology* (pp. 354–375). New York: Pergamon Press.

McGlashon, T. H. (1983). The borderline syndrome: I. Testing three diagnostic systems. *Archives of General Psychiatry, 40,* 1311–1318.

McGowan, B. G., & Mattison, M. (1998). Professional values and ethics. In M. A. Mattaini, C. T. Lowery, & C. H. Meyer (Eds.), *The foundations of social work practice: A graduate text* (2nd ed.). Washington, DC: NASW Press.

McLaughlin, M., Cormier, L. S., & Cormier, W. H. (1988). Relation between coping strategies and distress, stress, and marital adjustment of multiple-role women. *Journal of Counseling Psychology, 35*(2), 187–193.

McLaughlin, W. (1995). *The father's resource center: Executive Summary.* The Fathers Resource Center, Wishard Hospital, Indianapolis, Indiana.

Mead, L. (1986). *Beyond entitlement: The social obligations of citizenship.* New York: Free Press.

Meezan, W., & O'Keefe, M. (1998). Multifamily group therapy: Impact on family functioning and child behavior. *Families in Society, 79,* 32–44.

Mehrabian, A. (1972). *Nonverbal communication.* Chicago: Aldine Atherton.

Meichenbaum, D. (1983). *Coping with stress.* Somerset, NJ: John Wiley & Sons.

Meichenbaum, D., & Turk, D. C. (1987). *Facilitation treatment adherence: A practitioner's guidebook.* New York: Plenum Press.

Merbaum, M., & Rosenbaum, M. (1984). Self-control theory and technique in the modification of smoking, obesity, and alcohol abuse. In C. M. Franks (Ed.), *New developments in behavior therapy.* New York: Haworth Press.

Mersch, P. P., Breukers, P., & Emmelkamp, P. M. (1992). The simulated social interaction test. *Behavioral Assessment, 14,* 133–151.

Meyer, C. (1987). Direct practice with social work: Overview. *Encyclopedia of Social Work* (18th ed., pp. 409–422). Silver Spring, MD: NASW Press.

Meyer, C. H. (1976). *Social work practice: The changing landscape.* (2nd ed.). New York: Free Press.

Meyer, C. H. (Ed.). (1983). *Clinical social work in the ecosystems perspective.* New York: Columbia University Press.

Meyer, C. H. (1993). *Assessment in social work practice.* New York: Columbia University Press.

Meyer, C. H., & Mattaini, M. A. (1998). The ecosystems perspective: Implications for practice. In M. A. Mattaini, C. T. Lowery, & C. H. Meyer (Eds.), *The foundations of social work practice: A graduate text* (2nd ed., pp. 3–19). Washington, DC: NASW Press.

Meyer, R. G., Landis, E. R., & Hays, J. R. (1988). *Law for the psychotherapist.* New York: Norton.

Meyers, R., & Smith, J. (1995). *Clinical guide to alcohol treatment: The community reinforcement approach.* New York: Guilford.

Miers, T. C., & Raulin, M. L. (1985). *The development of a scale to measure cognitive slippage.* Unpublished manuscript. Available from M. Raulin, SUNY-Buffalo, Department of Psychology, Buffalo, NY 14260.

Milgram, G. G. (1987). Alcohol and drug education programs. *Journal of Drug Education, 17,* 43–57.

Miller, B. (1993, March). *Women's alcohol use and the connections to violent victimization.* Paper presented at the Working Group for Prevention Research on Women and Alcohol, Prevention Research Branch, Bethesda, MD.

Miller, D. (1994). Influences on parental involvement of African American adolescent fathers. *Child and Adolescent Social Work, 11*(5), 363–378.

Miller, P. M. (1981). Assessment of alcohol abuse. In D. H. Barlow (Ed.), *Behavioral assessment of adult disorders* (pp. 271–300). New York: Guilford Press.

Miller, P. M. (1987). Commonalities of addictive behaviors. In T. D. Nirenberg & S. A. Maisto (Eds.), *Developments in the assessment and treatment of addictive behaviors.* Norwood, NJ: Ablex.

Miller, W. R. (1985). Motivation for treatment: A review with special emphasis on alcoholism. *Psychological Bulletin, 98,* 84–107.

Miller, W. R., & Heather, N. (Eds.). (1986). *Treating addictive behaviors.* New York: Plenum.

Miller, W. R., & Hester, R. K. (1986). The effectiveness of alcoholism treatment: What research reveals. In W. R. Miller & N. Heather (Eds.), *Treating addictive behaviors.* New York: Plenum.

Miller, W. R., & Rollnick, S. (1991). *Motivational interviewing: Preparing people to change addictive behavior.* New York: Guilford.

Mills, F. B. (1996). The ideology of welfare reform: Deconstructing stigma. *Social Work, 41*(4), 391–395.

Millstein, K. H., Regan, J., & Reinherz, H. (1990, March 3–6). *Can training in single subject design generalize to non-behavioral practice.* Paper presented at the Council of Social Work Education Annual Program Meeting, Reno, NV.

Mintz, J., & Kiesler, D. J. (1982). Individualized measures of psychotherapy outcome. In P. C. Kendall & J. N. Butcher (Eds.), *Handbook of research methods in clinical psychology.* New York: Wiley.

Minuchin, P. (1995). Foster and natural families: Forming a cooperative network. In L. Combrinck-Graham (Ed.), *Children in families at risk: Maintaining the connections* (pp. 251–274). New York: Guilford.

Minuchin, S. (1974). *Families and family therapy.* Cambridge, MA: Harvard University Press.

Mishara, B. L., Robertson, B., & Kastenbaum, R. (1974). Self-injurious behavior in the elderly. *The Gerontologist, 14,* 273–280.

Monette, P. (1988). *Borrowed time: An AIDS memoir.* San Diego, CA: Harcourt, Brace and Jovanovich.

Monti, P. M., Abrams, D. B., Kadden, R. M., & Cooney, N. L. (1989). *Treating alcohol dependence: A coping skills guide.* New York: Guilford Press.

Moore, K. (1997). *Not just for girls: The roles of boys and men the teenage pregnancy prevention.* Washington, DC: National Campaign to Prevent Teen Pregnancy.

Morris, T. (1994). Alternative paradigms: A source for social work practice research. *Arete, 18*(2), 31–44.

Morrow-Bradley, C., & Elliott, R. (1986). Utilization of psychotherapy research by practicing psychotherapists. *American Psychologist, 41*(2), 188–197.

Mowbray, C. T., Plum, T. B., & Masterton, T. (1997). Harbinger II: Deployment and evolution of assertive community treatment in Michigan. *Administration and Policy in Mental Health, 25,* 125–139.

Munoz, R. (1997). The San Francisco depression prevention research project. In G. Albee & T. Gullotta (Eds.), *Primary prevention works* (pp. 380–400). Thousand Oaks, CA: Sage.

Murdach, A. D. (1996). Beneficence re-examined: Protective intervention in mental health. *Social Work, 41*(1), 26–32.

Muris, P., Merckelbach, H., Holdrinet, I., & Sijsenaar, M. (1998). Treating phobic children: Effects of EMDR versus exposure. *Journal of Consulting and Clinical Psychology, 66,* 193–198.

Murphy, G., & King, N. (1996). Australian data supporting validity claims of Azrin's Job Club program to reduce unemployment. *The Behavior Therapist, 19*(7), 104–106.

Murray, C. (1984). *Losing ground: American social policy from 1950–1980.* New York: Basic Books.

Myers, L. L., & Thyer, B. A. (1997). Should social work clients have the right to effective treatment? *Social Work, 42,* 288–298.

Naleppa, M. J., & Reid, W. J. (1998). Task-centered case management for the elderly: Developing a practice model. *Research on Social Work Practice, 8,* 63–85.

Nathan, P. E., & Gorman, J. M. (Eds.). (1998). *A guide to treatments that work.* New York: Oxford University Press.

National Association of Social Workers. (1987). *Impaired social worker program resource book.* Silver Spring, MD: National Association of Social Workers.

National Association of Social Workers (1996). *Code of ethics.* Washington, DC: Author.

National Center for Education Statistics (1993). *Drop out rates in the United States: 1993.* Washington, DC: National Center for Education Statistics, US Department of Education.

Navran, L. (1967). Communication and adjustment in marriage. *Family Process, 6,* 173–184.

Nay, W. R. (1979). Parents as real life reinforcers: The enhancement of training effects across conditions other than training. In A. P. Goldstein & F. H. Kanfer (Eds.), *Maximizing treatment gains: Transfer enhancement in psychotherapy* (pp. 249–302). New York: Academic Press.

Nelsen, J. C. (1978). Use of communication theory in single-subject research. *Social Work Research & Abstracts, 14,* 12.

Nelsen, J. C. (1981). Issues in single-subject research for the nonbehaviorist. *Social Work Research and Abstracts, 17*(2), 31–37.

Nelsen, J. C. (1984). Intermediate treatment goals as variables in single-case research. *Social Work Research and Abstracts, 20*(3), 3–10.

Nelsen, J. C. (1988). Single-subject designs. In R. M. Grinnell (Ed.), *Social work research and evaluation* (3rd ed.). Itasca, IL: Peacock.

Nelsen, J. C. (1993). Testing practice wisdom: Another use for single-system research. *Journal of Social Service Research, 18,* 65–82.

Nelson, H. F., Tennen, H., Tasman, A., Borton, M., Kubeck, M., & Stone, M. (1985). Comparison of three systems for diagnosing borderline personality disorder. *American Journal of Psychiatry, 142,* 855–858.

Neugarten, B. (1990). The changing meaning of age. In M. Bergener & S. Finkelhor (Eds.), *Clinical and scientific psychological geriatrics* (Vol. 1, Holistic approaches, pp. 1–6). New York: Springer.

Newman, J., Engel, R., & Jensen, J. (1991). Changes in depressive symptom experience among older women. *Psychology and Aging, 6*(2), 212–222.

Nicholls, G. (1956). Treatment of a disturbed mother-child relationship: A case presentation. *Smith College Studies in Social Work, 36,* 117–148.

Nierenberg, G. I., & Galero, H. H. (1973). *Meta-talk: Guide to hidden meanings in conversations.* New York: Simon and Schuster.

Nirenberg, T. D., & Maisto, S. A. (1987). *Developments in the assessment and treatment of addictive behavior.* Norwood, NJ: Ablex.

Norton, W. W., Weiss, R. L., Hops, H., & Patterson, G. R. (1973). A framework for conceptulizing marital conflict, a technology for altering it, some data for evaluating it. In L. S. Hamerlynck, L. C. Handy, & E. J. Mash (Eds.), *Behavior change: Methodology, concepts, and practice.* Champaign, IL: Research Press.

Novotny, D. (1998). *Mixed expressions and relationship quality amoung young expectant fathers.* Unpublished Dissertation Proposal, Committee on Human Development, University of Chicago.

Nowak, M. A., May, R. M., & Sigmund, K. (1995). The arithmetics of mutual help. *Scientific American, 272*(6), 76–83.

Nugent, W. (1991). An experimental and qualitative analysis of a cognitive-behavioral intervention for anger. *Social Work Research and Abstracts, 27,* 3–8.

Nugent, W. (1992a). Psychometric characteristics of self-anchored scales in clinical practice. *Journal of Social Service Research, 15,* 137–152.

Nugent, W. (1992b). The affective impact of a clinical social worker's interviewing style: A series of single-case experiments. *Research on Social Work Practice, 2*(3), 6–27.

Nugent, W., & Halvorson, H. (1995). Testing the effects of active listening. *Research on Social Work Practice, 5*(2), 152–175.

O'Farrell, T. J. (1987). Marital and family therapy for alcohol problems. In W. M. Cox (Ed.), *Treatment and prevention of alcohol problems.* New York: Academic Press.

Oetting, E. R., & Beauvais, F. (1990–1991). Orthogonal cultural identification theory: The cultural identification of minority adolescents. *The International Journal of the Addictions, 25,* 655–685.

O'Hare, T. (1996). Court-ordered versus voluntary clients: Problem differences and readiness for change. *Social Work, 41*(4), 417–423.

O'Looney, J. (1997). Marking progress toward service integration: Learning to use evaluation to overcome barriers. *Administration in Social Work, 21*(3/4), 31–65.

Olsen, L. (1978). *Focusing and self-healing* [Audio cassette].

Omer, H. (1985). Fulfillment of therapeutic tasks as a precondition for acceptance in therapy. *American Journal of Psychotherapy, 39*, 175–186.

O'Neil, M. (1984). Affective disorders. In F. Turner (Ed.), *Adult psychopathology: A social work perspective.* New York: MacMillian.

Ortiz, A. (1969). *The Tewa world: Space, time, being and becoming in a Pueblo society.* Chicago: University of Chicago Press.

Ost, L.-G., & Hugdahl, H. (1981). Acquisition of phobias and anxiety response patterns in clinical patients. *Behaviour Research and Therapy, 19*, 439–447.

Ost, L.-G., Mavissakalian, M. R., & Prien, R. F. (Eds.). (1996). *Long-term effects of behavior therapy for specific phobia.* Washington, DC: American Psychiatric Press.

Ostensen, K. W. (1981). The runaway crisis: Is family therapy the answer? *American Journal of Family Therapy, 9*, 3–12.

Paine, R. T., Jr. (1980). The work of volunteer visitors of the associated charities among the poor. *Journal of Social Science, 12*, 113.

Paine, S. C., Hops, H., Walker, H. M., Greenwood, C. R., Fleischman, D. H., & Guild, J. J. (1982). Repeated treatment effects: A study of maintaining behavior change in social withdrawn children. *Behavior Modification, 6*, 171–199.

Panel, N. E. G. (1997). *The national goals report: Building a nation of learners.* Washington, DC: US Government Printing Office.

Paone, D., & Chavkin, W. (1992). The impact of sexual abuse: Implications for drug treatment. *Journal of Women's Health, 1*(2), 149–153.

Patterson, G. R. (1982). *Coercive family process: A social learning approach.* (Vol. 3). Eugene, OR: Castalia.

Patterson, G. R., Chamberlain, P., & Reid, J. B. (1982). A comparative evaluation of a parent training program. *Behavior Therapy, 13*, 638–650.

Patterson, J. (1994). *America's struggle against poverty 1900–1994.* Cambridge, MA: Harvard University Press.

Patti, R. J., Poertner, J., & Rapp, C. A. (1987). *Managing for service effectiveness in social welfare organizations.* New York: Haworth Press.

Peele, S. (1989). *The diseasing of America: How the addiction industry captured our soul.* Cambridge, MA: Lexington.

Pegeron, J. P., Curtis, G. C., & Thyer, B. A. (1986). Simple phobia leading to suicide: A case report [letter]. *The Behavior Therapist, 9*, 134–145.

Pence, E., & Paymar, M. (1993). *Education groups for men who batter: The Duluth model.* New York: Springer.

Pendleton, B. F., Poloma, M. M., & Garland, T. N. (1980). *Scales for the investigation of the dual-career family. Journal of Marriage and the Family, 42*, 269–275.

Penka, C. E., & Kirk, S. A. (1991). Practitioner involvement in clinical evaluation. *Social Work, 36*, 513–518.

Penn, D. L., & Meuser, K. T. (1996). Research update on the psychosocial treatment of schizophrenia. *American Journal of Psychiatry, 153*, 607–617.

Pentz, M. A. (1985). Social competence skills and self-efficacy as determinants of substance use in adolescence. In S. Shiffman & T. A. Wills (Eds.), *Coping and substance use.* New York: Academic Press.

Perlman, H. H. (1965). Self-determination: Reality or illusion? *Social Service Review, 39*(4), 410–421.

Perlman, H. H. (1976). Believing and doing: Values in social work education. *Social Casework, 57,* 381–390.

Perry, J. C., & Klerman, G. (1980). Clinical features of the borderline personality disorder. *American Journal of Psychiatry, 137,* 165–173.

Pfeiffer, E. (1978). *Multidimensional functional assessment: The OARS methodology.* Durham, NC: Duke University Center for the Study of Aging and Human Development.

Phillips, E., Phillips, W., Fixsen, D., & Wolf, M. (1974). *The teaching-family handbook. Lawrence, KS: University of Kansas Press.*

Phillips, D. C. (1990). Postpositivistic science. In E. G. Guba (Ed.), *The paradigm dialog.* Newbury Park, CA: Sage Publications.

Phinney, J. S. (1992). The Multigroup Ethnic Identity Measure: A new scale for use with diverse groups. *Journal of Adolescent Research, 7,* 156–176.

Piaget, J. (1953). *The psychology of intelligence.* New Haven, CT: Yale University Press.

Pierce, R., & Drasgow, J. (1969). Teaching facilitative interpersonal functioning to psychiatric inpatients. *Journal of Counseling Psychology, 16,* 295–298.

Pikoff, H. B. (1996). *Treatment effectiveness handbook: A reference guide to the key research reviews in mental health and substance abuse.* Buffalo, NY: Data for Decisions.

Pinkston, E. M. (1994). Behavior-management training for caregivers of patients with dementia. *Seminars in Research and Language, 15,* 280–290.

Pinkston, E. M. (1997). A supportive environment for old age. In D. M. Baer & E. M. Pinkston (Eds.), *Environment and behavior* (pp. 258–268). Boulder, CO: Westview Press.

Pinkston, E. M., Howe, E. M., & Blackman, D. K. (1987). Medical social work management of urinary incontinence in the elderly: A behavioral approach. *Journal of Social Service Research, 10,* 179–194.

Pinkston, E. M., Levitt, J. L., Green, G. R., Linsk, N. L., & Rzepnicki, T. L. (1982). *Effective social work practice: Advanced techniques for behavioral intervention with individuals, families, and institutional staff.* San Francisco, CA: Jossey-Bass.

Pinkston, E. M., & Linsk, N. L. (1984a). *Care of the elderly: A family approach.* New York: Pergamon Press.

Pinkston, E. M., & Linsk, N. L. (1984b). Behavioral family intervention with the impaired elderly. *The Gerontologist, 24,* 576–583.

Pinkston, E. M., Linsk, N. L., & Young, R. N. (1988). Home-based behavioral family treatment of the impaired elderly. *Behavior Therapy, 19,* 331–344.

Plant, R. (1970). *Social and moral theory in casework.* London: Routledge & Kegan Paul.

Pleck, J. H. (1997). Father involvement: Levels, origins, and consequences. In M. E. Lamb (Ed.), *The father's role* (3rd ed., pp. 66–103). New York: Wiley.

Polich, J. M., Armor, D. M., & Braiker, H. B. (1981). *The course of alcoholism: Four years after treatment.* New York: Wiley.

Pollatsek, J. (1994). Grief, multiple loss, and burnout: Care for the care giver. *Leaders' guide.*

Poole, D. (1997). Building community capacity to promote social and public health: Challenges for universities. *Health and Social Work, 22,* 163–170.

Pope, K. S. (1988). How clients are harmed by sexual contact with mental health professionals: The syndrome and its prevalence. *Journal of Counseling and Development, 67,* 222–226.

Porterfield, J., Evans, G., & Blunden, R. (1985). Involving families in service improvement. *Journal of Organizational Behavior Management, 7*(1/2), 117–133.

Premack, D. (1959). Toward empirical behavior laws: Part 1: Positive reinforcement. *Psychological Review, 66,* 219–233.

Pumphrey, M. W. (1959). *The teaching of values and ethics in social work.* (Vol. 13). New York: Council on Social Work Education.

Quayle, J. D. (1983). American productivity: The devastating effect of alcoholism and drug abuse. *American Psychologist, 38,* 454–458.

Radloff, L. S. (1977). The CES-D Scale: A self-report depression scale for research in the general population. *Applied Psychological Measurement, 1,* 385–401.

Raine. (1989, April 1). Black American faces AIDS. *San Francisco Examiner.*

Raulin, M. L. (1984). Development of a scale to measure intense ambivalence. *Journal of Consulting and Clinical Psychology, 52,* 63–72.

Reamer, F. G. (1982). *Ethical dilemmas in social service.* New York: Columbia University Press.

Reamer, F. G. (1983). The concept of paternalism in social work. *Social Service Review, 57*(2), 254–271.

Reamer, F. G. (1987a). Values and ethics. In A. Minahan (Ed.), *Encyclopedia of social work* (18th ed., Vol. 2, pp. 801–809). Silver Spring, MD: National Association of Social Workers.

Reamer, F. G. (1987b). Informed consent in social work. *Social Work, 32*(5), 425–429.

Reamer, F. G. (1990). *Ethical dilemmas in social service.* (2nd ed.). New York: Columbia University Press.

Reamer, F. G. (1992a). The impaired social worker. *Social Work, 37*(2), 165–170.

Reamer, F. G. (1992b). Social work and the public good: Calling or career? In P. N. Reid & P. R. Popple (Eds.), *The moral purposes of social work* (pp. 11–33). Chicago: Nelson-Hall.

Reamer, F. G. (1994). *Social work malpractice and liability.* New York: Columbia University Press.

Reamer, F. G. (1995a). *Social work values and ethics.* New York: Columbia University Press.

Reamer, F. G. (1995b). Ethics and values. In R. L. Edwards (Ed.), *Encyclopedia of social work* (19th ed., Vol. 1, pp. 893–902). Washington, DC: NASW Press.

Reamer, F. G. (1995c). Ethics consultation in social work. *Social Thought, 18*(1), 3–16.

Reamer, F. G. (1997a). Ethical standards in social work: The NASW Code of Ethics. In R. L. Edwards (Ed.), *Encyclopedia of social work* (19th ed., Vol. Supp., pp. 113–123). Washington, DC: NASW Press.

Reamer, F. G. (1997b). Managing ethics under managed care. *Families in Society, 78,* 96–101.

Reamer, F. G. (1997c). Ethical issues for social work practice. In M. Reisch & E. Gambrill (Eds.), *Social work in the 21st century* (pp. 340–349). Thousand Oaks, CA: Pine Forge Press.

Reamer, F. G. (1998a). *Ethical standards in social work: A critical review of the NASW Code of Ethics.* (Vol. NASW Press). Washington, DC.

Reamer, F. G. (1998b). Social work. In R. Chadwick (Ed.), *Encyclopedia of applied ethics* (Vol. 4, pp. 169–180). San Diego, CA: Academic Press.

Reamer, F. G. (1998c). The evolution of social work ethics. *Social Work, 43,* 488–500.

Reamer, F. G. (1998d). Managed care: Ethical considerations. In G. Schamess & A. Lightburn (Eds.), *Humane managed care?* Washington, DC: NASW Press (pp. 293–298).

Reamer, F. G. (1999). *Social work values and ethics.* (2nd ed.). New York: Columbia University Press.

Reamer, F. G. (2000). Ethical issues in direct practice. In P. Allen-Meares & C. Garvin (Eds.), *Handbook of direct practice in social work.* Thousand Oaks, CA: Sage Publications.

Reamer, F. G. (2001a). *Tangled relationships: Managing boundary issues in the human services.* New York: Columbia University Press.

Reamer, F. G. (2001b). *Ethics education in social work.* Alexandria, VA: Council on Social Work Education.

Reamer, R. G., & Abramson, M. (1982). *The teaching of social work ethics.* Hastings-on-Hudson, NY: The Hastings Center.

Reamer, F. G., & Siegel, D. H. (1992). Should social workers blow the whistle on incompetent colleagues? In E. Gambrill & R. Pruger (Eds.), *Controversial issues in social work* (pp. 66–78). Boston, MA: Allyn & Bacon.

Redmon, W. K., & Wilks, L. A. (1991). Organizational behavioral analysis in the United States: Public sector organizations. In P. A. Lamal (Ed.), *Behavioral analysis of societies and cultural practices* (pp. 107–123). Washington, DC: Hemisphere.

Regehr, C., & Antle, B. (1997). Coercive influences: Informed consent in court-mandated social work practice. *Social Work, 42*(3), 300–306.

Reid, P. N., & Popple, P. (Eds.). (1992). *The moral purposes of social work.* Chicago: Nelson-Hall.

Reid, W. J. (1978). *The task-centered system.* New York: Columbia University Press.

Reid, W. J. (1979). The model development dissertation. *Journal of Social Research, 3,* 215–225.

Reid, W. J. (1985). *Family problem solving.* New York: Columbia University Press.

Reid, W. J. (1987). Service effectiveness and the social agency. In R. J. Patti, J. Poertner, & C. A. Rapp (Eds.), *Managing for service effectiveness in social welfare organizations* (pp. 41–58). New York: The Haworth Press.

Reid, W. J. (1992). *Task strategies.* New York: Columbia University Press.

Reid, W. J. (1993). Fitting the single-system design to family treatment. *Journal of Social Service Research, 18,* 83–99.

Reid, W. J. (1994). Reframing the epistemological debate. In E. Sherman & W. J. Reid (Eds.), *Qualitative research in social work.* New York: Columbia University Press.

Reid, W. J. (1997). Evaluating the dodo's verdict: Do all interventions have equivalent outcomes? *Social Work Research, 21,* 5–18.

Reid, W. J., & Fortune, A. E. (1992). Research utilization in direct social work practice. In T. Grasso & E. Epstein (Eds.), *Research utilization in social work.* New York: Haworth Press.

Reid, W. J., & Hanrahan, P. (1982). Recent evaluations of social work: Grounds for optimism. *Social Work, 27,* 328–340.

Reid, W. J., & Zettergren, P. (in press). *A perspective on empirical practice.* In I. Shaw & J. Lishman (Eds.). Thousand Oaks, CA: Sage Publications.

Resnick, H. (1978). Tasks in changing the organization from within (COFW). *Administration in Social Work, 2*(1), 29–42.

Resnick, M. D., Bearman, P. S., & Blum, R. W. (1997). Protecting adolescents from harm: Findings from the National Longitudinal Study on Adolescent Health. *Journal of the American Medical Association, 128–142.*

Reynolds, B. C. (1982/1934). *Between client and community.* Washington, DC: NASW Press.

Reynolds, M. M. (1976). Threats to confidentiality. *Social Work, 21,* 108–113.

Rhodes, M. (1986). *Ethical dilemmas in social work practice.* London: Routledge & Kegan Paul.

Rice, F. P. (1999). *Intimate relationships, marriages, and families.* Mountain View, CA: Mayfield Publishing.

Rich, R. F. (1977). Uses of social science information by federal bureaucrats: Knowledge for action versus knowledge for understanding. In C. H. Weiss (Ed.), *Using social research in public policy making* (pp. 115–128). Lexington, MA: Lexington Books.

Richan, W. C. (1996). *Lobbying for social change.* (2nd ed.). New York: Haworth Press.

Richardson, F. C., & Suinn, R. M. (1972). The Mathematics Anxiety Rating Scale. *Journal of Counseling Psychology, 19,* 551–554.

Richey, C. A., Blythe, B. J., & Berlin, S. B. (1987). Do social workers evaluate their practice? *Social Work Research & Abstracts, 23,* 14–20.

Richman, E. (1982). A comprehensive skills program for job finding with hardcore unemployed. In R. O'Brien (Ed.), *Industrial behavior modification.* New York: Pergamon.

Richmond, M. (1917). *Social diagnosis.* New York: Russell Sage Foundation.

Ridley, T. D., & Kordinak, S. T. (1988). Reliability and validity of the Quantitative Inventory of Alcohol Disorders (QIAD) and the veracity of self-report by alcoholics. *American Journal of Drug and Alcohol Abuse, 14,* 263–292.

Rife, J., & Belcher, J. (1994). Assisting unemployed older workers become re-employed: An experimental evaluation. *Research on Social Work Practice, 4,* 3–13.

Riley, K. C. (1988). Measurement of dissociation. *Journal of Nervous and Mental Disease, 176,* 449–450.

Rinsley, D. B. (1971). The adolescent inpatient: Patterns of depersonification. *Psychoanalytic Quarterly, 45,* 3–22.

Rivera, F., Sweeney, P., & Henderson, B. (1987). Risk of fatherhood among Black teenage males. *American Journal of Public Health, 77,* 203–205.

Rivera, F., Sweeney, P., & Henderson, B. (1996). Black teenage fathers: What happens when the child is born. *Pediatrics, 78,* 151–158.

Rivera, P., Rose, J., Futterman, A., Lovett, S., & Gallagher-Thompson, D. (1991). *Psychology and Aging, 6*(2), 232–237.

Robin, A. L. (1982). A controlled evaluation of problem-solving communication training with parent-adolescent conflict. *Behavior Therapy, 12,* 593–609.

Robins, L. E., & Regier, D. A. (1991). *Psychiatric disorders in America.* New York: Free Press.

Robins, L. N., et al. (1984). Lifetime prevalence of specific psychiatric disorders in three sites. *Archives of General Psychiatry, 41,* 949–958.

Robinson, J. P., & Shaver, P. R. (1973). *Measures of social psychological attitudes.* (revised ed.). Ann Arbor, MI: Institute for Social Research.

Rooney, R. H. (1992). *Strategies for work with involuntary clients.* New York: Columbia University Press.

Rooney, R. H., & Bibus, A. A. (1996). Multiple lenses: Ethnically sensitive practice with involuntary clients who are having difficulties with drugs or alcohol. *Journal of Multicultural Social Work, 4*(2), 59–73.

Rorty, R. (1979). *Philosophy and the mirror of nature.* Princeton, NJ: Princeton University Press.

Rose, S. D., & Edelson, J. L. (1987). *Working with children and adolescents in groups.* San Fransisco, CA: Jossey-Bass.

Rosen, A., & Proctor, E. K. (1978). Specifying the treatment process: The basis for effectiveness. *Journal of Social Service Research, 2,* 25–26.

Rosenfarb, I., Becker, J., & Khan, A. (1994). Perceptions of parental and peer attachments by women with mood disorders. *Journal of Abnormal Psychology, 103*(4), 637–644.

Rosica, T. C. (1995). AIDS and boundaries. *Focus: A Guide to AIDS Research and Counseling, 10*(2), 1–4.

Ross, E. C., & Croze, C. (1997). Mental health service delivery in the age of managed care. In T. R. Watkins & J. W. Callicutt (Eds.), *Mental health policy and practice today* (pp. 346–361). Thousand Oaks, CA: Sage Publications.

Ross, R. (1996). *Returning to the teachings: Exploring aboriginal justice.* Toronto, Canada: Penguin Books Canada.

Rossiter, A., de Boer, C., Narayan, J., Razack, N., Scollay, V., & Willette, C. (1998). Toward an alternative account of feminist practice ethics in mental health. *Affilia, 13*(1), 9–30.

Roth, A., & Foragy, P. (1996). *What works for whom? A critical review of psychotherapy research.* New York: Guilford Press.

Rotheram-Borus, M. J., & Tsemberis, S. J. (1989). Social competency training programs in ethnically diverse communities. In L. S. Bond & B. E. Compas (Eds.), *Primary prevention and promotion in the schools.* Newbury Park, CA: Sage.

Rothery, M. A. (1980). Contracts and contracting. *Clinical Social Work Journal, 8,* 179–187.

Rothman, J. (1989). Client self-determination: Untangling the knot. *Social Service Review, 63*(4), 598–612.

Rothman, J., Smith, W., Nashima, J., Paterson, M. A., & Mustin, J. (1996). Client self-determination and professional intervention: Striking a balance. *Social Work, 41*(4), 396–405.

Rothman, J., & Thomas, E. J. (Eds.). (1994). *Intervention research: Design and development for human service.* New York: The Haworth Press.

Rothman, J., & Thyer, B. A. (1984). Behavioral social work in community and organizational settings. *Journal of Sociology and Social Welfare, 11,* 294–326.

Roy-Byrne, P., & Cowley, D. (1998). Pharmacological treatment of panic, generalized anxiety, and phobic disorders. In P. Nathan & J. Gorman (Eds.), *A guide to treatments that work* (pp. 319–338). New York: Oxford University Press.

Royse, D., & Thyer, B. A. (1996). *Program evaluation: An introduction.* Chicago: Nelson-Hall.

Rubin, A. (1985). Practice effectiveness: More grounds for optimism. *Social Work, 30,* 469–476.

Rubin, A., & Knox, K. S. (1996). Data analysis problems in single-case evaluation: Issues for research on social work practice. *Research on Social Work Practice, 6*(1), 40–65.

Ruble, D., Greulich, F., Pomerantz, E., & Gochberg, B. (1993). The role of gender-related processes in the development of sex. *Journal of Affective Disorders, 29*(2–3), 97–128.

Rzepnicki, T. L. (1991). Enhancing the durability of intervention gains: A challenge for the 1990s. *Social Service Review, 65*(1), 92–111.

Sackett, D. L., Robinson, W. S., Rosenberg, W., & Haynes, R. B. (1997). *Evidence-based medicine: How to practice and teach EBM.* London: Churchill-Livingstone.

Saenz, J. (1978). The value of a humanistic model in serving families. In M. Monteil (Ed.), *Hispanic families.* Washington, DC: COSSMHO.

Safren, S. A., Turk, C. L., & Heimberg, R. G. (1998). Factor structure of the Social Interaction Anxiety Scale and the Social Phobia Scale. *Behaviour Research and Therapy, 36,* 443–453.

Saleeby, D. (1997). *The strengths perspective in social work practice.* (2nd ed.). New York: Longman.

Salter, W., & Johnson, W. (1997). *Paternal involvement among poor, nonresident fathers: National concern, local solution.* Paper presented at the Social Service Administration's Friends' Luncheon.

Saltzman, A., & Proch, K. (1990). *Law in social work practice.* Chicago: Nelson-Hall.

Sands, R., & Nuccio, K. (1992). Postmodern feminist theory and social work. *Social Work, 37*(6), 489–494.

Santrock, J. W. (1996). *Adolescence.* Madison, WI: Brown & Benchmark.

Saulnier, C. (1996). *Feminist theories and social work practice.* Chicago: Haworth Press.

Saxton, W. (1979). Behavioral contracting. *Child Welfare, 63,* 523–529.

Schaef, A. W. (1987). *When society becomes an addict.* San Francisco, CA: Harper & Row.

Schafer, W. (1996). *Stress management for wellness.* Fort Worth, TX: Harcourt Brace Jovanovich.

Schamess, G., & Lightburn, A. (Eds.). (1998). *Humane managed care?* Washington, DC: NASW Press.

Schare, M. L., & Milburn, N. G. (1996). Multicultural assessment of alcohol and other drug use. In L. A. Suzuki (Ed.), *Handbook of multicultural assessment* (pp. 453–473). San Francisco, CA: Jossey-Bass.

Schatz, B., & O'Hanlan, K. (1994). *Anti-gay discrimination in medicine.* San Francisco, CA: American Association of Physicians for Human Rights.

Scheid-Cook, T. L. (1993). Controllers and controlled: An analysis of participant constructions of outpatient commitment. *Sociology of Health and Illness, 15*(2), 179–198.

Schinke, S. P., Blythe, B. J., & Gilchrist, L. D. (1981). Cognitive behavioral prevention of adolescent pregnancy. *Journal of Counseling Psychology, 28,* 451–454.

Schlesinger, S. E. (1988). Cognitive-behavioral approaches to family treatment of addictions. In N. Epstein, S. E. Schlesinger, & W. Dryden (Eds.), *Cognitive behavioral therapy with families.* New York: Brunner/Mazel.

Schnelle, J., Kirchner, R., MaCrae, J., McNees, M., Eck, R., Snodgrass, S., Casey, J., & Uselton, P. (1978). Police evolution research: An experimental and cost-benefit analysis of a helicopter patrol in a high crime area. *Journal of Applied Behavior Analysis 11,* 11–21.

Schreter, R. K., Sharfstein, S. S., & Schreter, C. A. (Eds.). (1994). *Allies and adversaries: The impact of managed care on mental health services.* Washington, DC: American Psychiatric Press.

Schrumpf, F., Crawford, D., & Usadel, H. C. (1991). *Peer mediation: Conflict resolution in the schools.* Champaign, IL: Research Press.

Schuerman, J. R. (1982). Debate with authors: The scientific imperative in social work research. *Social Service Review, 56,* 144–146.

Schultz, B. M. (1982). *Legal liability in psychotherapy.* San Francisco, CA: Jossey-Bass.

Schutte, N. S., & Malouff, J. M. (1995). *Sourcebook of adult assessment strategies.* New York: Plenum.

Schwartz, E. B., & Waetjen, W. B. (1976). Improving the self-concept of women managers. *Business Quarterly, 41*(4), 20–27.

Scopetta, M. A., & Alegre, C. (1975). *Clinical issues in psychotherapy research with Latins.* Paper presented at the Third National Drug Abuse Conference, New Orleans, LA.

Segal, R., & Sisson, B. V. (1985). Medical complications associated with alcohol use and the assessment of risk of physical damage. In T. E. Bratter & G. G. Forrest (Eds.), *Alcoholism and substance abuse* (pp. 137–175). New York: Free Press.

Sekaran, U. (1986). *Dual-career families.* San Francisco, CA: Jossey-Bass.

Seligman, L. (1998). *Selecting effective treatments: A comprehensive guide to treating mental disorders.* San Francisco, CA: Jossey-Bass.

Senna, J. J. (1974). Changes in due process of law. *Social Work, 19,* 319–324.

Shadish, W., Matt, G., Navarro, A., Siegle, G., Crits-Christoph, P., Hazelrigg, M., Jorm, A., Lyons, L., Nietzel, M., Prout, H., Robinson, L., Smith, M., Svartberg, M., & Weiss, B. (1997). Evidence that therapy works in clinically representative conditions. *Journal of Consulting and Clinical Psychology, 65,* 355–365.

Shaffer, H., & Kauffman, J. (1985). The clinical assessment and diagnosis of addiction: Hypothesis testing. In T. E. Bratter & G. G. Forrest (Eds.), *Alcoholism and substance abuse* (pp. 225–258). New York: Free Press.

Shapiro, M. B., & Zifferblatt, S. M. (1976). Zen meditation and behavioral self-control: Similarities, differences, and clinical applications. *American Psychologist, 31,* 519–532.

Shapiro, T. (1989). Psychoanalytic classification and empiricism with borderline personality disorder as a model. *Journal of Consulting and Clinical Psychology, 57,* 187–194.

Sharp, T., Brown, M., & Crider, K. (1995). The effects of a sportmanship curriculum intervention on generalized positive social behavior of urban elementary school students. *Journal of Applied Behavior Analysis, 28,* 401–416.

Sheafor, B., Horejsi, C., & Horejsi, G. (1988). *Techniques and guidelines for social work practice.* Boston, MA: Allyn and Bacon.

Sheafor, B., Horejsi, C., & Horejsi, G. (1997). *Techniques and guidelines for social work practice.* Boston, MA: Allyn and Bacon.

Sheehy, M., Goldsmith, L., & Charles, E. (1980). A comparative study of borderline patients in a psychiatric out-patient clinic. *American Journal of Psychiatry, 137,* 1374–1379.

Shelby, R. D. (1992). *If a partner has AIDS.* New York: Harrington Press.

Shelton, J. L., & Levy, R. L. (1981). *Behavioral assignments and treatment compliance.* Champaign, IL: Research Press.

Sherman, W. R., & Wenocor, S. (1983). Empowering public welfare workers through mutual support. *Social Work, 28,* 375–379.

Sidman, M. (1989). *Coercion and its fallout.* Boston, MA: Authors Cooperative.

Sidman, M. (1993). Reflections on behavior and analysis and coercion. *Behavior and Social Issues, 3*(1/2), 75–85.

Siegel, D. (1984). Defining empirically based practice. *Social Work, 29,* 325–331.

Silko, L. M. (1996). *Yellow woman and a beauty of the Spirit.* New York: Simon and Schuster.

Silver, D. (1985). Psychodynamics and psychotherapeutic management of self-destructive character disordered patients. *Psychiatric Clinics of North America, 8,* 357–375.

Silverman, W. K., & Nelles, W. B. (1988). The Anxiety Disorders Interview Schedule for Children. *Journal of the American Academy of Child and Adolescent Psychiatry, 27,* 772–778.

Simkin, J. S., & Yontef, G. M. (1984). Gestalt therapy. In R. Corsini (Ed.), *Current psychotherapies.* Itasca, IL: Peacock.

Simons, R. L., & Aigner, S. M. (1985). *Practice principles: A problem-solving approach to social work.* New York: Macmillan.

Siporin, M. (1975). *Introduction to social work practice.* New York: Macmillan.

Siporin, M. (1992). Strengthening the moral mission of social work. In P. N. Reid & P. R. Popple (Eds.), *The moral purposes of social work* (pp. 71–99). Chicago: Nelson-Hall.

Sisson, R. W., & Azrin, N. H. (1986). Family member involvement to initiate and promote treatment of problem drinkers. *Journal of Behavior Therapy and Experimental Psychiatry, 17,* 15–21.

Skeel, J. D., & Self, D. J. (1989). An analysis of ethics consultation in the clinical setting. *Theoretical Medicine, 10,* 289–299.

Skinner, B. F. (1981). Selection by consequences. *Science, 213,* 501–504.

Skinner, H. A. (1982). The drug abuse screening test. *Addictive Behaviors, 7,* 363–371.

Slonim-Nevo, & Anson. (1998). *Research in Social Work, 22,* 66–74.

Slot, N., van Bilsen, H., & Kendall, P. (1995). Competency based treatment for antisocial youth. In H. V. Bilsen (Ed.), *Behavioral approaches for children and adolescents* (pp. 77–86). New York: Plenum.

Smart, J. J. C., & Williams, B. (1973). *Utilitarianism, for and against.* Cambridge, England: Cambridge University Press.

Smith, A., & Reid, W. (1986). *Role-sharing marriage.* New York: Columbia University Press.

Smith, C., Lizziotte, A. J., Thornberry, T. P., & Krohn, M. D. (1995). *Resilient youth: Identifying factors that prevent high risk youth from engaging in delinquency and drug use. 4,* 217–247.

Smith, E. M. (1993). Race or racism? Addiction in the United States. *Annals of Epidemiology, 3,* 165–170.

Smith, J., & Meyers, R. (1995). The community reinforcement approach. In R. Hester & W. Miller (Eds.), *Handbook of alcoholism treatment approaches* (2nd ed., pp. 251 266) Boston, MA: Allyn & Bacon.

Smith, J., Meyers, R., & Delaney, H. (1998). The community reinforcement approach with homeless alcohol-dependent individuals. *Journal of Consulting and Clinical Psychology, 66,* 541–548.

Sobell, L. C., Sobell, M. B., & Nirenberg, T. D. (1988). Behavioral assessment and treatment planning with alcohol and drug abusers: A review with an emphasis on clinical application. *Clinical Psychology Review, 8,* 19–54.

Sobell, M. B., & Sobell, L. C. (1993). *Problem drinkers: Guided self-change treatment.* New York: Guilford.

Social Casework. (1989). *Social Casework, 70*(6), Entire issue.

Soloff, T. H. (1981). Concurrent validation of a diagnostic interview for borderline patients. *American Journal of Psychiatry, 138*(691–693).

Solomon, P., & Draine, J. (1995). One-year outcomes of a randomized trial of case management with seriously mentally ill clients leaving jail. *Evaluation Review, 19,* 256–273.

Specht, H., & Courtney, M. (1994). *Unfaithful angels: How social work has abandoned* its *mission.* New York: Free Press.

Spielberger, C. D. (1977). *The Test Anxiety Inventory.* Palo Alto, CA: Consulting Psychologists Press.

Spielberger, C. D., Jacobson, A., Russell, S., & Crane, R. S. (1983). Assessment of anger: The State Trait Anger–Scale. In J. N. Butcher & C. D. Spielberger (Eds.), *Advances in personality assessment* (Vol. 2). Hillsdale, NJ: Lawrence Erlbaum.

Sprock, J., Blashfield, R., & Smith, B. (1990). Gender weighting of DSM-III-R personality disorder criteria. *American Journal of Psychiatry, 147,* 586–590.

Staab, S., & Lodish, D. (1985). Reducing joblessness among disadvantaged youth. In L. D. Gilchrist & S. P. Schinke (Eds.), *Preventing social and health problems through life skills training.* Seattle, WA: Center for social Welfare Research, University of Washington.

Stalley, R. F. (1975). Determinism and the principle of client self-determination. In F. E. McDermott (Ed.), *Self-determination in social work* (pp. 93). London: Routledge and Kegan Paul.

Stangl, D., Pfhol, B., Zimmerman, M., Bowers, W., & Corenthal, C. (1985). A structural interview for the DSM-III personality disorders. *Archives of General Psychiatry, 42*(591–596).

Stanley, J., & Goddard, C. (1993). The association between child abuse and other family violence. *Australian Social Work, 46*(2), 3–8.

Steketee, G. S. (1987). Behavioral social work with obsessive compulsive disorders. *Journal of Social Service Research, 10*(2/3/4), 53–72.

Stidham, H., & Remley, T. (1992). Job club methodology applied to a work fare setting. *Journal of Employment Counseling, 29,* 69–76.

Stine, G. (1998). AIDS and society: Knowledge, attitudes and behavior. *AIDS update: 1998.* Upper Saddle River, NJ: Prentice Hall.

Stitzer, M. L., Bigelow, G. E., & McCaul, M. E. (1983). Behavioral approaches to drug abuse. In M. Hersen (Ed.), *Progress in behavior modification* (Vol. 14,). New York: Academic Press.

Stouthard, M., Hoogstraten, J., & Mellenbergh, G. (1995). A study on the convergent and discriminant validity of the Dental Anxiety Inventory. *Behaviour Research and Therapy 33,* 589–595.

Strayhorn, J., Jr. (1977). *Talking it out: A guide to effective communication and problem-solving.* Champaign, IL: Research Press.

Strick, A. (1996). *Injustice for all: How our legal system betrays us.* New York: Barricade Books.

Strom-Gottfried, K., & Corcoran, K. (1998). Confronting ethical dilemmas in managed care: Guidelines for students and faculty. *Journal of Social Work Education, 34,* 109–119.

Stuart, R. B. (1980). *Helping couples change: A social learning approach to marital therapy.* New York: Guilford.

Suarez, Z., Lewis, E., & Clark, J. (1995). In N. Van Den Bergh (Ed.), *Feminist practice in the 21st century.* Washington, DC: NASW Press.

Sullivan, M. (1985). *Teen fathers in the inner city: An exploratory ethnographic study.* A report to the Ford Foundation, Urban Poverty Program.

Sullivan, M. (1986). *Ethnographic research on young Black fathers and parenting: Implications for public policy.* New York: Vera Institute of Justice.

Summers, A. B. (1989). The meaning of informed consent in social work. *Social Thought, 15*(3/4), 128–140.

Sweetland, R. C., & Keyser, D. J. (1983). *Tests: A comprehensive reference.* Kansas City, MO: Test Corporation of America.

Swigonski, M. (1993). Feminist standpoint theory and the questions of social work research. *Affilia, 8*(2), 171–183.

Swigonski, M. (1994). The logic of feminist standpoint theory for social work research. *Social Work, 39*(4), 387–393.

Szapocznik, J., & Kurtines, W. (1980). Acculturation, biculturalism, and adjustment among Cuban Americans. In A. Padilla (Ed.), *Psychological dimensions on the acculturation process: Theories, models, and some new findings.* Boulder, CO: Westview Press.

Szapocznik, J., Santiesteban, D., Kurtines, W., Perez-Vidal, A., & Hervis, O. (1984). Bicultural effectiveness training: A treatment intervention for enhancing intercultural adjustment in Cuban American families. *Hispanic Journal of Behavioral Sciences, 6*(4), 317–344.

Szapocznik, J., & Truss, C. (1978). Intergenerational sources of conflict in Cuban mothers. In M. Montiel (Ed.), *Hispanic families.* Washington, DC: COSSMHO.

Tarasoff v. Board of Regents of the University of California, C. d., 529 P. 2d 553 (1974), 17 Cal. 3d 425 (1976), 131 Cal. Rptr. 14. (1976).

Tarnopolsky, A., & Berelowitz, M. (1987). Borderline personality: A review of recent research. *British Journal of Psychiatry, 151,* 724–734.

Taylor, D., Barry, P., & Block, C. (1958). Does group participation when using brainstorming facilitate or inhibit creative thinking? *Administrative Science Quarterly, 3,* 23–47.

Taylor, J., & Jackson, B. (1990). Factors affecting alcohol consumption in black women. *International Journal of the Addictions, 25*(11), 1287–1300.

Taylor, J., & Jackson, B. (1991). A holistic model for understanding and predicting depressive symptoms in African American women. *Journal of Community Psychology, 19,* 306–321.

Taylor, S. (1996). Meta analysis of cognitive-behavioral treatment for social phobia. *Journal of Behavior Therapy and Experimental Psychiatry, 27,* 1–9.

Teel, K. (1975). The physician's dilemma: A doctor's view: What the law should be. *Baylor Law Review, 27,* 6–9.

Teicher, M. (1967). *Values in social work: A re-examination.* New York: National Association of Social Workers.

Test, M. A. (1998). Community-based treatment models for adults with severe and persistent mental illness. In J. B. W. Williams & K. Ell (Eds.), *Advances in mental health research: Implications for practice.* Washington, DC: NASW Press.

Tetenbaum, T. J., Lighter, J., & Travis, M. (1981). Educator's attitudes toward worker mothers. *Journal of Educational Psychology, 73,* 369–375.

Thibaut, J. W., & Kelly, H. H. (1959). *The social psychology of groups.* New York: Wiley.

Thomas, E. J. (Ed.). (1967). *The socio-behavioral approach and applications to social work.* New York: Council on Social Work Education.

Thomas, E. J. (1987). Design and development in organization innovation. In R. J. Patti, J. Poertner, & C. A. Rapp (Eds.), *Managing for service effectiveness in social welfare organizations.* New York: The Haworth Press.

Thomas, E. J., Santa, C., Bronson, D., & Oyserman, D. (1987). Unilateral family therapy with the spouses of alcoholics. *Journal of Social Service Research, 10*(2/3/4), 145–162.

Thomas, E. J., & Yoshioka, M. R. (1989). Spouse interventive confrontation in unilateral family therapy for alcohol abuse. *Social Casework, 70,* 340–347.

Thomas, N., & O'Kane, C. (1998). *Children and decision making: A summary report.* University of Wales Swansea: International Centre for Childhood Studies.

Thompson, C. E., & Carter, R. T. (1997). Race, socialization, and contemporary racism manifestations. In C. E. Thompson & R. T. Carter (Eds.), *Race identity theory: Applications to individual, group, and organizational interventions* (pp. 1–14). Mahwah, NJ: Lawrence Erlbaum.

Thompson, M., & Heller, K. (1990). Facets of support related to well being: Quantitative social isolation and perceived family support in a sample of elderly women. *Psychology and Aging, 5*(4), 535–544.

Thompson, R., Smith, G., Osgood, D., Dowd, T., Friman, P., & Daly, D. (1996). Residential care: A study of short- and long-term educational effects. *Children and Youth Services Review, 18,* 139–162.

Thyer, B. A. (1981). Prolonged in-vivo exposure therapy with a 70-year-old woman. *Journal of Behavior Therapy and Experimental Psychiatry, 12,* 69–71.

Thyer, B. A. (1987). *Treating anxiety disorders: Guidelines for human service professionals.* Newbury Park, CA: Sage.

Thyer, B. A. (1992). Should all social workers be well trained in behavioral principles? In E. Gambrill & R. Pruger (Eds.), *Controversial issues in social work* (pp. 79–84). Boston, MA: Allyn & Bacon.

Thyer, B. A. (1995). Promoting an empiricist agenda in the human services: An ethical and humanistic imperative. *Journal of Behavior Therapy and Experimental Psychiatry, 26,* 93–98.

Thyer, B. A. (1998). Promoting research on community practice: Using single-system research designs. In R. H. MacNair (Ed.), *Research strategies for community practice.* Binghamton, NY: Haworth Press.

Thyer, B. A., Baum, M., & Reid, L. D. (1988). Exposure techniques in the reduction of fear: A comparative review of the procedure in animals and humans. *Advances in Behavior Research and Therapy, 10,* 105–127.

Thyer, B. A., & Curtis, G. C. (1983). The repeated pretest-post-test single subject experiment: A new design for empirical clinical practice. *Journal of Behavior Therapy and Experimental Psychiatry, 14,* 311–315.

Thyer, B. A., & Himle, J. (1987). Phobic anxiety and panic anxiety: How do they differ? *Journal of Anxiety Disorders, 1,* 59–67.

Thyer, B. A., Himle, J., & Santa, C. (1986). Applied behavior analysis in social and community action: A bibliography. *Behavior Analysis and Social Action, 5,* 14–16.

Thyer, B. A., & Larkin, R. (1998). Promoting community through group work: Developing a research agenda. *Journal for Specialists in Group Work, 23,* 454–459.

Thyer, B. A., Papsdorf, J. D., Davis, R., & Vallecorsa, S. (1984). Autonomic correlates of the Clinical Anxiety Scale. *Journal of Behavior Therapy and Experimental Psychiatry, 15,* 3–7.

Thyer, B.A., Parrish, R.T., Himle, J., Cameron, O. G., Curtis, G. C., & Nessi, R. (1986). Alcohol abuse among clinically anxious patients. *Behavior Research and Therapy, 24,* 357–359.

Thyer, B. A., & Stocks, J. T. (1986). Exposure therapy in the treatment of phobic blind persons. *Journal of Visual Impairment and Blindness, 80,* 1001–1003.

Thyer, B. A., & Wodarski, J. S. (Eds.). (1998). *Handbook of empirical social work practice.* (Vol. 1, Mental Disorders). New York: Wiley.

Timms, N. (1983). *Social work values: An inquiry.* London: Routledge and Kegan Paul.

Tolson, E. (1977). Alleviating marital communication problems. In W. J. Reid & L. Epstein (Eds.), *Task-centered practice.* New York: Columbia University Press.

Towle, C. (1965). *Common human needs.* Washington, DC: National Association of Social Workers.

Tripodi, T., & Epstein, I. (1980). *Research techniques for clinical social workers.* New York: Columbia University Press.

Tuma, J. M. (1989). Mental health services for children: The state of the art. *American Psychologist, 44,* 188–199.

Turnbull, J., & Dietz-Uhler, B. (1995). The Boulder model: Lessons from clinical psychology to social work training. *Research on Social Work Practice, 5,* 411–429.

Turner, J. (1986). *The structure of sociological theory.* Chicago: Dorsey Press.

Tyson, K. B. (1992). A new approach to relevant scientific research for practitioners: The heuristic paradigm. *Social Work, 37*(6), 541–556.

Ulali. (1997). *All my relations, Mahk Jchi* [sound recording].

United Nations (1948). *The universal declaration of human rights.* New York: Author.

United States Census Bureau (1997). *Statistical abstract of the United States: 1997.* Washington, DC: US Government Printing Office.

United States Department of Health, Education and Welfare (1979). *Background papers for healthy people: The surgeon general's report on health promotion and disease prevention* (DHEW Publication 79–55072). Washington, DC: Government Printing Office.

US Department of Health and Human Services (1998). *SACWIS (Statewide Automated Child Welfare Information System).* http://www.acfdhhs.gov/programs/oss/sacwis/status.htm.

Van Den Bergh, N. (1991). Having bitten the apple: A feminist perspective on addictions. In N. V. D. Bergh (Ed.), *Feminist perspectives on additions* (pp. 3–30). New York: Springer Publishers.

Van Den Bergh, N. (1992). Feminist treatment for people with depression. In K. Corcoran (Ed.), *Structuring change.* Chicago: Lyceum Books, Inc.

Van Den Bergh, N. (1995). *Feminist practice in the 21st century.* Washington, DC: NASW Press.

Van Den Bergh, N., & Cooper, L. (1986a). Introduction. In N. V. D. Bergh & L. Cooper (Eds.), *Feminist visions for social work* (pp. 1–28). Silver Spring, MD: NASW Press.

Van Den Bergh, N., & Cooper, L. (1986b). Feminist social work practice. In T. Tripodi (Ed.), *Encyclopedia of social work* (18th ed., pp. 610–618). Washington, DC: NASW Press.

Van Den Bergh, N., & Cooper, L. B. (1995). Introduction to feminist visions for social work. In J. E. Tropman, J. L. Erlich, & J. Rothman (Eds.), *Tactics and techniques of community intervention* (pp. 79–93). Itasca, IL: Peacock.

Van Hook, M. (1996). Challenges to identifying and treating women with depression in rural primary care. *Social Work in Health Care, 23*(3), 73–92.

Varley, B. K. (1968). Social work values: Changes in value commitments from admission to MSW graduation. *Journal of Education for Social Work, 4,* 67–85.

Vega, W., Valle, R., Kolody B., Hough, R., & Munoz, R. (1987). The Hispanic social network prevention intervention study: A community-based randomized trial. In R. Munoz (Ed.) *Depression prevention: Research directions* (pp. 217–291). Washington, DC: Hemisphere.

Videka-Sherman, L. (1988). Meta-analysis of research on social work practice in mental health. *Social Work, 33,* 325–338.

Vigilante, J. (1974). Between values and science. *Journal of Education for Social Work, 10,* 107–115.

Wade, W. A., Treat, T. A., & Stuart, G. L. (1998). Transporting an empirically-supported treatment for panic disorder to a service clinical setting. *Journal of Consulting and Clinical Psychology, 66,* 231–239.

Wahler, R. G. (1969). Setting generality: Some specific and general effects of child behavior therapy. *Journal of Applied Behavior Analysis, 2,* 239–246.

Wakefield, J. C., & Kirk, S. A. (1997). Science, dogma, and the scientist-practitioner model. *Social Work Research, 21*(3), 201–205.

Waldinger, R. J. (1987). Intensive psychodynamic therapy with borderline patients: An overview. *American Journal of Psychiatry, 144,* 267–274.

Waldron, H. B. (1997). Adolescent substance abuse and family therapy outcome: A review of randomized trials. *Advances in Clinical Child Psychology, 19,* 199–234.

Wartenberg, A. A., & Liepman, M. R. (1987). Medical consequences of addictive behaviors. In T. D. Nirenberg & S. A. Maisto (Eds.), *Developments in the assessment and treatment of addictive behaviors.* Norwood, NJ: Ablex.

Washington, E. M., & Pinkston, E. M. (1986). Positive consequences of helping for informal caregivers: A conceptual model for research. In E. M. Pinkston, P. Hanrahan, & E. M. Washington (Eds.), *Proceedings of the Charlotte Towle symposium on behavioral gerontology.* Chicago: The Charlotte Towle Foundation.

Watzlawick, P. (1978). *The language of change.* New York: Basic Books.

Watzlawick, P., Beavin, J. H., & Jackson, D. D. (1967). *Pragmatics of human communication: A study of interactional patterns, pathologies, and paradoxes.* New York: W. W. Norton.

Watzlawick, P., Weakland, J., & Fisch, R. (1974). *Change: Principles of problem formation and problem resolution.* New York: W. W. Norton.

Way of the Spirit (The) (1997). Chicago: Time-Life Custom Publishing.

Weakland, J. H., Jordan, L., & Dimmock, B. (1992). Working briefly with reluctant clients: Child protective services as an example. *Journal of Family Therapy, 14*(3), 231–254.

Webb, E. J., Campbell, D. T., Schwartz, R. D., Sechrest, L., & Grove, J. B. (1981). *Unobtrusive measures: Non-reactive research in social sciences.* Boston, MA: Houghton Mifflin.

Webster-Stratton, C. (1997). From parent training to community building. *Families in Society, 78,* 156–171.

Weeks, G. (1977). Toward a dialectical approach to intervention. *Human Development, 20,* 277–290.

Weeks, G., & L'Abate, L. (1982). *Paradoxical psychotherapy.* New York: Brunner/Mazel.

Weinrott, M., Jones, R., & Howard, J. (1982). Cost effectiveness of teaching family programs for delinquents: Results of a national evaluation. *Evaluation Review, 6,* 173–201.

Weisner, S., & Silver, M. (1981). Community work and social-learning theory. *Social Work, 26,* 146–150.

Weiss, C. H., & Bucuvalas, M. J. (1980). *Social science research and decision-making.* New York: Columbia University Press.

Weiss, R. L., Hops, H., & Patterson, G. R. (1973). A framework for conceptualizing marital conflict, some data for evaluating it. In L. S. Hamerlynck, L. C. Handy, & E. J. Mash (Eds.), *Behavior change: Methodology, concepts, and practice.* Champaign, IL: Research Press.

Weissman, A. L. (1976). Industrial social services: Linkage technology. *Social Casework, 55,* 50–54.

Weissman, M., & Klerman, G. (1987). Gender and depression. In R. Formanek & A. Gurian (Eds.), *Women and depression: A lifespan approach.* New York: Springer Publishers.

Wells, E. A., Hawkins, J. D., & Catalano, R. F. (1988a). Choosing drug use measures for treatment outcome studies, I: The influence of measurement approach on treatment results. *The International Journal of the Addictions, 23,* 851–873.

Wells, E. A., Hawkins, J. D., & Catalano, R. F. (1988b). Choosing drug use measures for treatment outcome studies, II: Timing baseline and follow-up measurement. *The International Journal of the Addictions, 23,* 875–885.

Wells, R. A., Figurel, J. A., & McNamee, P. (1975). Group facilitative training with conflicted marital couples. In A. S. Gurman & D. G. Rice (Eds.), *Couples in conflict.* New York: Jason Aronson.

Welton, G., Pruitt, D., & McGillicuddy, N. (1988). The role of caucusing in community mediation. *Journal of Conflict Resolution, 32,* 181–202.

Westbrook, D., & Hill, L. (1998). The long-term outcome of cognitive behavior therapy for adults in routine clinical practice. *Behaviour Research and Therapy, 36,* 635–643.

Westhuis, D. J., & Thyer, B. A. (1989). Development and validation of the Clinical Anxiety Scale. *Educational and Psychological Abstracts, 49,* 153–163.

Westin, A. (Ed.). (1981). *Whistle blowing? Loyalty and dissent in the corporation.* New York: McGraw-Hill.

Westney, O., Cole, O., & Munford, T. (1986). Adolescent unwed prospective fathers: Readiness for fatherhood and behaviors toward the mother and the expected infant. *Adolescence, 21*(8), 901–911.

Wetzel, J. (1986). A feminist world view conceptual framework. *Social Casework, 67,* 166–173.

Wetzel, J. (1994). Depression: Women at risk. *Social Work in Health Care, 19*(3/4), 85–108.

Wetzel, J. (1987). *American youth: A statistical snapshot.* Washington, DC: William T. Grant Foundation Commission on Youth and America's Future.

White, G., Paine-Andrews, A., Mathews, R., & Fawcett, S. (1995). Home access modifications: Effects on community visits by people with physical disabilities. *Journal of Applied Behavior Analysis, 28,* 457–463.

Whittington, C. (1975). Self-determination re-examined. In F. E. McDermott (Ed.), *Self-determination in social work* (pp. 81–92). London: Routledge & Kegan Paul.

Widiger, T., & Weissman, M. (1991). Epidemiology of borderline personality disorder. *Hospital and Community Psychiatry, 42,* 1015–1019.

William T. Grant Foundation. (1988). *The forgotten half: Pathways to success for America's youth and young families.* Washington, DC: William T. Grant Foundation Commission on Work, Family and Citizenship.

Williams, J. (1984). *The psychological treatment of depression.* New York: Free Press.

Williams, M., Thyer, B., Bailey, J., & Harrison, D. (1989). Promoting safety belt use with traffic signs and prompters. *Journal of Applied Behavior Analysis, 22,* 71–76.

Williams, O. J. (1992). Ethnically sensitive practice to enhance treatment participation of African American men who batter. *Families in Society, 73,* 588–595.

Wills, T. A., Weiss, R. L., & Patterson, G. R. (1974). A behavioral analysis of the determinants of marital satisfaction. *Journal of Consulting and Clinical Psychology, 42,* 802–811.

Wilsnack, S. (1993, March). *Patterns and trends in women's drinking: Recent findings and some implications for prevention.* Paper presented at the Working Group for Prevention Research on Women and Alcohol, Prevention Research Branch, NIAAA, Bethesda, MD.

Wilson, S. J. (1978). *Confidentiality in social work.* New York: Free Press.

Wilson, W. (1996). *When work disappears: The world of the new urban poor.* New York: Alfred Knopf.

Wine, J. D. (1981). From defects to competence models. In J. D. Wine & M. D. Smye (Eds.), *Social competence.* New York: Guilford Press.

Winiarski, M. (1991). *AIDS-related psychotherapy.* New York: Pergamon.

Winkler, E. R. (1998). Applied ethics, overview. In R. Chadwick (Ed.), *Encyclopedia of applied ethics* (Vol. 1, pp. 191–196). San Diego, CA: Academic Press.

Winnicott, D. W. (1969). The use of an object. *International Journal of Psychoanalysis, 41,* 594–595.

Witkin, S. (1991). If empirical practice is the answer, then what is the question? *Social Work Research, 20*(2), 69–75.

Witty, C. (1980). *Mediation and society: Conflict management in Lebanon.* New York: Academic Press.

Wodarski, J. S., & Thyer, B. A. (Eds.). (1981). *The role of research in clinical practice: A practical approach for the human services.* Baltimore: University Park Press.

Wolf, M., Kirigin, K., Fixsen, D., Blase, K., & Braukmann, C. (1995). The Teaching Family Model: A case study in databased program development and refinement (and dragon wrestling). *Journal of Organizational Behavior Management, 15,* 11–68.

Wolf, M., Phillips, E., Fixsen, D., Braukman, C., Kirigin, K., Willner, A., & Schumaker, J. (1976). Achievement place: The Teaching Family Model. *Child Care Quarterly, 5,* 92–103.

Wood, K. M. (1978). Casework effectiveness: A new look at the research evidence. *Social Work, 23,* 437–459.

Woods, M. E., & Hollis, F. (1990). *Casework: A psychosocial approach.* (4th ed.). New York: McGraw-Hill.

Woolfolk, R. L., Carr-Kaffashan, L., McNulty, T. F., & Lehrer, P. M. (1976). Mediation training as a treatment for insomnia. *Behavior Therapy, 7,* 359–365.

Work on clinical guides begins. (1998), February. *NASW News, 42*(2), 13, ch. 4.

Working definition of social work practice. (1958). *Social Work, 3*(2), 5–8.

Yamaguchi, K., & Kandel, D. B. (1984). Patterns of drug use from adolescence to young adulthood: III. Prediction of progression. *American Journal of Public Health, 74,* 673–681.

Younghusband, E. (1967). *Social work and social values.* London: Allen and Unwin.

Zarit, S. H., Reever, K., & Bachman-Peterson, S. (1980). The burden interview. *The Gerontologist, 20,* 649–656.

Zaslow, M. J. (1989). Sex differences in children's response to parental divorce: Samples, variables, ages, and sources. *American Journal of Orthopsychiatry, 59,* 118–140.

Zetzel, E. R. (1971). A developmental approach to the borderline patient. *American Journal of Psychiatry, 172,* 867–871.

Ziarnik, J., & Bernstein, G. (1982). A critical examination of the effect of in-service training on staff performance. *Mental Retardation, 20*(3), 109–114.

Zillman, D. (1993). Mental control of angry aggression. In D. Wegner & J. Pennebaker (Eds.), *Handbook of mental control* (pp. 370–392). Englewood Cliffs, NJ: Prentice Hall.

Zlotnick, J. L. (1997). *Preparing the workforce for family-centered practice: Social work education and public human services partnerships.* Alexandria, VA: Council on Social Work Education.

Index

Social workers
  ability to work at all system levels, 23
  ability to work with systems of all
    sizes, 23
  academic-based researchers, 45
  agency-based researchers, 44–45
  case individualization and, 22
  client's right of self-determination
    and, 91
  clients with HIV/AIDS and, 258–260
  clinical social workers, ethical
    dilemmas for, 88–90
  community-based, 59
  dual/multiple relationships and,
    92–93
  ethical dilemmas for, 85–86
  ethical frameworks for, 95–97
  impairment of, 102–103
  legal complaints against, 101–103
  managed care dilemmas and, 94–95
  managing ethical risks and, 100–103
  practice models for, 24–25
  professional/personal values of,
    93–94
    as researchers, 40
  sources of knowledge for, 23–24
  stress and AIDS work, 262
  whistle blowing by, 94
Social work practice. *See also* Family-
    centered practice; Feminist social
    work practice
  core processes, 25–26
  ecomaps for, 33–35
  establishing treatment contracts for,
    11
  ethical dilemmas in, 88–90
  evaluation measurement of, 72–77
  evaluation of, 67–68
  evaluation process for analyzing
    changes and goal attainment,
    77–82; measurement selection and
    use, 72–77; specifying target
    behaviors and setting goals, 68–72
  evaluation versus research, 67–68
  integrating evaluation into, 82–84
  maintaining treatment gains in,
    11–12
  models for, 24–25
  monitoring and evaluating clients, 11
    as network of transactions, 29–32
  processes of, 25–26
  professional knowledge and, 23–24
  reasons for evaluating, 66–67

selecting interventions for, 8–9
setting client objectives for, 5–7
setting goals for, 3–5
shared power principles for, 121–122
social justice and, 18–20
structuring interventions for, 9–11
with unmarried, nonresident fathers,
    335–336
Solomon, Phyllis, 59
Spanier Dyadic Adjustment Scale,
    174–175
Specific phobias (SPPs), 148–150
  defined, 148
  exposure therapy for, 156
Splitting, 268, 269
Splitting Scale, 272
Spousification. *See also* Acculturation;
    Acculturation stress; Adultification;
    Biculturation
  case study of, 292–294
  clinical manifestations of, 290–292
  defined, 287–288, 289–290
  successful treatment of, 294–301
Standardized scales, 75–76
  for substance abuse, 224
Standards of care, 101, 102
State-Trait Anger Scale, 306
Stop-action approach, for
    communication skills training,
    183–184
Stress
  acculturation, 285–286
  AIDS caregiving and, 262–264
  control training, for substance abuse,
    232–233
  coping skills for, 180
  couples' functioning and, 173
  management techniques, for marital
    discord treatment, 193–194
  rapid assessment instruments for, 177
Structural family therapy techniques, for
    acculturation stress, 295–296
Structured behavioral observations, for
    anxiety-evoking stimulus (AES), 152
Structured Clinical Interview for the
    DSM-IV (SCID), 150
Stuart Clinical Aids, 174
Subjectivity, feminist practice and,
    144–145
Substance abuse
  adolescents and, 201
  basic principles of assessment
    methodologies for, 220–221